REHABILITATION STUDIES HANDBOOK

REHABILITATION STUDIES HANDBOOK

Edited by

BARBARA A. WILSON, BA, MPhil, PhD
Senior Scientist, Medical Research Council Applied Psychology Unit, Cambridge

and

D. LINDSAY McLELLAN, MA, MB, PhD, FRCP
Professor of Rehabilitation, University of Southampton Rehabilitation Research Unit, Southampton General Hospital

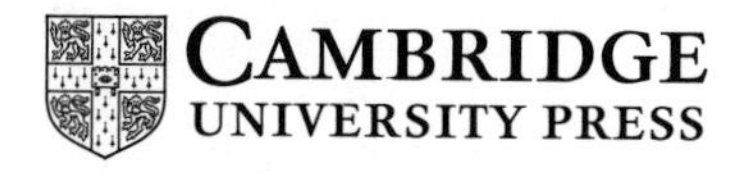

PUBLISHED BY THE PRESS SYNDICATE OF THE UNIVERSITY OF CAMBRIDGE
The Pitt Building, Trumpington Street, Cambridge CB2 1RP, United Kingdom

CAMBRIDGE UNIVERSITY PRESS
The Edinburgh Building, Cambridge CB2 2RU, United Kingdom
40 West 20th Street, New York, NY 10011-4211, USA
10 Stamford Road, Oakleigh, Melbourne 3166, Australia

First published 1997

Printed in the United Kingdom at the University Press, Cambridge

Typeset in Times 11/14 pt

A catalogue record for this book is available from the British Library

Library of Congress cataloguing in publication data

Rehabilitation studies handbook / edited by Barbara A. Wilson and D. Lindsay McLellan.
p. cm.
Includes index.
ISBN 0 521 43713 X (pbk.)
1. Medical rehabilitation. I. Wilson, Barbara A. II. McLellan, D. Lindsay.
RM930.R367 1997
617'.03 – dc20 96-22502 CIP

ISBN 0 521 43713 X paperback

Contents

Contributors

Dr Keith Andrews
Royal Hospital for Neuro-disability, West Hill, Putney, London SW15 3SW, UK

Professor Roger Briggs
Geriatric Medicine, University of Southampton, Level E, Centre Block, Southampton General Hospital, Tremona Road, Southampton SO16 6YD, UK

Ms Eva Bower
University of Southampton, Rehabilitation Research Unit, Southampton General Hospital, Tremona Road, Southampton SO9 4XY, UK

Dr Trevor M. Bryant
Department of Medical Statistics and Computing, Southampton General Hospital, Tremona Road, Southampton, SO9 4XY, UK

Dr Ted Cantrell
University of Southampton, Rehabilitation Research Unit, Level C, West Wing, Southampton General Hospital, Tremona Road, Southampton SO9 4XY, UK

Dr Colin Coles
Centre for General Practice, Institute for Health and Community Studies, Royal London House, Christchurch Road, Bournemouth BH1 3LT, UK

Dr Stephen Duckworth
Disability Matters Ltd, Berkeley House, West Tytherley, Salisbury SP5 1NF, UK

Dr Caroline Glendinning
NPCRDC, 5th Floor, Williamson Building, University of Manchester, Oxford Road, Manchester M13 9PL, UK

Mrs Sandra Horn
Department of Psychology, University of Southampton, Highfield, Southampton SO9 5NH, UK

Dr P. Jane Lones
'Mandai', 7 Winters Close, Portesham, Weymouth DT3 4HP, UK

Dr David Machin
MRC Cancer Trials Office, 5 Shaftesbury Road, Cambridge, CB2 2BW, UK

Professor D. Lindsay McLellan
University of Southampton, Rehabilitation Research Unit, Level C, West Wing, Southampton General Hospital, Tremona Road, Southampton SO9 4XY, UK

Professor John P. Martin
3 Gordon Place, Withington, Manchester M20 9LR, UK

Mr Allan Read
Chartered Clinical Psychologist, Southampton Community Health Services, Knowle Hospital, Fareham PO17 5NA, UK

Dr Barbara A. Wilson
MRC Applied Psychology Unit, Rehabilitation Research Group, Box 58, Addenbrooke's Hospital, Cambridge CB2 2QQ, UK

1

Introduction to rehabilitation

D. LINDSAY McLELLAN

This chapter reviews some of the basic factors that determine the direction and effectiveness of rehabilitation and which are important for its scientific development. Many of the issues touched on here are dealt with in greater depth later in the handbook.

The word 'rehabilitation' can be applied to many things: crumbling buildings, disgraced politicians, convicted burglars, frail old ladies and soldiers injured in battle. This book is about the type of rehabilitation that people with biological impairments and disabilities often seek to achieve in order to attain the kind of lifestyle of their choice. It discusses some of the approaches used both by them and the various rehabilitation professions which help bring this about. This inevitably requires an understanding of the cultural and physical environment in which disabled people are living.

Rehabilitation can be defined in two quite different ways.

1. A process of active change by which a person who has become disabled acquires the knowledge and skills needed for optimal physical, psychological and social function.
2. The application of all measures aimed at reducing the impact of disabling and handicapping conditions and enabling disabled and handicapped people to achieve social integration

The first definition recognises that rehabilitation involves a personal journey in which the disabled person not only has to choose the destination and the route taken, but also to do most of the work. This process is much closer to education and training than to medical treatment with drugs or surgery.

The primary purpose of medicine is to relieve suffering caused by disease. To this end, medicine seeks to cure or to prevent pathological changes and thus to restore the patient to a biologically and psychologically 'normal' condition. The primary purpose of rehabilitation is to help disabled persons achieve the lifestyle they would like to have. This is likely to involve far more than a passive response to medical or surgical treatment and it does not necessarily involve any biological change in the individual.

The second World Health Organization (WHO) definition of rehabilitation is formulated from a standpoint outside the disabled person, from which rehabilitation is seen as a set of influences, procedures and resources to be applied both to the disabled person and to the environment. It covers not only people with acquired disabilities where impairment is diminishing but those with progressive conditions in which impairment is increasing with time. In such cases, the 'measures' that are applied may have to be updated continually to ensure an optimal outcome. Rehabilitation thus defined involves **the prevention of disability and the maintenance of social role**, and not simply recovery of or improvement in function.

At this stage we need to define some more terms. The definitions advocated by the WHO will be adopted here, despite the fact that some of them do not have universal approval, because the *concepts* at least are generally recognised.

Impairment is the lack of a body part or function.

Disability is a lack of ability to undertake an activity to a level or in a manner that is considered normal for a human being.

Handicap is a disadvantage for a given individual resulting from impairment or a disability that limits or prevents the fulfilment of a role that is normal (depending on age, sex, social and cultural factors) for that individual.

To achieve successful rehabilitation, handicap could thus theoretically be minimised through a combination of three approaches:

1. Reducing the disability
2. Acquiring new strategies and skills through which the impact of the disability could be minimised
3. Altering the environment, including the behaviour of non-disabled people, so that impairment and disability no longer confer a handicap.

Consider the following example of a housewife with three children who in her mid-thirties has to use a wheelchair for most outdoor mobility because of multiple sclerosis. What might these three approaches achieve?

1. Her disability could be reduced by adopting a regular muscle strengthening and stretching programme and by taking medication to help the bladder retain urine.
2. She could learn a number of strategies such as ascending and descending stairs safely, pacing her activities to minimise the effects of fatigue, adapting the family menu to increase the use of the microwave oven and encourage the

children to help, using a message and appointment reminder pad by the telephone and establishing new recreational interests that do not rely on her ability to walk.

3. Her bathroom and kitchen could be adapted for periods when she is too weak to stand, access to the garden and street could be improved and her car could be adapted for manual controls. The family could accept the probability of a lower income. Her husband could move to a job with more flexible hours, their children could take on a number of regular tasks to help with the physical work involved in running a household while a home-help could do the heavy cleaning so that the family can spend recreational time together. Friends could recognise her disability and do their best to develop their friendship by spending time engaging in activities and going to venues that are accessible.

If you felt an increasing sense of scepticism as you read the last paragraph, you were no doubt recognising the fact that changes in the environment and the behaviour of non-disabled people in it are not only crucial elements in the minimisation of handicap, but also the hardest to bring about.

Outcomes

In general terms the outcome of rehabilitation is the disabled person's situation at the end of it, or, for those in whom rehabilitation has a maintenance function, their situation at the time that services are monitored. Thus for some people, rehabilitation will have an 'end-point' that can be measured but, for many others, regular surveys will be needed to check on their situation.

In most areas of medical practice, the hope is to understand the pathology of the patient's condition and to find the means to cure it so that there is no residual impairment of function. If this is the purpose and expectation of treatment, then it is reasonable to use the 'biological norm' as a measure of the treatment's success. Many biological norms tend to hold true across our species irrespective of cultural or social factors.

In rehabilitation, it is usually inappropriate to use the biological norm as an outcome standard. Each individual will be starting from a different situation, and will be identifying (consciously or unconsciously) different objectives that relate to physical, cognitive and social functions and that are influenced by personal, cultural and environmental factors. In children whose capacities are still developing, disability may give a progressive divergence from their peers, irrespective of whether the disabled child's function worsens or not (Figure 1.1). The kind of measures used to locate an individual or group of people within the general population (such as general indices of impairment, disability or handicap) may be quite unsuitable for testing the effectiveness of

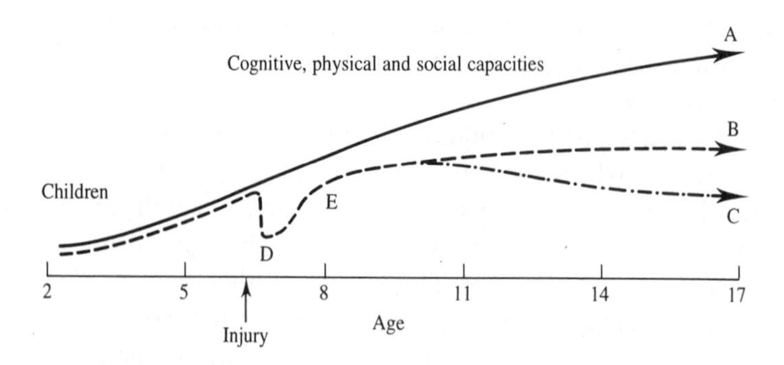

Figure 1.1. Trajectories of recovery and personal development.
A, uninjured children – peers;
B, head injured child who adjusts well but fails to make the same progress as uninjured peers and progressively diverges from them;
C, head injured child who cannot adjust and becomes despondent and excluded from peers and family;
D, immediate loss of function after the injury;
E, Six to 12 months : stage of rapid biological recovery. Note that at E, the discrepancy between the injured child and peers is improving compared with the position of D, but from this point their paths increasingly diverge.
Even in adults, and particularly in teenagers and young adults, the injured person's peers are moving through personal and social changes that leave the injured person behind, and progressively excluded from peer group and family. The family may respond by stopping its own clock and becoming isolated from others.

therapies, especially when the therapy has a very precise or restricted objective. In trials of therapy, therefore, outcome measures are needed that precisely reflect **the objectives of the therapy**. It may be possible to study the mechanisms involved in therapy at the same time and if this is the case, measures that test or explore the mechanisms may also be used but these will only be interpretable in the light of the achievement or non-achievement of the therapy's objectives.

Individualised specific treatment goals should meet the 'SMART' criteria and be:

Specific
Measurable
Activity-related
Realistic
Time-specified.

Such goals or objectives can be plotted on a graph in which 100% represents the measured function aimed at, with shortfalls or overshoots scoring less or more than 100%. Thus if the objective were to sit unsupported on a potty for two minutes, an ability to do this for one minute scored 50% or three minutes

150%. Such graphs allow the rate of achievement to be plotted and changes in the slope correlated with different therapeutic inputs and with other relevant events.

An example of the **poor** use of outcome measures would be the use of a general dependency scale such as the Barthel Index or Functional Independence Measure to test the effectiveness of 'physiotherapy' in an undifferentiated group of elderly people with stroke. Without knowing precisely what the physiotherapy was attempting to achieve or what outcomes were being predicted for individuals, it would be impossible to arrive at a useful interpretation of the change or lack of change in the outcome measure.

Are there circumstances in which objectives can be predicted from a knowledge of the person's disability? It may be reasonably assumed that no-one wants to be incontinent. Therefore the demonstration of incontinence can usually be taken as implying an objective: the gaining of continence; but this will not *always* be appropriate. For example, an elderly demented person may be permanently incapable of continence, in which case the objective might be to prevent him or her from being uncomfortable or wet and soiling the furniture.

Needs

If a knowledge of the disability cannot predict rehabilitation objectives it can still less identify *need*. In the context of a service that is being provided, a **need** may be defined as an intervention or resource that would confer a gain or achieve an objective relevant to the purpose of the service. An incontinent housewife with multiple sclerosis in whom continence is a reasonable objective could have any one (or a combination) of different health and social care *needs*, for example: (1) treatment of a urinary tract infection; (2) drugs to improve detrusor instability; (3) a downstairs toilet; (4) physiotherapy to preserve the ability to transfer quickly and independently to the toilet; and (5) a live-in carer. Needs are the means to an end rather than objectives themselves. If it is proposed to monitor needs then this must be done directly and specifically – surrogate or proxy methods will not do.

In assigning a value or priority to needs, different scores may be given by the patient, the main carer and by service providers. How can needs best be prioritised? Disabled people themselves may use the word 'need' to identify their objectives rather than the means needed to reach their objectives. In the above example, when asked what her needs were the housewife with multiple sclerosis might reply 'I desperately need to be continent' indicating that, to her, continence is a high-priority objective.

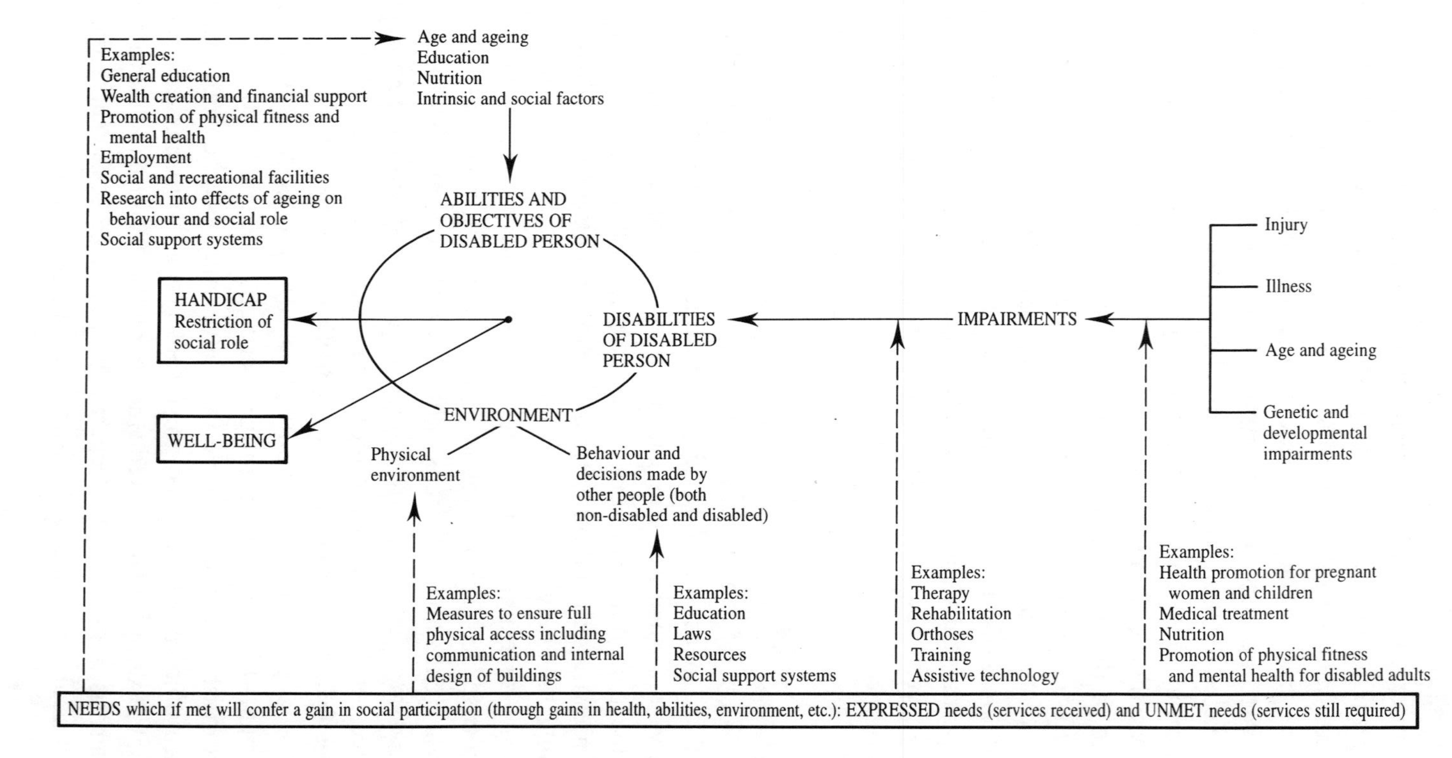

Figure 1.2. Conceptual 'map' of rehabilitation linking impairment, handicap, the environment and needs.

To prioritise a need, it is nearly always necessary to know what the objective is, and what gain will actually be conferred. The priority afforded to the need will reflect the importance of the objective and the cost of reaching it. The importance of the objective may be difficult to judge out of context and so it is often necessary to define disability, objectives *and* needs to be able to arrive at a decision about the priority to be afforded to the needs. The relationships between disability, handicap and needs are shown in Figure 1.2.

Many studies of needs have been flawed by a failure to take into account the necessity for gaining the disabled person's perspective, and also the difficulty of doing this. The context in which questions are posed will influence the answers given. When surveyed about disability, elderly people may, for example, under report the disability they have because they assume that what they are being asked is whether their capacities are within acceptable limits for their age. If the interviewer is a doctor, disabled people may say that they have 'no particular needs' meaning they are not ill, but they may nevertheless have considerable rehabilitation and social needs. Identifying the frame of reference is an essential and intuitive element in all conversation. Interviewers may simply not be able to conceal their own assumptions and thus unintentionally bias the answers received. For example, occupational therapists place a high value on physical personal independence and may unintentionally invite the identification of needs relating to independence at the expense of other needs, for example those relating to fatigue or loneliness. When helping someone to identify their own needs it is often helpful to start the interview by a general conversation about their likes and dislikes, how they spend their time and what their hopes and expectations are for the future. This sets out a wider context, embracing social activity and the dimension of handicap as well as impairment and disability.

Medicine: the biomedical model and rehabilitation

In the United Kingdom (UK), medical rehabilitation had its origins in the treatment given to soldiers in the First World War. Lower ranks who received psychological and social encouragement to resume physical activity soon after their injury recovered faster than the officers who had received gentler treatment. This result was startling at the time, showing that social and educational advantages were not determinants of biological recovery and could be upstaged by training.

Since this time, both medicine and rehabilitation have developed but medical advances have greatly outstripped those of rehabilitation. So many pathological processes can now be cured that the relief of suffering and rehabilitation *in their own right* have become relatively sidelined, a kind of 'fall back' option to be invoked only when medical treatment has failed. By regarding disability as evidence of failed treatment, medicine is of course being intentionally rigorous with itself, signalling that medical science must not rest until restoration of the biological norm can be guaranteed for all.

Unfortunately this laudable mission has contaminated the approach of some medical practitioners towards individual disabled patients whose pathology and impairments cannot be reversed. 'Alas poor fellow, I am afraid there is nothing I can do!' expresses the physician's dismay at his own powerlessness, lack of awareness of the value of the patient's way of life for which the word 'Alas' may be completely inappropriate, and a preoccupation with pathology at the expense of rehabilitation and the relief of suffering. Indeed, the very success of medical advances in reducing impairment adds to the status of other measures that affect impairment. Some therapists too concentrate their efforts on impairments at the expense of disability and handicap. This has led to difficulties not only in rehabilitation practice but also in research, where outcome measures appropriate to impairment have been used inappropriately to test the effectiveness of therapy that was not aimed at altering impairment.

Rehabilitation team work

There are many potential problems in working closely and harmoniously with people trained in different disciplines. Each discipline or profession has its own theoretical framework, traditions, sense of mission, priorities and rules. The hard work that goes into obtaining a professional qualification and scrambling eventually to the battlements of one's own profession has a personal cost, and we all look forward to a good clear view when we get there. To protect the public by maintaining high standards, and to make certain that others cannot reach the high ground more easily than we did, we protect our professions with moats and drawbridges such as entrance qualifications, minimum duration of training, schedules, examinations and legal protection of title. Moreover, it is enjoyable to meet together in our professional societies to talk about our work and perhaps share a meal afterwards. Such social systems are both pleasant to belong to and effective in maintaining the commitment that is essential for reliability and advances in practice. They run the risk, however, of reinforcing a reluctance to look for ideas from elsewhere, and they can also encourage competition and friction between professional groups, as well as between professions and patients. This is a well-recognised problem both in traditional medicine and in rehabilitation.

Rehabilitation is such a broad and complex activity that a wide range of expertise is essential. A consensus should always be reached about what the disabled person's objectives and needs actually are, the best way of meeting them, the timetable and programme that will be implemented and how the implementation is to be monitored. Some issues are relatively straightforward or fall within the competency of a single profession and in such cases the question of deploying a multi-disciplinary team does not arise. For people with particularly complex disabilities and rehabilitation needs, however, a team approach is needed.

Within a single profession such as medicine, the term 'multi-disciplinary' tends to be used to denote the grouping of doctors from different specialties or medical disciplines. In rehabilitation the term implies a much wider mixture of different rehabilitation professions including some or (theoretically) all of the following alphabetical list: arts-related therapies, clinical psychology, education, employment training, medicine, nursing, occupational therapy, orthotics, physiotherapy, podiatry, prosthetics, psychotherapy, rehabilitation engineering, social work, and speech and language therapy.

Team work

Theoretical models (i.e. ideas) for team work have generated some new terms. In this context 'multi disciplinary' implies that each member of the team operates within the boundaries of the objectives and competencies adopted by his or her own profession.

'Interdisciplinary' means that each member operates across these boundaries by agreement with a neighbouring discipline, but retains primary responsibility for the areas central to his or her own discipline. Many individuals from the team will thus need to be personally involved with a disabled person whose needs are complex. 'Transdisciplinary' means that team members take on a much wider role, calling on their colleagues only when they have problems. This has the advantage of reducing the number of different rehabilitation professionals with whom an individual disabled person has to interact. A possible but unproven disadvantage is that consistent standards are harder to maintain. Transdisciplinary working is professionally more threatening because of the fear that one species of professional would become more successful than the rest and threaten their food supply, i.e. their status and employment.

Rehabilitation teams must always meet in person regularly, otherwise they are not teams at all but simply loose conglomerates. They need to be led effectively by someone whose authority is accepted by the team members, by the disabled people to whom services are being provided and to the service's general management.

In the UK at the present time, the management of many rehabilitation services is fragmented. Teams include members drawn from different service providers whose management structures and practices unintentionally impede team working. A quirky example from the writer's experience occurred at Christmas 1994, when some members of our rehabilitation team received a £5 token from our hospital Trust as a symbol of the high regard in which their year's work was viewed by management. Leaving aside the question of whether this symbol was appropriate, the exercise was resented because although we function as a team with shared objectives and resources, our occupational therapists, speech and language therapists and clinical psychologist received no token (because their contracts of employment were with a different Trust) whereas our cleaners likewise received nothing because their services had been privatised. More important matters, such as resourcing and service development, are equally vulnerable to fragmented management structures.

To provide a service that appears 'seamless', it is necessary to simplify the contact point for the disabled person, whether patient or client, and the responsibility for the individual's programme to rest with a single person. Ideally, of course, this would be with the disabled person himself or herself. This had been developed successfully in relation to care, where some disabled people have been funded to run self-operated care schemes (SOCS) because they have (or have been helped to acquire) the skills needed to hire and fire their own care staff and manage their own budget. Such schemes are unlikely to be so widely applicable to rehabilitation but the SOCS model remains a valuable ideal against which alternatives should be tested. The ideal should not be used, however, to disempower people with cognitive impairments by preventing them from receiving the help that they need.

Case management

This was pioneered by the medical profession developing the British system of general medical practice or 'primary medical care' in the late 1940s. The general practitioner, or GP, is a personal family doctor who acts as a point of first contact or 'health case manager' for the patient. This relationship is a continuous one spanning all episodes of illness and including a monitoring function. Patients are assessed and treated by their GP and the primary health care team. If necessary, they are admitted to hospital at the request of their GP, returning to the same GP's care when discharged. When it is working well, this system ensures that an individual's social context is taken into account when they are being assessed or treated for medical conditions. Ideally, a personal relationship of trust and understanding develops that improves the quality of care.

Traditionally the GP was employed by the National Health Service and did not hold a budget. The GP would thus act as an advocate for the patient as well as gatekeeper to the treatment. This role has become blurred with the recent introduction of 'fund holding' for GPs and it is too early to say whether patients will regard them as warmly in their new role as they did in the old one.

Rehabilitation is not currently included in the training of British GPs and in most cases they are not equipped to fulfil this role in relation to rehabilitation. In recent years, the case management model has been developed by social sciences in relation to care, especially for disabled people living in the community rather than in residential institutions. **Care** may be defined as the term most often used for tending, involving physical contact for daily living activities, and for the assumption of responsibility for making decisions on behalf of people with disabilities, in the light of their expressed and of their perceived wishes and needs. It often overlaps with **support** which is the term most often used for activities that do not involve making decisions on behalf of people with disabilities, but includes undertaking simpler physical activities to help them and in providing social and psychological support both for them and for informal carers and other members of the family.

The community case management model includes the control of a budget that usually covers part at least of the costs of the service and of the coordinating function of the case manager.

Brokerage

An alternative system of mediation between the funding for a service (the **purchaser**) and the people providing the service (the **provider**) is brokerage. A **broker** is an independent agent who works on behalf of the disabled person to bring together the services required and the funds necessary to provide them (including the salary of the broker). Theoretically, a broker is in a better position than a case manager to act as an advocate for the disabled person. A broker has to have considerable experience and expertise, however, to be taken seriously by clients, purchasers or providers, and the complexity and paperwork involved probably explain why this model is more a theoretical concept than a popular practical option.

Key worker

Probably the most widespread means of coordinating a team's focus on an individual is to designate, by negotiation with the patient or client, a member of the team to be the individual's 'key worker'. The key worker's role is to get to know the disabled person very well, to be responsible for ensuring that progress is monitored and reviewed by the team, and to negotiate as necessary with the other team members involved in the programme and to act as advocate and coordinator for that individual.

It is clear from this brief theoretical discussion that there are overlaps between medicine, therapy, health care, rehabilitation and social care. There are also potential overlaps between advocacy, key working, case management, team management and general management.

Support of team members

Members of rehabilitation teams need to be supported through their own professional systems as well as through the team; but there is a dark side to professionalism. Sandra Horn, (Chapter 4) and Allan Read (Chapter 13) draw attention to the influences that govern behaviour of members of the 'caring' professions. In his analysis of the abuse of patients in long-stay psychiatric hospitals, Martin (1984) drew attention to the emotional and social stresses involved in caring for disturbed and disabled people and the catastrophic consequences of failing explicitly to provide for this. Staff who become professionally isolated, who perceive themselves as undervalued by the organisation, and who are in a position to exercise control and power over their patients, face serious risks of sliding into abusive patterns of behaviour.

Many of us who work in rehabilitation are motivated by a wish to help, which depends on our role as a helper being complemented by patients acquiescing in their role of those needing help. When under stress, we may mount powerful psychological defences against any erosion of these complementary and balancing roles, which of course prevents the disabled person from achieving rehabilitation at the same time as preventing us from seeking the help we need. These important issues should be addressed pro-actively so that individual team member's problems do not become team problems or, worst of all, a patient's problems. Such psychotherapeutic support is best provided prophylactically to the team from a fully trained psychotherapist who is not a member of the team.

The social model of disability

We have seen that the biomedical model of disability views impairment and disability as something that is intrinsically undesirable and inviting correction. In contrast, the social model of disability construes handicap neutrally as a mismatch between the functional ability of a disabled person and the environment. Many aspects of the environment, especially in cities in developed countries are man-made. Steps, narrow corridors, doors that are hard to open, lifts whose controls are out of reach of wheelchair users, newspapers whose print is too small for visually impaired people to read and theatres in which people whose hearing is impaired cannot hear, are all there by choice and design : a choice that excludes disabled people from participation. These choices may not have been made specifically to bring about exclusion, but have usually gone through on the assumption that the environment should expect to meet the needs only of 'normal' people. Yet, as life expectancy increases, many of us who survive to old age will have disabilities of many kinds. What range of ability is 'normal' for an elderly person?

Culturally-determined concepts of normality exist in all cultures, excluding different subsections of the population in each. Disability is a commonly encountered criterion but others, such as gender, sexuality, wealth, racial origin and religious belief, are also widespread. In the social model of disability, disability is simply one of the many forms of socially or culturally-determined disadvantage that places the onus of exclusion on those who are excluded despite the fact that the decision to exclude them has been made almost entirely by those who are *not* excluded. Such behaviour could be interpreted as evidence of the operation of psychological defences against disability, such as denial and projection. The 'biomedical model' of disability is perceived not only as differing from the social model but as directly opposed to it through its focus on abnormality. Its enthusiasm for converting disabled people into 'able-bodied' ones exposes the biomedical model to the charge of reinforcing prejudice against disabled people and maintaining their exclusion from society. These issues are dealt with in more depth by Stephen Duckworth (Chapter 3) and Sandra Horn (Chapter 4).

Disability, like other forms of disadvantage, is an integral part of the human condition. Many disabled people's difficulties could be solved by political and cultural changes rather than by medical and therapeutic ones. This faces all of us with difficult choices about how we wish our society to develop, how we should formulate rehabilitation objectives and needs, and how we should share and deploy our resources.

Clinical audit and research

The word 'science' means 'systematic and formulated knowledge' especially in relation to 'branches of knowledge . . . that can be conducted on scientific principles' (Concise Oxford Dictionary). The word 'scientific' means 'according to rules laid down in exact science for performing observations and testing the soundness of conclusions' (Concise Oxford Dictionary). Accuracy of observation and a systematic approach can increase the *certainty* of a conclusion so that it can be accepted as a provisional truth, all scientific truth being of a provisional nature.

Research is 'the endeavour to discover new or collate old facts by scientific study of a subject or course of critical investigation' (Concise Oxford Dictionary). Again the emphasis is on a systematic approach to increase the certainty that the new facts will be closer to the truth, or will illuminate previously hidden areas of knowledge.

Given the breadth of focus involved in rehabilitation, it is self-evident that the techniques of natural, medical and social sciences will all need to be used to increase the certainty of knowledge in this area. Some research will be generalisable, i.e. it will establish general truths that apply across a wide range of different contexts. For example, regular muscular exercise increases the strength of a muscle irrespective of where the subject lives or who measures the strength of the muscle, provided that standard and systematic procedures are employed to select, train and measure the subjects.

By contrast, some knowledge is only of local validity. For example, to establish how many people with traumatic head injury are admitted to hospital X per annum, those admitted can be systematically and prospectively counted with reasonable certainty of an accurate total after a year's observation. This result will be true in so far as hospital X and that year is concerned, but will not be directly generalisable to other hospitals or other years; applying the same methodology to them would be likely to give different results.

Clinical audit

This is a process by which the effectiveness of a clinical service can be repeatedly tested by critical observation and intervention using a systematic methodology, the results being fed back leading directly to an improvement in practice. Carried out well, it is a form of scientific research, the results of which have local rather than general relevance. The methodology of clinical audit for rehabilitation teams is still being worked out, but it is already clear that a number of elements are important:

1. The effectiveness with which specific individual techniques are applied or specific interactions take place.
2. The overall effectiveness of the individual team members' contribution.
3. The effectiveness and efficiency of the team as a whole in meeting its patients or clients needs.

All audit work involves a systematic cycle in which the results are fed back to change practice. The **audit cycle** is illustrated in Figure 1.3. The clinical standards should be set prospectively but if this is not possible, because criteria are unknown, an initial turn of the cycle may be needed to establish a standard before proper audit begins.

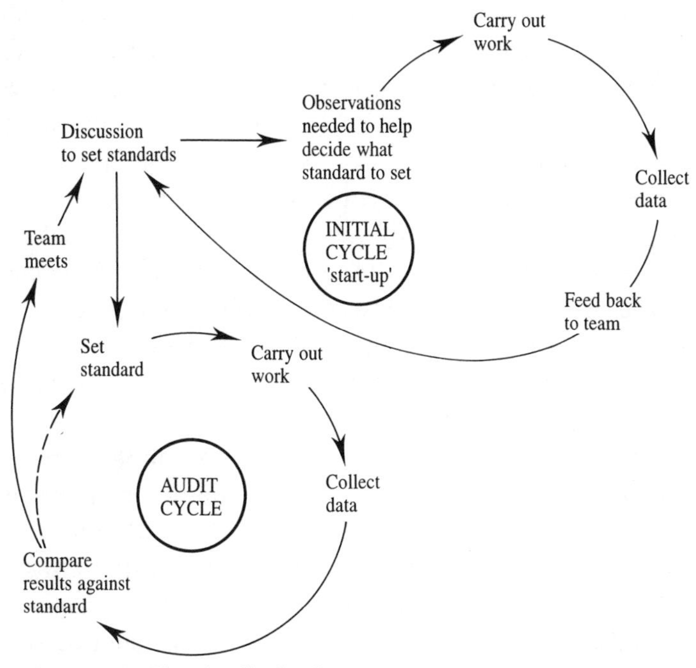

Figure 1.3. The Audit Cycle.

Data collected should ideally relate to **outcomes**, i.e. results for the service or individual. Sometimes proxy measures such as **process** standards have to be used. The disadvantage of process measures is that they tend to focus on the team rather than the patient or client, and their relevance to outcome is often questionable.

Research in rehabilitation

A conceptual framework for rehabilitation is a necessary component in its evolution, enabling question to be posed, hypotheses to be developed and appropriate methodologies to be applied. Its traditional links with medicine have helped with some aspects of scientific advance, but there are fundamental differences between the methodologies needed to develop and test practice in rehabilitation and those needed to test movement towards a biological norm in patients whose only contribution to treatment is acquiescence in it. The conceptual framework shown in Figure 1.2 brings together some of the important principles summarised in this chapter.

Research strategy in rehabilitation

Part of the erratic progress made by rehabilitation research reflects a tendency to attempt to answer inappropriate questions. Consider a project to study the effect of 15 drugs in alleviating the symptoms of 15 illnesses. No-one would tackle this by mixing a handful of each of 15 drugs in a pot and feeding the contents to a crowd in which all 15 illnesses were randomly distributed. The first stage would be to ascertain which drug is active for each condition. Then, the factors determining the strength of activity and any unwanted effects in different patients would be established one by one for each drug and each patient. Finally, the cost-effectiveness and optimal model of delivering appropriate drugs routinely to appropriate patients would be tested. It would be impossible to design effective experiments for the second or third stages until the first and second had been completed.

In rehabilitation there have been many examples of attempts to measure the outcome of a rehabilitation service in which the inputs are unknown and unmeasured, the objectives of the patients and therapists are unknown, and the outcome measures used thus had no proven relationship either to the objectives of therapy or to the therapy itself. It is hardly surprising that the results of such studies have often been inconclusive. In clinical trials, the ability to predict outcomes is extremely valuable. Once the factors that determine outcome are known, they can be controlled. This greatly reduces the variance of the outcome so that definitive results can be obtained with fewer subjects and there is much less risk of obscuring an effect through having too heterogenous a sample (Chapters 8 and 9).

Most of the published attempts to predict the outcome of disabling conditions have tested biological variables that are more likely to influence biological outcome or natural recovery than the response to rehabilitation. For example, attempts to predict the outcome of stroke have studied factors such as age, sex, side of lesion, previous stroke, presence of cardiac disease, incidence of consciousness and incontinence, and the electroencephalogram.

Factors actually used by therapists in day-to-day practice when selecting patients and rationing their therapy, such as willingness to collaborate with therapy, enthusiasm for independence, stamina and the ability to remember instructions from one day to the next, have never been formally and prospectively tested as predictors of rehabilitation outcome after stroke.

Controversy repeatedly surfaces about research methodology and rehabilitation. Sometimes it is claimed that some methodologies are better or 'more scientific' than others. The proposition that randomised double-blind prospective quantitative group trials are better and more scientific than qualitative observational studies is of course absurd. Both methods, when used properly, are scientific (carried out in a systematic way so as to maximise the degree of certainty of the results). The questions that are best addressed by these two methodologies are, however, quite different from each other. Using the wrong methodology would be most unscientific, however systematically the methodology itself were applied.

In a group of people recovering from stroke, different individuals will inevitably identify specific and different objectives. If their therapists successfully establish a therapeutic relationship with them, progress can be expected towards these objectives, but not necessarily towards the objectives that have been selected by *other* individuals and *their* therapists. Observational and qualitative methods (which are often more difficult to plan and implement than quantitative ones) are very helpful in establishing the context for rehabilitation and in evaluating such things as fears, beliefs, hopes, determination, behaviour and the ability to communicate. Controlled single case experimental designs can then help to establish the effectiveness of specific techniques replicating results over a representative sample of subjects as in series of 'n=1' group trials. Just as in conventional group trials, these studies need to be prospective, to define precisely the selection of subjects and the objectives of treatment, and they usually need to employ the principle of randomisation of subjects (or treatments) because this is one of the most helpful mechanisms for controlling bias. As a general principle, the outcome of treatment should always be assessed by someone who has not been involved in its delivery and is masked or 'blind' to its nature. Once the salient factors controlling response have been identified, the focus can shift from proving that a type of therapy is effective in specific circumstances to testing whether its influence modified outcomes more generally, and can realistically be incorporated and afforded in routine rehabilitation practice.

Vague entities such as 'exposure to speech and language therapy' are almost meaningless until the identity and effectiveness of the constituents of therapy are known. Moreover, studies of such entities cannot facilitate the development of new techniques.

Sometimes the difficulties involved in rehabilitation research appear to divert people from studying what is difficult but important to studying what is easy but less important. Surveys in which questionnaires are filled in by therapists on how they feel about various aspects of their role will tell us no more than that. They will not establish whether the therapists' work is effective or worthwhile.

Multi-disciplinary research

Even a tightly focused study of a specific therapy technique is likely to require not only the clinical and analytic skills of the therapist but the participation of a social scientist and a statistician. The more complex the study or the more it crosses disciplinary boundaries, the more essential it is to involve those with relevant expertise. Many bad rehabilitation trials have been designed by physicians who failed to enlist the knowledge or clinical skills that therapists could have provided and who therefore ended up with an expensive ambiguity instead of a clear outcome.

When setting out on a career in research, it is not uncommon for people to be secretive about their ideas because of an anxiety that they will be stolen and used by others. Of course, the whole point of researching good ideas is to ensure that they *are* adopted by others, but it is natural to hope that when this happens, their provenance will be recognised. Institutional pressures may intensify the need for secrecy and discourage people (especially in those professions that are newly emerging in the research field) from developing ideas in a multi-disciplinary way. The importance of overcoming these natural reservations cannot be overemphasized. The days are long past when an individual could expect to formulate a first class research project on his or her own. All that has been said above in relation to clinical practice applies with even greater force to research in rehabilitation.

Environment and the behaviour of non-disabled people

There are innumerable accounts of the handicapping effects of the environment and the behaviour of the other people in it. These issues are covered in depth in Chapters 2, 3, 6 and 10. A conceptual framework of rehabilitation should include the political, social and cultural influences and the measures that are capable of changing the way that people behave. The essence of rehabilitation is, perhaps, the purposeful changing of behaviour – of individuals and of societies.

Reference

Martin, J. P. (1984). *Hospitals in Trouble*, Oxford : Blackwells.

2

Disabled people in society

JOHN MARTIN

Can there be an objective measure?

It is fatally easy to fall into the trap of talking as if there were some 'correct' number of disabled people in a country. It is natural enough for concerned people, members of healing professions, politicians and others who have to provide resources and services to want a target figure at which to aim. They want simple answers to questions such as 'how many people need hearing aids, or wheelchairs, or special education or adaptations to their homes'? Once they have such numbers they can attempt to meet the 'demand' thus quantified.

Part of this chapter will indeed discuss these kinds of estimates, but at best they are approximations and at worst they can be misused to give a rather spurious statistical basis to arguments about the needs of individuals and the adequacy or inadequacy of service provision. Moreover, there is a school of thought among some disabled people which holds that such calculations imply a philosophy which overlooks the extent to which social customs and inadequate facilities create handicaps for people with impairments. They even use the word 'oppression' to describe the restricting effects of some features of social organisations (Oliver, 1986; Abberley, 1987; Bynoe *et al.*, 1991).

Computations about numbers of people with disabilities inevitably rest on a whole series of assumptions and definitions. People fall into two broad categories: those who in some way identify their own disability and those identified by others. Self-identification starts from individual perceptions of impairment about which the person feels strongly enough to consult someone else, say a teacher, a psychologist or a doctor, about it. Even if they do raise the matter it does not follow that they will decide to take any further action. It may be that little that is effective can be done about their condition, or they may feel the benefits will be outweighed by the costs, whether medical, financial or social. For example, the act of registering as disabled may make certain benefits or services available, but have the disadvantage of attaching to them a 'label' of disability which, for other purposes, they may not wish to have. There is a large sociological literature about the processes by which people take decisions to seek professional help; some of its findings will be discussed below.

On another level, however, people with impairments may be identified by others, usually doctors or public officials, because of something that strikes their attention. This is often the case with impairments diagnosed at birth or in childhood. Rather different, and more numerous, are disabilities that become conspicuous through the behaviour associated with them. Such people, whose problems tend to stem from mental illness or impairment of learning abilities, may be seen as dangerous to themselves or others, and this is taken to legitimise 'official' action. What action is actually taken depends on how people feel about the behaviour, and this is strongly influenced by the setting in which it occurs. Reactions may range from tolerance and tacit acceptance, to the immediate detention of the person concerned. In rural societies such deviance might be accommodated, and in the past the existence in English of the phrase 'the village idiot' implied that it was normal for the obviously mentally handicapped person to occupy a recognised social role albeit a stigmatised one. In an urban industrial setting dangers may be greater, and public tolerance less, so that official action becomes more likely and incarceration in an institution is liable to be seen as necessary (Barnes, 1991: 18).

Public action, however, is not solely in response to perceived dangers; all too often it derives from embarrassment and a desire to remove from public view people whose condition or behaviour provides a disturbing reminder of what life can be like when things go wrong. In the UK this has applied particularly to people with mental difficulties, whether due to illness or impaired development. For example, in the last years of the nineteenth century a pressure group was set up to campaign for the lifetime segregation of disabled people (The National Association for the Care and Control of the Feebleminded). It survived well into the twentieth century. More recently the case for not caring for mentally ill people in the community was argued by the National Schizophrenia Fellowship that was set up in response to problems arising from the lack of adequate community care for such patients.

It was and is all too easy for powers to incarcerate people to be misused. For example, it is absolutely clear that at least up until the Second World War young women who had illegitimate babies were liable to be labelled moral defectives and placed in institutions for people with mental handicaps. In the UK in the early 1990s numbers of such women, now of pensionable age, have appeared on television talking perfectly coherently about how they were 'put away' for behaviour that today would do no more than earn them the label of single parents, and actually make them eligible for various state-funded benefits. Indeed, *Put Away* was aptly used as the title of the first major study of mental handicap institutions to be published during the 1960s (Morris, 1969). Whereas not everyone would use the term oppression to apply to the treatment of all people with disabilities it would be hard to deny its aptness to such procedures.

Many people with impairments, however, may not attract attention by their behaviour yet be significantly handicapped. Perhaps the clearest example is afforded by people who are wholly or partially deaf. They have no distinguishing physical characteristics, and no behavioural ones either until they fail to respond to sounds clearly audible to others. Nowadays a good screening system should detect hearing defects in babies but adults, particularly as they become elderly, may develop hearing loss without realising it, or possibly simply regarding it as a normal, if regrettable, stage of old age. This point is well illustrated by the important early study by Leslie Wilkins (1948) made by the then Government Social survey to assess the likely demand for the rather primitive hearing aids being made available for the first time under the National Health Service (NHS).

Wilkins found that many people took a fatalistic view of the onset of deafness. Others may not have realised that hearing aids were available that might help to solve the problem (once the backlog of unmet demand had been satisfied). Hearing aids were not regarded as relevant; as Wilkins said they were not 'fashionable'. Interestingly enough their public acceptability was markedly enhanced when it became obvious that public figures, including the Prime Minister, Sir Winston Churchill, and the popular singer Johnny Ray, were using them (Wilkins, 1948; Martin, 1957).

The same point is made on a more general basis in the most recent Office of Population Censuses and Surveys (OPCS) survey when comparing its findings with those of the General Household Survey : 'many elderly people do not think of themselves as having health problems or being disabled; they consider limitations in activities a normal consequence of old age' (Martin *et al.*, 1988: 21). It is all too easy, however, for this line of thinking to be used, sometimes tacitly, to deny older people screening for treatable conditions (Henwood, 1990: 53). Thus discrimination creeps in.

In recent years, however, a more sinister form of non-recognition has appeared in the form of an official policy that people should not be assessed as having a need unless official provision exists to meet such needs. It is not clear how such a policy will be implemented as it is liable to make government organisations vulnerable to political and legal attack, but in essence this could be a legalistic way of making need invisible. The situation is obscure, but if its use develops as a method of conducting official business it could lead to abuse and cynical disregard of individual needs (Cervi, 1993).

Handicap and impairment in the 1960s

Despite the arguments about 'oppression' and the difficulties of measuring disabilities, the practical purposes of government require the effort to be made. Clinicians and others have, of course, made many attempts to estimate the prevalence of various disabling diseases, for example multiple sclerosis (Roberts *et al*., 1991). There have also been attempts to combine the results of specific surveys to produce more general estimates (Royal College of Physicians, 1986; Bradshaw, 1980). Inevitably, however, only the government has the resources to undertake the national surveys required to give a comprehensive picture covering all disabilities throughout the country. Two such attempts have been made in the UK. The first major official study was undertaken in the late 1960s by the Social Survey Division of the OPCS. It was published under the title of *Handicapped and Impaired in Great Britain* (Harris, 1971). It was a massive survey

> designed to give reliable estimates of the number of handicapped people aged 16 and over, living in private households in Great Britain, and to examine what local authority health and welfare services were being made available to the handicapped aged 16 and over and living in private households to assist them to overcome their disablement as far as possible. (Harris, 1971: 1).

Large though this pioneering survey was, it omitted children under 16 years of age, those living in institutions and all those who, though impaired, did not wish to admit to the fact (it relied on respondents being prepared to define themselves as impaired and handicapped). The survey found a total of 'just over three million people aged 16 or over living in private households who have some physical, mental or sensory impairment, about one and a quarter million men, and just over one and three-quarter million women' (Harris, 1971: 4). They represented about one in 13 of people aged 16 years or over, approximately 7.7%.

Surveying disabilities in the 1980s

The Harris survey was used for official purposes until it inevitably became out of date. By the mid-1980s new figures were needed, so in 1984 the then Department of Health and Social Security (DHSS) commissioned a new series of surveys. Once again they were carried out by the Social Survey Division of the OPCS and the results have been published in a series of volumes of which the first was *The prevalence of disability among adults* (Martin *et al.*, 1988).

As a matter of DHSS policy the new survey was to differ from its predecessor in two important respects: it was to cover more categories of people, and the key concept would be disability rather than impairment or handicap. The new categories to be included were:

children
people living in communal establishments
people with *all* types of *disabilities*.

The first two of these were obviously important because of their potential demands on resources, whereas the third was an attempt to avoid some of the anomalies produced by the Harris definitions. For example, Harris had commented that 'A man who is totally deaf, or blind, or mentally impaired, would not be included unless he feels his impairment limits in some way his getting about, working, or taking care of himself, or he has some physical impairment. The same conditions apply to disorders such as diabetes or epilepsy' (Martin *et al.*, 1988: 4). In the new survey people were asked questions about their ability to perform various acts, irrespective of whether they would have described themselves as disabled.

Definitions of disability

The pros and cons of various possible definitions are fully discussed in Chapter 2 of the first report of the 1980s series of surveys (Martin *et al.*, 1988). The prime considerations informing the choice of method were to reconcile, as far as possible:

1. The International Classification of Impairments Disabilities and Handicaps (ICIDH) (World Health Organization, 1980).
2. The terminology used relating to social security benefits. These were 'roughly equivalent' to 'impairment' as defined in the ICIDH.
3. The fact that 'disabled people themselves and organisations representing their interests generally found questions about disability easier to answer and more relevant than questions about impairment' (Martin *et al.*, 1988 : 8).
4. The fact that a single disability may be caused by more than one impairment, and vice-versa.

Taking all these considerations into account it was decided to focus on disabilities, and to ignore impairments except when ensuring that 'people with disabilities such as those caused by mental or psychological problems were not missed' (Martin *et al.*, 1989: 9). Generally the descriptive emphasis of the questions asked should have made them easy to understand but no form of wording could probably overcome strong reluctance to admit to a disability on the part of the person completing the form used in the initial postal screening.

The survey was notable for the care taken to establish the levels of disability, ranking each on a scale, and developing a method for combining scores relating to more than one area of disability. The processes by which this was carried out were elaborate and need not be described here in any detail. The result was that answers to a range of questions asked in interviews with each disabled person (or in some cases with a person who answered for them), were combined to give scores on 13 areas of disability. These were: Locomotion; Reaching and Stretching; Dexterity; Personal Care; Continence; Seeing; Hearing; Communication; Behaviour; Intellectual Functioning; Consciousness; and Eating, Drinking and Digestion.

If a person had more than one form of disability the scores were combined according to a formula; the final result placed them in one of ten severity categories, one being least severe and ten most severe. In the lowest category, for example, might be someone deaf in one ear who had difficulty in hearing a person talking in a normal voice in a quiet room. In an intermediate category (severity category 4) was a man more severely deaf who could not use a telephone, follow the sound of a TV programme at a volume others found acceptable, and who found it very difficult to understand strangers. The most severe degrees of disability (category 10) involved, say, a stroke victim totally unable to walk, to care for himself, to do anything involving holding, gripping or turning, very limited capacity to reach or stretch, difficult for strangers to understand and incontinent at least once a month.

Locating disabled adults

The plan was for the main survey to be based on interviews with at least 10 000 disabled adults and 2000 disabled children. Adults were defined as being 16 years or older. To locate this sample of disabled units it was necessary to screen a large number of the adult population. This was carried out using a postal questionnaire; those selected from the responses to this were then interviewed about their disabilities. Altogether 14 308 adults in private households were approached as a result of the postal screening, but 3273 had a short form of the main interview (which was broken off if it became apparent that they were not sufficiently disabled to include in the survey). The level of cooperation was high; in only 11% was there a complete non-response at the interview stage. The sample was stratified in various ways to ensure adequate coverage of the types of disabilities and regions of the country.

Disabled adults were also to be found living in various forms of communal establishment. These included general hospitals, nursing and residential homes, hospitals for the mentally ill and a range of establishments for mentally handicapped people. In the end, interviews were undertaken in a total of 570 institutions; they yielded a total of 3533 full and 242 short interviews. As in the household survey, interviews were discontinued if it were found that there were 'no long-term health problems'.

Normally the interviews were with the disabled people themselves, but where the disability severely hindered communication, as with many of those in communal settings, the information was gained from a relative, carer or staff member.

Locating disabled children

The methods used to locate disabled children were similar to those used with adults, although after the initial screening it was the parents rather than the children who were approached. Separate surveys were, however, required because young children, even if not disabled, might not be able to do the things used to identify disability in adults. In practice two sets of questions were devised: the first covered school age children from 5–15 years (which was only different from the adult questionnaire in a few, but important, respects), the second was for children under the age of 5 years, who would normally be developing rapidly. The methods of devising standards of judgement were similar to those used for adults, but with special features. It is clearly difficult in some respects to judge whether a child is actually disabled or merely developing slowly. Hence it was important to take age into account when assessing position on the severity scales relating to locomotion, seeing, continence, personal care, intellectual functioning and behaviour in the 5–15 age group, and for virtually all areas when the age was below 5.

Disability among adults

The total population of disabled adults in Great Britain was estimated to be 6.2 million. They represented 14.2% of the adult population. Of these 5780 000 (93%) were living in private households, while the remaining 422 000 (7%) were in establishments of one kind or another.

The fact that the figure of 6.2 million was just over twice the 3 071 000 found in the 1971 survey reflects the wider scope of the more recent study, together with its broader definitions of disability. A proportion of this increase could probably be attributed to greater expectation of life in the population in general which has also led to somewhat higher proportions falling into the most elderly category of people of 75 years or more. A more pertinent comparison might be made with the estimates obtained from the General Household Survey (GHS) (Office of Population Censuses and Surveys, 1985). The GHS figures were more oriented towards long-standing illness or disability recognised as limiting the person's activities in some way. The somewhat surprising result was that up to the age of 74 years, the GHS rates of disability per thousand of the private household population were higher than those obtained from the OPCS survey, but for age 75 years and above the survey figures were higher. The differences were probably due to the fact that the OPCS survey focused on specific activities and only where these were limited was disability recorded; the GHS had a broader scope but was dependent on subjective judgement. It is likely that at older ages people would not regard themselves disabled so much as elderly and therefore incapable of doing things listed in the severity scales. By 75 years of age their aspirations would be less, and their feelings of frustration might have died down. The disability survey was inevitably rather mechanistic in its approach and would count the disabilities that the GHS respondents came to ignore. Its importance was that it could demonstrate areas of need that respondents might have played down through ignorance of what might have been done for them had resources been devoted to them.

Interpreting national surveys

On its own an aggregate figure such as that of 6.2 million disabled adults in the population is useless. Before such figures can be of any value they have to be broken down to relate to subgroups about whom meaningful things can be said. Disabled people may fall into many subgroups that have little in common with each other beyond what they may feel to be a stigmatising and misleading label. When analysing statistics from a major survey such as the 1985 OPCS one it is important, therefore, to consider what relatively homogeneous subgroups may exist and to consider their situations in turn.

Subgroups may be identified either because their members can be observed from outside to have characteristics in common that differentiate them from the rest of the population, or because their disabilities create a common consciousness, so that they are aware of belonging to the group and expressing feelings and views about shared experiences, or possibly both. People with severe brain injury, for example, may fairly easily be classified by outside observers without themselves necessarily being aware of their common experience. Blind or deaf people on the other hand, are likely to be aware of their shared disabilities and may form associations or pressure groups to lobby on their behalves. They may not necessarily get together physically, but linkages between them are such that it makes sense to talk of them as social groups.

Perhaps the first set of distinctions that can be applied for policy purposes are those based on what Topliss (1981: 4) has referred to as the 'three ages of disability' : 'children, adults of working age and the elderly'. The 1985 survey showed that children below the age of 15 years formed 5.5% of the total disabled population; those aged 16–59 years formed 29.4%, whereas the remaining 65.1% consisted of those of 60 years and above. Not only were approximately two-thirds in the elderly category, but approaching one-third (28%) of all disabled people were aged 75 years or over.

Topliss' discussion shows that, even though the distinction is an administrative one, it is based on a reasonable perception that the needs of disabled people in these age groups differ. It is a robust if not refined distinction. It takes in the differences in expectations and histories of those of various ages but it also reflects existing patterns of service provision.

This set of distinctions can be refined by looking at what happens at the various ages with a slightly more clinical eye. Some children have congenital impairments that may limit expectations of lifespan, or may be expected to endure throughout a life of average duration. Children with spina bifida exemplify the former category, while those with learning difficulties are in the second. Psychologically such children have always been seen, and may have seen themselves, as disabled. There are, of course, those who grow out of disabilities or otherwise overcome their disadvantages, but when they do they fall outside the scope of surveys of disabled people. Trends in disabilities among children are subject to paradoxical influences: on the one hand, health education and improvements in antenatal diagnosis may reduce the risk of impaired children being born but on the other, once alive improved medical technology may increase the survival of children with severe and multiple impairments who, ten years ago, might not have survived.

Among those of working age there are those who become disabled in adult life relatively suddenly, sometimes as a result of illness, such as poliomyelitis, or a traumatic event, such as an accident at work or a war wound. Many of these may establish an equilibrium, different from their earlier lives, but not implying an obvious or immediate decline in health, although in the longer term their expectation of life may be somewhat affected. Improvements in preventive medicine and in health and safety measures should lead to a reduction in the numbers of such casualties, but any such improvements can be overwhelmed by the effects of war and social conflicts.

Moreover, in adult life there are also those who develop progressive conditions, such as motor neurone disease, or multiple sclerosis, which may imply a long-term decline in health with increasing disability. Sometimes as with psychoses such as schizophrenia, the disability will be varying and unpredictable. The increased capacity to save people from death has as its corollary higher levels of chronic and disabling illnesses.

Finally, there are the diseases and declining powers that affect the elderly. There is no exact chronological dividing point, but many elderly people become disabled to some extent. The proportion rises steeply with age; OPCS found that 714 per thousand of the population aged 80 years and over had some form of disability, and 35% were in severity categories 6–10, i.e. experiencing multiple forms of severe and lasting disability. This compared with 5.7% of the 60–69 year age group. Many old people tend to expect their abilities to be limited in old age and therefore their attitude may be one of philosophical resignation that may make them less demanding of medical and social care than would be the case with younger people with similar levels of disability. Unfortunately this possibility is too often taken as a reason for not providing allowances (available for younger people) on the ground that there is no need for them. This tacit acceptance may not persist; attitudes and expectations are socially determined and it may well be that generations of elderly people who have grown up since the establishment of the NHS in 1948 will expect more positive policies than their predecessors.

The roles of private households and communal establishments

One of the most fundamental findings of the OPCS survey was the fact that 93% of disabled adults were living in private households. Whether it is called community care or not, the fact remains that at all but the highest level of severity more disabled people were living in private households than in institutions. Only at severity level 10, restricted to those who cannot care for themselves at all and who have major difficulty with almost every activity of daily living, was the number of adult women in communal establishments slightly higher than those in private households: 77 000 as against 69 000. At no level of severity were the majority of disabled men in communal establishments. This situation is largely explained by women's greater expectation of life; most women in residential care are very elderly, single or widowed. It is still a fact of vital importance that such a great majority of disabled people live and are cared for in private households.

Types of disability among adults

By a wide margin the most frequent type of disability was that of locomotion, reported by 99 out of a 1000 adults, almost exactly 10% Next in frequency came difficulties in hearing (59 per 1000), and in personal care (57 per 1000). Dexterity was a problem for 40 per 1000. Difficulties with seeing affected 38 per 1000. After these came problems of intellectual functioning (34) and behaviour (31). Unfortunately the analysis did not consider how the various disabilities were linked. It did, however, find comparatively slight differences in the types of disability affecting those in private households compared with those in institutions, although one would imagine there might be considerable differences in degree.

What were conspicuous were the differences between age groups. For almost all forms of disability the rate among the elderly (75 years and over) was at least ten times that for people of working age. In both groups difficulties of locomotion were the most frequent form of disability, but the rate for the elderly was 15 times as high as for those of working age. Problems of continence, rare between the ages of 16 and 59 years (8 per 1000), increased 30-fold to a rate of 120 per 1000 among the elderly, not much talked about but likely to be an embarrassment for more than one in ten. Other contrasts affected perception, with the prevalence of seeing and hearing difficulties increasing sharply 28 and 19 times, respectively.

The disabilities of the working age group were also headed by those of locomotion (31 per 1000), but were followed by a group (behaviour, intellectual functioning and personal care) which suggest the effects of mental illness, learning difficulties and possibly multiple handicaps. Indeed, the survey commented that 'Communication, behavioural and intellectual functioning disabilities are more common among those aged under 60 years than among the older disabled. This is because conditions such as mental handicap do not increase with age and are a major cause of disability at younger ages' (Topliss, 1981 : 31). Hearing disabilities were twice as prevalent as problems with seeing (16 as against 8 per 1000).

Severity of disability of people living in private households

The survey showed that there were important differences between the sexes in terms of the severity of their disabilities, and their age distribution (Topliss, 1981, table 4.2). Men with disabilities tended to be younger than disabled women. Whereas 29% of disabled women in private households were of working age, for men the proportion was 36%. Adding in those in the 60–74 year age group showed that 77% of disabled men were under 75 years, whereas the corresponding proportion for women was 62%. Disabilities among women were, therefore, more likely to be associated with old age than were the disabilities of men.

The disabilities of women living in private households were also more likely to be in the higher categories of severity. Only a third (34%) of disabled men were in severity categories 5–10, whereas approaching a half (46%) of women were in these groups. These figures, incidentally, imply that the majority of both sexes were in categories 1–4. This was particularly evident in the case of men, of whom 41% were in categories 1 and 2, compared with 30% of women.

Severity of disability of people in communal establishments

As over 90% of disabled people were living in private households, and only a minority (422 000 out of 6202 000 or 6.8%) in communal establishments, it was likely that those in institutions would be the most severely disabled. This was indeed so: 77% of men and 83% of women were in the more severely disabled categories 5–10.

Once again there were differences between men and women. Women were more concentrated in the most severely disabled categories (47% were in groups 9 and 10 and 70% in categories 7–10) whereas for men the corresponding proportions were 39% and 61%. There was also a difference in their ages. Nearly a third of the men were of working age (32%) compared with only 10% of women. Just over three-quarters of women (77%) were aged 75 years or above, compared with only 44% of men.

Complaints causing disabilities

Informants were asked what conditions caused the disabilities that they reported. The answers were often given in lay terms, and may not have been entirely accurate (although when given by the staff of communal establishments they should have been based on case notes). Moreover, the disabilities mentioned might have more than one cause, so the picture painted below is inevitably an over simplified one. Nevertheless it is worth sketching, both to show the broad impact of various diseases/conditions, and to indicate the quite significant differences between the populations of disabled adults living in private households and in communal establishments.

Among *adults living in private households* the largest single category of complaints causing disability related to the **musculoskeletal system**; 46% of disabled people were so affected. Two-thirds of this group (67%) had some form of **arthritis**. Where the type was specified two-thirds mentioned osteoarthritis. Next in frequency came **diseases of the ear** (38%), almost all involving some form of deafness (Martin *et al.*, 1989).

The third group of complaints in terms of frequency among those living in private households affected **eyes** (22%). Apart from 6% attributed to cataracts or glaucoma the details of these conditions were unspecified. The fourth largest group (20%) were those affected by diseases of the **Circulatory system**. A slight majority of these specified heart conditions, principally coronary artery disease, with the remainder having various problems with arteries or veins.

Three groups of complaints came next, each affecting 13% of disabled adults living in private households. They affected the **Respiratory system**, the **Nervous system** and what was loosely termed **Mental**.

The **respiratory** complaints were largely due to bronchitis and emphysema, asthma and allergies which together accounted for nine of the 13%. Curiously, no respondents cited 'industrial diseases', possibly because of the way the questions were asked. It is hard to believe that none of the above conditions was related to employment circumstances.

Complaints under the heading of the **Nervous system** accounted for only 13% of disabilities in private households spread over a range of conditions of which strokes/hemiplegia accounted for 5%. Diseases such as multiple sclerosis or Parkinson's, which are often the subject of prominent appeals for support, accounted for no more than 1% each.

The 13% of complaints in private households cited under the **Mental** heading covered a range of conditions of which depression (5%) was the most common. What was described as mental retardation accounted for 2%. The rate quoted for schizophrenia was zero. In view of the known prevalence of this disease this is surprising, and perhaps indicates the limitations of the method of self-completed questionnaires when applied to such a delicate area. No other specific type of complaint accounted for more than 2% of disabilities among adults living in private households.

People living in *communal establishments* were mainly affected by the same conditions but the balance between physical and neurological or psychological problems was rather different. Musculoskeletal complaints were prominent (37%) but were not the most common cause of disability. Arthritis, however, was still the prime form of musculoskeletal problem.

Problems relating to ears and eyes were less prominent as causes of disabilities: 13% and 17%, respectively. Circulatory conditions accounted for 16%, of which a slight majority were heart conditions. Respiratory complaints were cited in only 6% of cases, half of them being specified as bronchitis or emphysema. Endocrine and metabolic conditions were apparent in 8% of cases, the majority of which were diabetes. Cancers accounted for 4%.

In communal establishments, in contrast to private households, conditions classed as **Mental** accounted for the largest single group of disabilities (56%). Almost half of these (26%) were due to senile dementia. The next largest subgroup (15%) consisted of those who were mentally handicapped or severely mentally handicapped. Virtually all the remainder suffered from some form of mental illness, of which schizophrenia (7%) and depression (6%) were the most common.

Whereas complaints under the heading of the **Nervous system** accounted for only 13% of disabilities in private households they were quite prominent in the communal establishments (30%). Strokes/hemiplegia formed the largest subgroup (14%), followed by epilepsy as the second most common cause of reported disability associated with disease of the nervous system (7%). Parkinson's disease accounted for 4% of those in communal establishments and multiple sclerosis 1%.

We can, perhaps, summarise these findings by saying that disability in adults was shown, above all, to be related to the diseases and deterioration of old age. At every level of severity the rate of disability among women was higher than among men. Overall there were 161 disabled women per 1000 of the population compared with 121 men. The great majority of people with disabilities, even serious ones, were living in private households. Nevertheless, other features were important: firstly, was the large element of care in communal establishments related to mental conditions; secondly, the very rarity (in national terms) of many conditions serious in themselves means that services will have to be provided in sensitive and imaginative ways if those individuals are not to be overlooked.

The disabilities of children

The OPCS survey of disabled children was undertaken in two stages. Private households were surveyed in 1985 and communal establishments in 1988 (Meltzer *et al.*, 1989). The methods were broadly similar to those used for adults, except that special care had to be taken to distinguish between those activities that children could not do because of impairments from those which they could not do because of their ages. This was particularly difficult with children under 5 years of age.

The total number of disabled children was found to be 360 000, or just over 3% of all children under 16 years in the UK. This was a much smaller proportion than the corresponding figure of 14% for adults. The number living in communal establishments was approximately 5565, or just over 1.5% of all disabled children. This compares with the corresponding proportion of 7% among adults. It should be remembered that as this was a sample survey, all numbers were subject to sampling errors that are liable to be higher when the size of samples is small.

Disabilities among children were distributed in quite different ways from those of adults. The first point was that the numbers in the different categories of severity did not vary in any systematic way, whereas with adults numbers decreased as severity increased. The numbers of children in the various categories of severity ranged from 19 000 to 46 000, but not in a regular way. In particular the least severe group only included about 10% of disabled children whereas the corresponding proportion for adults was nearly 20%. Altogether, 'younger children are over-represented in the lower severity categories and under-represented in the higher ones' (Bone & Meltzer, 1989: 27).

The cumulative prevalence of disability among children below the age of 5 years was 21 per 1000, but rose to 38 per 1000 in the 5 to 9-year-old group. It was slightly lower for the 10 to 15-year-old group. This decline was attributed to a reduction in the prevalence of disabilities concerned with continence and personal care. The jump in prevalence from the 0–4 to 5–9 age groups was thought to result from 'an increase in the identification of disabilities as children encounter the demands of school life' (Bone & Meltzer, 1989: 19).

Again in contrast to the position with adults, the prevalence of disability was substantially higher among boys than girls. The cumulative rate for boys was 37 per 1000 population, whereas for girls it was only 26 per 1000. The position is reversed in the adult population, with women becoming the majority in the 20 to 24-year-old group and increasingly so in older age groups.

The types of disability recorded among children were significantly different from those of adults. They were dominated by what were probably multiple problems of behaviour, communication, intellectual functioning, continence and personal care. The highest rate was for behaviour problems, 24 per 1000 between 5 and 15 years. Communication disabilities also remained constant at 13 per 1000, but problems of personal care and continence dropped considerably by the time the age of 10 years was reached. It is also noticeable that by the ages of 16–19 years, the first age group in the adult survey, almost all figures for disabilities were notably lower; this suggests that the figures for children were higher because they derived from adult views of their behaviour, whereas from 16 years onwards, on more of a self-report basis, these disabilities were not admitted.

Difficulties of locomotion were also fairly prevalent, at 11 per 1000 for the 10 to 15-year-old group, but again the proportion was suspiciously lower in the 16 to 20-year-old group, suggesting a difference in reporting standards.

The only other form of disability with a fairly high prevalence related to hearing (8 per 1000 for the 5 to 9-year-old group).

When parents were asked about causes of their children's disabilities the replies given were often vague and 'the value of evidence about the causes of disability is very limited' (Bone & Meltzer, 1989: 27). Almost 40% of children had disabilities arising from **'mental complaints**'; within this category slightly more than half referred specifically to mental retardation or learning and development problems, with an equal size of group just described as 'other mental illness'. The next largest category of complaint related to the **Respiratory system**, predominantly asthmas and allergy (15%). **Ear** complaints accounted for 18%, primarily conductive deafness. Epilepsy (12%) was the principal subgroup of the complaints of the **Nervous system** which, including cerebral palsy, head injury and migraine, totalled 18%. It should be noted that with children multiple disabilities tended to be common: 'nearly two-thirds had more than one type of disability' (Bone & Meltzer, 1989: 22).

Disabled children living in communal establishments

It is important to note that only a very small proportion of disabled children, even in the most severely disabled category, were living in communal establishments. The survey in fact excluded children under 5 years of age who were living in them. This was because 'the census of children's establishments which preceded the survey revealed some 150 disabled children in the age group who were residents' (Bone & Meltzer, 1989: 19). As these would have been too few for separate analysis in the sample survey it was decided to exclude them; the 150 would have made little difference to the overall total of 5565 children in communal establishments.

The great majority (88%) of children living in communal establishments were in the age group 10–15 years, and this was true for both boys and girls. Boys formed a substantial majority (60%) of both age groups. The concentration in this older age group was the result of the policies of the 1970s and 1980s which aimed to get disabled children out of institutional care; they did not really succeed with those already there, but numbers entering institutions were substantially reduced. With the passage of time children in the 10- to 15-year-old group will grow out of it and not be replaced in such numbers. Given that the vast majority of disabled children were cared for in private households it is not surprising that the reasons for being in communal establishments were predominantly social. Almost exactly a third (32%) were there because the parents could not cope with the child's problems; this was largely unrelated to the severity of the disability. Unsuitable home conditions affected a further

30%, with this being the leading factor for those in the least seriously disabled category (56%). Unspecified problems at home accounted for a further quarter (26%), and this 'cause' became more prominent as the severity of disability increased (Bone & Meltzer, 1989, table 4.9). Fortunately less common, although still evident, was sexual abuse which affected 8% overall, and 14% of those in categories of severity 5–6. Physical cruelty or neglect affected 7%, spread fairly widely over the range of severity of disability.

Information about the types of disability experienced by children in communal establishments was limited in quantity and reliability. It is probably sufficient here to say that they were dominated by behavioural problems (94%). 'Half the children were disabled in intellectual functioning, a third had communication disabilities and a quarter each had problems with continence and personal care' (Bone & Meltzer, 1989: 31, table 4.13). It was, moreover, recognised that being in residential care might itself exacerbate such problems.

On the other hand, it should not be overlooked that 22% of disabled children in communal establishments experienced problems with locomotion and probably about half of these also had difficulties with reaching, stretching and dexterity.

Despite the predominance of these emotional and behavioural disabilities among children in communal establishments some 26% had physical complaints either in conjunction with behavioural problems or on their own. They were, however, scattered over such a wide range, in such small numbers, that generalisation is almost impossible. Apart from mental retardation the only specific conditions mentioned which accounted for more than 2% of cases were epilepsy (9%), cerebral palsy (6%) and head injury (3%).

We can, perhaps, summarise the account of disabled children in communal establishments by emphasising a number of points. Firstly, the proportion **not** being cared for in a private home is remarkably small. Secondly, the distribution of disabilities seen in communal establishments is not very different from that in private households, and the causes of children being in communal care seem to be largely social. Thirdly, the majority display multiple disabilities, almost all of which include behavioural and emotional aspects. Fourthly, although numerically small, of those in the two most severe categories of disability, significant proportions had complaints described as mental, or of the nervous system. Sixteen per cent were described as congenital.

Demographic implications

The OPCS and GHS surveys discussed above provide almost the only substantial body of national data about disability in the UK, but this has mainly been used as a basis for discussions of the wider problems of, to quote the title of McGlone's (1992) study, *Disability and Dependency in Old Age*. Nevertheless, in view of the dominance of age as a factor in the prevalence of disability, his findings are of major importance. The effects of ageing are undeniable : nearly a half of those aged 75 years and above have a 'limiting long-standing illness'. This, however, did not mean they were institutionalised or incapable of independent living : 'it is still only a minority of elderly people who are unable to cope . . . even among very elderly people, large proportions are not dependent on other people for everyday domestic and personal care' (McGlone, 1992: 14–15). He draws attention, however, to the influences not only of gender but social class, which is related to the existence of chronic illness : 'professional groups have the lowest prevalence of chronic sickness, and unskilled groups the highest. This applies to all age groups, except children, and is particularly striking among women' (McGlone, 1992: 13).

The main research by demographers appears to have been carried out in the United States (USA) where considerable attention has been paid to the effects of changes in life expectancy (Crimmins *et al.*, 1989). The value of such work may be greatest at a macroeconomic level when considering likely developments in the cost of pensions and health care.

For example, the types of conclusion drawn from their analyses were, for the USA population, that 'in age groups below 65 less than one per cent of the population was institutionalised. Above age 65 the proportion institutionalised rose sharply, so that for those aged 85 and over in 1980 one out of four women was institutionalised for a physical or mental instability (Crimmins *et al.*, 1989: 238). Although, no doubt, it would be possible to produce comparable figures from the OPCS data they are not contained in the first published report. Such estimates depend on prevailing practices in providing care for elderly people in institutions. In the UK, with policies which purport to emphasise community care, the results might well be different. The whole question of the provision of residential care is contentious; it can be argued that some people in institutions need not be there, and would not be, except for the perverse effects of the social security system (McGlone, 1992: 27). The financial circumstances of disabled adults living in private homes have been described by Martin & White (1988).

Crimmins *et al.*, (1989) also use data obtained from the National Heath Interview Survey to make a whole series of calculations of periods of life free of all disability, free of long-term disability, with short-term disability, with long-term disability and institutionalised. From a comparison of data for 1980 with that for 1970 they conclude that 'additions to life expectancy between 1970 and 1980 were concentrated in the disabled years – primarily of long-term disability. On the other hand this did not mean bed-ridden. The implications for health planners were that 'future gains in life expectancy could be accompanied by increased demands on the health care system as more years of life are spent with chronic disability. It is also possible that gains in life expectancy over age 85 may result in particularly heavy use of institutional services . . . in planning for future health care needs, trends in disability as well as mortality should be considered' (Crimmins *et al.*, 1989: 255). While this interpretation depends on USA practices with regard to institutional care it seems likely that the same principles would apply in the UK.

Although rather generalised studies may have macroeconomic value, for practical purposes the best data seem to have been assembled by actuaries. They indicate that, even if life risks can be calculated for specific diseases, judgements still depend on fairly close clinical observation. Those who have to advise disabled people on their long-term prospects would, as a starting point, find it useful to consult *Medical Selection of Life Risks* (Brackenridge & Elder, 1992).

Informal carers

It would be wrong to finish an account of the numbers of people with disabilities without drawing attention to the many people linked with them through caring relationships. Although, as has been said earlier, many people with disabilities are fully or largely able to look after themselves, others cannot manage without help. The great majority of these depend on informal carers, i.e. people who are not employed professionally as carers.

The OPCS has twice published information about informal carers derived from questions in the GHS (Green, 1988; OPCS, 1992*b*). The 1990 survey (published in 1992*b*) showed that there were about 6.8 million carers in the UK (2.9 million men and 3.9 million women) aged 16 years or over. They represented 15% of the population aged 16 years and over. The peak age for caring was 45–64 years; about three-quarters of the carers in this age group were looking after parents or parents-in-law.

While the majority of carers (57%) spent less than 10 hours a week caring, a substantial minority (23%) spent 20 or more hours a week. In numerical terms this meant that in 1990 1.5 million adults were spending 20 or more hours a week on caring activities. Almost half of this group (11% of all carers) actually spent 50 hours or more caring each week.

Carers were divided into those who looked after someone in the same, or another, household. In 15% of households the carer was looking after someone in another household; 5% were looking after someone in the same household. The great majority (66%), however, of those who spent 20 or more hours a week caring did so for someone in their own household; in ten times out of ten they were the main carer. Care within the same home included personal care, e.g. with washing, in over 50% of cases. Those who were caring for someone elsewhere usually took fewer hours and tended to cover a less intimate type of help, mainly keeping company, taking out, shopping and generally keeping an eye on the dependent person.

Discrimination and 'oppression'

The convenient label 'the disabled', with its associated international symbol of a person in a wheelchair, has advantages and disadvantages. It readily brings to mind the notion of physical disability, and generates a degree of sympathy in many people. It justifies making allowances for all manner of things from providing disability pensions to ramps and parking spaces. It has, however, the unfortunate effect of casting the disabled person in what medical sociologists call 'the sick role', i.e. a role in which they are seen primarily as patients, excused many things on account of their disabilities but on the implied condition of being required to submit to medical direction. This tends to have at least four bad consequences:

1. It implies that all people with disabilities have medical problems, and that doctors are the best people to help them : an attitude sometimes known as the 'medicalisation' of disability.
2. It stereotypes even physical disablement as involving wheelchairs, whereas many impairments have different, or no, visible signs. It totally overlooks disabling mental conditions.
3. It obscures the true circumstances of the disabled person and often leads to the (perhaps unconscious) treatment of disabled people as if they were totally incapable, an attitude neatly encapsulated in the title of the BBC programme 'Does he take sugar?' It fosters unwarranted assumptions about dependency.
4. It treats the disabled person as the possessor of a problem (often true) but ignores the extent to which societies can ease or hinder both specific activities and the integration of disabled people into the community.

It may come as a surprise to some readers of this book that some disabled people talk of themselves as belonging to an 'oppressed' group. To doctors, nurses, therapists and professional carers at first sight it may seem ridiculous to apply a political term to people whom they seek to help; yet it is important to understand the thinking and feelings that lie behind the rhetoric. Those who wish to explore the arguments in detail should consult, for example, the works of Abberley (1987), Oliver (1986, 1990), Finkelstein (1980), McEwen (1990), Barnes (1991) and Bynoe *et al.*, (1991) and Stephen Duckworth (Chapter 3). What follows is an attempt to state the essence of that position as simply as possible.

The disabled person is at a disadvantage compared with an otherwise similar individual without his or her particular set of disabilities. Some of those disadvantages are unavoidable, the blind cannot see, the injured sportsman can no longer compete with former opponents, but some disabilities can, or could, be reduced by social action. The argument turns on how much? The answers lie on a continuum with, at one end, the 'official' or 'conventional' view that underpins studies such as the OPCS' disability survey and, at the other, the 'oppression' view expressed, for example, by Oliver (1990). He maintains that official classifications 'while acknowledging that there are social dimensions to disability, do not see disability as arising from social causes' (Oliver, 1990: 6). He goes on to devise a list of 'alternative questions' which range from the rather vague 'can you tell me what is wrong with society?' to the more specific 'do you have problems at work because of the physical environment or the attitudes of others?'

The difficulty with Oliver's position lies with the assumption on which it depends. It is what might be called a 'level playing field' theory; in other words that somehow society, physically and culturally, should be organised so that everyone has an equal chance to do what they want. As a matter of practical politics that is not convincing, but it does point to the vital question of whether enough is done to make the playing field sufficiently level for more to be able to play on it. Inevitably this is a matter of balancing costs and benefits; the balance that is struck cannot be determined automatically, but depends on the values of all with powers to take decisions. Each decision involves attaching a value to the human dignity of *others* as individuals, and to the importance of having a society without degrading inequality. In the last resort it is a matter of how society interprets the notion of citizenship as applied to its less able members. Whether it is helpful, or politically wise, to use the term 'oppression' in the present UK context is a matter of opinion.

Conclusions

This attempt to consider the situation in the UK regarding disability leads inevitably to the conclusion that no families can for long be untouched by the problems associated with disability. All are subject to the fundamental influence of the age structure of the population. The prevalence of disability can be seen as the product of two distinct frequency distributions: the major one being primarily age-related, and the lesser being dependent on events which are more independent such as congenital conditions, accidents and epidemics. Health policy can do little to alter the former, except bear its implications in mind, but should do as much as possible to prevent, or at least mitigate, the effects of the latter. Prevention and mitigation raise issues of citizenship beyond immediate health care. This is not a revolutionary observation; our Victorian ancestors achieved their greatest successes through prevention. It is unfortunate that the lessons of that period are having to be relearned a century later because modern politicians have had selective memories of what actually happened at that time.

References

Abberley, P. (1987). The concept of oppression and the development of a social theory of disability. *Disability, Handicap and Society*, **2**, pp 5–19.
Barnes, C. (1991). *Disabled People in Britain and Discrimination.* London: Hurst.
Bone, M. & Meltzer, H. (1989). *The prevalence of disability among children.* (OPCS surveys of disability in Great Britain: Report 3). London: HMSO.
Brackenridge, R. D. C. & Elder, W. J. (1992). *Medical Selection of Life Risks.* Basingstoke: Macmillan.
Bradshaw, J. (1980). *The Family Fund.* London: Routledge & Kegan Paul.
Bynoe, I., Oliver, M. & Barnes, C. (1991). *Equal Rights for Disabled People*: the case for a new law. London: Institute for Public Policy Research.
Cervi, Bob (1993). Trail of confusion. *Community Care*, **18**, March, 6.
Crimmins, E. M., Saito, Y. & Ingegneri, D. (1989). Changes in Life Expectancy and Disability-Free Life Expectancy in the United States. *Population and Development Review*, **15**, 235–65.
Finkelstine, V. (1980). *Attitudes and Disabled People.* New York: World Rehabilitation Fund.
Green, H. (1988). *Informal Carers.* Series GHS no. 15 Supplement A. London: HMSO.
Harris, A. J. (with Cox, E. & Smith, C. R. W.) (1971). *Handicapped and Impaired in Great Britain.* Office of Population Censuses and Surveys: Social Survey Division. London: HMSO.
Henwood, M. (1990). No sense of urgency: age discrimination in health care. In E. McEwen ed. *Age: The Unrecognised Discrimination.* London: Age Concern.
McEwen, E. (1990). *Age: The Unrecognised Discrimination.* London: Age Concern.
McGlone, F. (1992). *Disability and Dependency and Old Age: A Demographic and Social Audit.* London: Family Policy Studies Centre.
Martin, J. P. (1957). Notes on the use of statistics in social administration. *British Journal of Sociology*, **8**, 208–23.
Martin, J., Meltzer, H. & Elliot, D. (1988). *The prevalence of disability among adults.* OPCS surveys of disability in Great Britain: Report 1. London: HMSO.
Martin, J. & White, A. (1988). *The financial circumstances of disabled adults living in private households.* OPCS surveys of disability in Great Britain: Report 2. London: HMSO.

Martin, J., White A. & Meltzer, H. (1989). *Disabled adults: services, transport and employment*. OPCS surveys of disability in Great Britain: Report 4. London: HMSO.

Meltzer, H., Smyth, M. & Robins, N. (1989). *Disabled children: services, transport and education*. OPCS surveys of disability in Great Britain: Report 6. London: HMSO.

Morris, P. (1969). *Put Away. A Sociological Study of Institutions for the Mentally Retarded*. London: Routledge & Kegan Paul.

Office of Population Censuses and Surveys. (1986). *General Household Survey 1985*. London: HMSO.

Office of Population Censuses and Surveys. (1992a). *General Household Survey 1990 Report*. London: HMSO.

Office of Population Censuses and Surveys. (1992*b*). *OPCS Monitor: General Household Survey: Carers in 1990*. London: OPCS.

Oliver, M. (1986). Social policy and disability: some theoretical issues. *Disability, Handicap and Society*, **1**, 5–17.

Oliver, M. (1990). *The Politics of Disablement*. Basingstoke: Macmillan.

Roberts, M., Martin, J. P., McLellan, D. L., McIntosh-Michaelis, S. A. & Spackman, A. J. (1991). The prevalence of multiple sclerosis in the Southampton and South West Hampshire Health Authority. *Journal of Neurology, Neurosurgery and Psychiatry*, **54**, 55–9.

Royal College of Physicians. (1986). *Physical Disability in 1986 and Beyond*. London: Royal College of Physicians.

Smyth, M. & Robus, N. (1989). *The financial circumstances of families with disabled children living in private households*. OPCS surveys of disability in Great Britain: Report 5. London: HMSO.

Topliss, E. (1981). *Social responses to Handicap*. London: Longman.

Wilkins, L. T. (1948). *Survey of the Prevalence of Deafness in the Population of England, Scotland and Wales*. The Social Survey, Reports (New Series) No. 109. London: The Social Survey.

World Health Organization. (1980). *International classification of Impairments, Disabilities and Handicaps*. Geneva: WHO.

3

Disability equality training

STEPHEN DUCKWORTH

Introduction

The primary focus of this chapter is to describe the philosophy behind Disability Equality Training (DET) and its use in challenging employment discrimination. DET is a short training programme of one or two days that has been developed by disabled people for employers. The training aims to provide delegates with an understanding of the social model of disability. This will help them improve their organisations' policies and procedures in order to reduce the impact of institutional discrimination on disabled applicants and employees.

Previous alternative attempts to reduce this discrimination have not worked. Legislation which has imposed a quota of disabled people on employers and attitude modification programmes designed in the USA have failed to combat discrimination. Alternative approaches are needed (Duckworth, 1995). This chapter introduces one such approach that is based on the social model of disability. This model rejects the assumption that employment discrimination results solely from the negative attitudes of employers as being too simplistic. It favours viewing discrimination as a process institutionalised within social organisation.

Initially the experience of discrimination is considered with reference to the changing nature of work. Then the construction of the 'disability category' is described with regard to the development of the social model of disability as based on the underlying ideology. The utility of the social model in challenging employment discrimination is considered by contrasting its application with the individual (medical and tragedy) model. Next the social model is developed to suggest a new and probably more realistic reason for the failure of the quota scheme. This discussion concludes by presenting a new definition of disability. Next a balance is sought between the polar views expressed by the individual and social models. This concludes by arguing that the social model provides a more useful framework to understand and challenge employment discrimination.

Following this the application of anti-discrimination legislation to challenge racism and sexism is considered and the campaign to gain similar protection for the rights of disabled people in the UK is described. Next an international comparison is drawn between the two principal approaches selected by a variety of countries to address employment discrimination.

The chapter continues by describing the relationship between the development of the social model and disability politics. Finally, the findings of a five year research project to evaluate the effectiveness of Disability Equality Training are described. It is revealed that training based on the social model of disability can be of value in challenging employment discrimination and is more appropriate than attitude change based training.

The changing nature of work

During early industrialisation, impairment probably did exclude many disabled people from the labour force. Work typically involved heavy physical labour in large and small factories, mines and on the land. Conditions were harsh and demanding, often resulting in the disablement of the workforce, who were then unable to perform their work tasks. Since the Second World War, however, the nature of work itself in industrialised nations has changed substantially with the steady decline of heavy manufacturing industry, the introduction of new technology to replace human labour and the expansion of the service sector. In addition, new technologies, particularly information technology, and the emergence of new science-based industries have dramatically transformed the labour markets of modern societies (Cornes,1984).

Thus there are many more kinds of jobs, requiring different sets and levels of skill, in the workforce. For a whole range of jobs, some sort of technology is required in the conduct of work. It is this kind of technological development which has transformed the potential of people with impairments, as modern technology can eliminate most functional limitations in employment. It is, however, difficult to envisage how all impairment-related difficulties, such as the fatigue experienced by some people with multiple sclerosis and the cognitive problems of people after a head injury, can be overcome by technology alone. Other changes such as flexible working hours and support workers may also be required.

Notwithstanding this, some writers have heralded these technological developments as paving the way for a significant expansion in the range and number of jobs that disabled people might undertake (Bowe, 1980). This was expected to occur through the development of a new generation of equipment and adaptations, through technologies which reduced the need for physical strength and through increased opportunities for remote working brought about by developments in communications. In addition to changes in the economic base and developments in new technology, legislation has ensured a shorter working week and improvements in working conditions that are favourable to all.

Finkelstein (1980) anticipated the impact of the benefits above in an idealised three phase account of disability. Phase I refers to feudal society, seen as a cooperative community of agriculture and small scale industry which did not preclude most disabled people from participating, in some way, in the process of production. With industrialisation, i.e. Phase II, the nature and speed of factory work and the hours and discipline required resulted in many disabled people being excluded from the labour market, not to mention disabling many others in the process. Disabled people came to be seen as a social and educational problem resulting in their segregation within institutions of various kinds. Finally, Finkelstein believed that the late 1980s would be characterised by an emerging Phase III. He anticipated that during this period disabled people would be liberated from the segregating practices of society by new technologies and by closer partnership between professionals and disabled people.

In some respects Finkelstein was right to anticipate the distinctiveness of Phase III. It is difficult to find a class of employment that is not currently being carried out by a person with some kind of impairment. This is supported both by reference to disabled luminaries, in fields ranging from cosmology to politics, and to numerous examples in the literature on successful employment projects involving disabled people (Tackney, 1989; Murray & Kenny, 1990).

Even where a job requires the most rigorous selection tests of physical and intellectual ability, disabled people need not necessarily be excluded and may actually offer some advantages as demonstrated by Rogers (1991) in his only partially tongue in cheek 'Case for the Amputee Astronaut'. This is not to say that every disabled person can do any job, or that impairment will not be a factor for some in certain employment options, but that the changing nature and conditions of work should mean that disabled people could become more adequately represented among all occupations than is presently the case.

The range of employment and the new opportunities afforded by technology, however, have not yet mitigated the position of disabled people as the most marginal in the labour force. Indeed, technology may even further contribute to the disadvantage experienced by disabled people. Over a decade ago, Schworles (1983) identified an emerging 'culture gap' in the expertise of using new technology between disabled people and their non-disabled peers.

In the light of these technological developments it is worth considering the additional cost to employers of employing disabled people. This is important when trying to justify the expenditure of scarce resources. For example, it would be difficult to defend significant investments in employing one disabled person when the same resources could have been used to create three jobs for three 'less expensive' disabled people. A review of these cost implications (RADAR, 1994) reveals little concern as the total cost of complying with antidiscrimination and making 'reasonable accommodation' in employment in the UK is about £16 million. Most of this sum is available from the Employment Service to support disabled people in work so the issue of cost should rarely, if ever, be a factor.

If Finkelstein's Phase III has failed to materialise for most disabled people, this is less likely to result from the failed promise of technology than from deficiencies in training and the resistance provided by other barriers. Nor can blame be laid at the door of disabled people's ability.

It has previously been demonstrated that within UK employment legislation the principal barrier identified is that of discrimination which is implicitly and explicitly assumed, as defined by policy, to be resulting from the negative attitudes of individual employers (Duckworth, 1995). Success is held to be dependent on changing those employer attitudes by persuasion to bring about non-discriminatory employment practices. Such a claim has never been demonstrated as being achievable and its utility has been challenged (Duckworth, 1995).

This incumbent approach contrasts with an evolving alternative explanation for the disadvantage experienced by disabled people in employment which views discrimination as institutionalised within society's beliefs and practices rather than as a function of individual attitudes. The inequality resulting from institutionalised discrimination has led some commentators to view the disadvantage experienced by disabled people as a particular form of oppression (Abberley, 1987).

Advocates of the view that disability is institutionalised express their views both nationally and internationally through such organisations as the British Council of Disabled People (BCODP) and Disabled Peoples' International (DPI). The utility of this approach which encompasses the social model of disability in combating the employment discrimination experienced by disabled people is contrasted next with the individual model approach.

The individual model

There are always a variety of ways that can be used to explain particular situations. Historically, disability has been conceptualised as a problem of the individual. The approach is underpinned by an assumption that there is something intrinsically wrong with disabled people which results in their experience of limited opportunities. This model positions the impairment as the primary focus of concern for employers. Candidates for jobs are often judged according to their impairment rather than the skills, aptitudes and qualifications that they have to do particular tasks.

The individual deficiency, as defined by this model, can be viewed as a personal tragedy resulting in people who need to be looked after and cared for. It can also be seen as a medical problem requiring therapeutic intervention to help resolve the situation. The tragedy approach has assumed that the experience of disability devastates the individual to such a degree that there is little hope of participating as an active citizen. The individual is deemed to have become dependent and is defined in terms of their diagnostic label. Charities were established, based on impairment categories, to help these 'unfortunate' individuals and their fund-raising efforts have often adopted an approach based on the tragedy model. This sociological phenomenon has had a significant impact on the employment prospects of disabled people and does not measure up to the facts about the ability of disabled people in employment.

The medical model also positions the impairment as the primary focus of concern. It has been underpinned by an assumption that the quality of life of disabled people can be best improved by resolving or limiting the impairment through treatments aimed at curing the individual. While these are laudable expectations, there are problems in maintaining this approach as the only, or even the primary, focus is that when interventions do not 'cure' the individual, disabled people are likely to be perceived as having a permanent medical problem, or illness, that will result in limiting their opportunities.

Notwithstanding the inadequacies of the medical model, it is difficult to challenge for a variety of reasons. Firstly, for any individual who has just lost a degree of motor, sensory or intellectual functioning their initial desire would be to regain it as fully and rapidly as possible. Research by Martin *et al.* (1988; 1989), however, demonstrates that this is not an option for 6.2 million adults in the UK as 14.2% of the adult population who experience an impairment through accident or illness will not be cured.

The second problem in challenging the medical model results from the considerable level of expertise developed by practitioners working in this field. They have gained a great deal of knowledge about impairment through research and practice and have been vested with considerable power over disabled people's lives by society. Any challenge to the status of the medical model is a challenge to this knowledge and the power that underlies it.

The challenges to this model, however, can be illustrated by specific examples. For instance, people with spinal injuries are often instructed and encouraged by medical practitioners to use a 'standing-frame' two or three times a week for an hour at a time. This frame is a device that helps a paralysed individual stand in one position with the assistance of straps and posts. People with high level injuries require the help of two assistants to achieve this and the process can be quite painful and time consuming. People with spinal injuries are advised that this will help with kidney function, reduce bladder infections, improve psychological well-being and reduce spasms, yet there is no evidence to support this.

This 'therapy' is expensive not only in terms of the cost of the standing frame but also in paying for the personal assistants that would be required. The pain experienced and time needed adds a personal component to the cost involved for participating in a 'therapeutic' process that has dubious scientific merit. There is a possibility that the whole regimen may be based on a deep rooted assumption that it is 'normal' to be upright and that attempts have been made to validate this position through scientific theory and medical research. Similar problems can arise when people with mobility impairments are encouraged to walk with the assistance of a cane or crutches rather than using a wheelchair which is often considered as the solution of last resort. In addition, a powered wheelchair is often perceived less favourably than a manual wheelchair.

These ideas may be based on assumptions which presume that quality of life can best be enhanced by attempting to approximate 'able-bodiedness' rather than equipping disabled people with the most effective tool to get them from one place to another while leaving the person with enough energy to complete a day's work.

No model is capable of providing all the answers to a particular situation but it is clear from the discussion above that the individual model, encapsulated by the tragedy and medical approaches, is very problematic when considering how best to improve opportunities in employment. The scenarios outlined above could deny employment for a variety of reasons. Firstly, disabled people may be too busy undergoing therapy to have time to work or train for work; secondly, they may be too tired to work competitively on their arrival at the job because of the high energy used getting to work; thirdly, employers may associate disability with illness; and fourthly, the tragic images of charity fund-raising may encourage corporate donations while limiting employment opportunities.

Under these particular circumstances it is not surprising than at employment policy to promote opportunities for disabled people that seeks to change negative attitudes has not been fruitful. It is clear that an alternative approach is required which is discussed below as the social model of disability.

Developing the social model of disability

To shift the focus in the definition of disability has been the driving aim behind sociologists working with the disabled (Finkelstein, 1980; Abberley, 1987; Morris, 1989; Oliver, 1990). They have set themselves the task of applying sociological perspectives to the issue of disability as the basis for producing a new social theory of disability. They have identified the 'Grand Theory' implicitly underpinning almost all previously mentioned studies of disability as 'personal tragedy theory' leading to the medicalisation and individualisation of disability (Oliver, 1990). More recently, the socially created 'dependency model' of disability current in social theory and policy which has resulted in institutionalised discrimination in our society has also been introduced (Barnes, 1991).

A recent, refined version of this approach (Oliver, 1990) explores the roots of personal tragedy theory. Oliver argues that disability as a category can be understood only within a framework that suggests that it is both culturally produced and socially structured. Central to this framework is the mode of production and the way in which the production process is organised. This does not however imply straightforward historical materialism. As Oliver asserts, the core or central values of a society, such as superstitious, religious or philosophical values, also have a role to play.

The existence of cultural factors explains the variation in the experience of disabled people in different societies noted by anthropologists (Hanks & Hanks, 1980). There is, however, a relationship between the mode of production and the prevailing mode of thought within society. This results from the requirement to redistribute the economic surplus according to the needs of the mode of production and social perceptions about how this should be appropriately achieved. Social practices are therefore underpinned by a set of values or beliefs which, according to Oliver, comprise 'ideology'.

In describing the ideological construction of disability, Oliver adapts the work of Gramsci (1971) to distinguish between interrelated core and peripheral aspects of ideology. Core aspects are those historically necessary to the mode of production. They are equivalent to Gramsci's 'organic' ideologies which have a psychological validity in that they organise human masses and create the terrain on which people move (Gramsci, 1971). Peripheral ideologies are related but more equivalent to movements or trends.

Under capitalism one core aspect of ideology is that of individualism because of the requirement for individuals to sell their labour in the open market. This necessitates a break from collectivist notions of work as a product of family or group involvement. The construction of the disabled identity was a corollary of this development as an idea of individual able-bodiedness or able-mindedness was thought of as being essential to the development of individual wage labour (Stone, 1984). Applying Foucault's (1965) work on madness, Oliver stated that it is only this idea of individual 'able-bodiedness' which makes possible the idea of disability as an individual pathology justifying exclusion with the focus on the body. This, combined with the scientific revolution in medicine, has contributed to the 'medicalisation' of disability.

Various theories have been put forward to explain the dominance of the medical model of disability, including Finkelstein's (1980) structural explanation which linked 'medical control' with the rise of institutions and the success of hospital-based medicine. To this Oliver added the influence of 'germ theory; and, latterly, the ability of the medical profession to expand its activities into the field of rehabilitation.

One of the consequences of the medicalisation of disability and its consequent definition as an individual pathology was the widespread acceptance of the concept of adjustment. This emphasised the requirement for the disabled individual to undergo medical treatment and rehabilitation in order to be as 'normal' as possible and also presupposed a process of psychological adjustment or coming to terms with the disability.

Oliver contends, however, that if the ideological construction of disability has been determined by the core ideology of capitalism, i.e. individualism and the peripheral ideologies associated with medicalisation and underpinned by personal tragedy theory, this is not the whole story. Disability has also been socially created. In ideological terms, disability has been defined as an individual disadvantage requiring a set of particular social policies, rather than incorporating provision into general social and environmental planning. The effect of special policies has been increasingly to create or reinforce dependency among disabled people.

This process is traceable to the origins of the welfare state. Prior to the Second World War, the position of disabled people in society was predominantly a picture of institutionalisation or isolation within the family. The proliferation of war time and post-war legislation, of which the 1944 Disabled Person's Employment Act was part, appeared to offer the promise to disabled people of full citizenship. The welfare state as envisaged by the Beveridge Report was based on a philosophy of active citizenship within a framework of entitlements, providing cradle to the grave security for all individuals. In translating this philosophy into practice, the welfare state became side-tracked into a form of provision that emphasised need, and created passive rather than active citizens (Ignatieff, 1983).

For example, the Chronically Sick and Disabled Persons Act (1970) extended services for disabled people but, in its style of provision, also facilitated the emergence of a dependency creating professional/client relationship. Oliver (1990) documented the factors that trap both professionals and disabled people in this relationship:

> economic structures determine the roles of professionals as gatekeepers of scarce resources, legal structures determine their controlling functions as administrators of services, career structures determine their decisions about whose side they are actually on and cognitive structures determine their practice with individual disabled people who need help – otherwise why would they be employed to help them. (Oliver, 1990: 90-1).

Barnes (1991) points out that even the recent Disabled Person's (Services, Consultation and Representation) Act 1986, in spite of its rhetoric, extends this approach to disability through its statementing procedures. The Act originally afforded disabled people the right to be assessed, consulted and represented, and included in its provisions reference to meaningful collaboration between users and providers of services.

Subsequently, it has been announced that important aspects of the Act regarding the right to an advocate, the right to have a written statement on needs assessment and the right to ask local authorities for services are not to be implemented. There is also evidence that there has been little attempt by local authorities to interpret their obligations towards consultation within the spirit of the Act (Barnes, 1991).

Institutionalised discrimination is also evident in housing policy where accessible homes form only a tiny percentage of total housing stock. Much of what exists forms ghettos in public sector 'special needs' developments leading to homelessness among disabled people, often masked by disabled people remaining with families. Housing difficulties will compound the employment disadvantages of disabled people by decreasing their occupational mobility.

Disabled people also experience institutionalised discrimination in transport policy. Adaptation of production cars is often prohibitively expensive for disabled people while most urban 'public' transport, buses and local rail systems are inaccessible to many, leading to a reliance on more expensive methods, such as taxis, or segregated transport provision, e.g. Dial-A-Ride which is not sanctioned for regular journeys such as to the work place.

Problems in the built environment for disabled people have been somewhat ameliorated recently with building regulations stipulating that structures erected after 1987 should be accessible. However, the voluntarist approach to buildings erected before that time means that disabled people will continue to experience institutionalised discrimination in the built environment restricting access to both work, leisure, social and political life.

In this way, therefore, disability is not merely socially constructed but also socially created and 'dependency' has supplemented 'personal tragedy' as a prevailing peripheral aspect of ideology in service provision.

The creation and reinforcement of dependency has a political basis in the way in which the legislative approach to disability is locked into a professional and service based approach rather than a civil rights approach. This is perpetuated by the way in which political discourse about disability is conducted in a particular linguistic form illustrated by such descriptors as 'community care', 'care attendants' and even 'carers'.

The political context determines the professional basis for the creation of dependency which is apparent in modes of service provision incorporating little consultation, unequal professional/client relationships and inflecting patronising social attitudes.

The influence of the medicalisation of disability, the personal tragedy thesis and the creation of dependency are all reflected in modern cultural and media images of disability. The Broadcasting Research Unit (BRU, 1990) reported that the most common feature of factual reporting in broadcasting on disabled people concerned medical treatment, particularly 'cures' for impairment. Other disability issues tend to be referred to specialist slots.

Broadsheet newspapers similarly tend to report on even non-medical disability issues in the health section. The influence of the personal tragedy thesis is especially evident in, but by no means confined to, tabloid newspapers reporting, particularly if some celebrity can be seen to be intervening on behalf of a particular group of disabled people. Intrinsic to the personal tragedy approach and also popular in 'human interest' style reporting is the 'brave cripple' approach which applauds any disabled individual who is deemed to overcome personal tragedy often by accomplishing perfectly normal acts (Reiser & Mason, 1990).

Fictional representations of disabled people, television programmes, films and literature demonstrate the ideological content of cultural images of disability. Many have the historical, religious or superstitious roots also identified by attitude theorists. Only rarely in any of these areas, however, is disability treated realistically, i.e. incidentally, as a situation occurring naturally in a percentage of the population. It is more often employed as a symbolic device for a range of metaphors. Disability has been used to portray or enhance a variety of characterisations ranging from malevolence to helplessness (Thurer, 1980; Kent, 1987) or to convey a parable on adjustment (Longmore, 1987) ultimately conveying the essential soundness of prevailing social norms.

The failure to use realistic images of disabled people is also obvious in advertising which is the section of the media most directly targeting our behaviour. UK advertising agencies have so far generally declined to 'risk' using disabled people in general advertising to sell their products, implying assumptions of negative association.

The impact of ideological representations of disability is readily apparent in charity advertising. Historically, charities have commonly made quite aggressive use of both the personal tragedy and dependency images in their efforts to raise funds. Reiser & Mason (1990) point to the reliance placed by the former Spastics Society on pathetic and pitiable images of disabled children begging outside shops. The Winged Fellowship, a charity providing holidays for disabled people, has emphasised the perceived burden that disabled people place on their families and hence assumptions about their dependent position. This approach has been moderated in recent years to suggest that readers focus on 'ability not disability'. Campbell (1990) noted that this is still misleading for it retains the focus on the disabled individual rather than on society.

Other charities, particularly those seeking funds for medical research, still rely heavily on the personal tragedy image with an emphasis on the solution being provided by a cure. This is seen, for example, in recent Multiple Sclerosis Society advertisements or the Schizophrenia – A National Emergency campaign.

Finally, ideological definitions of disability are also reflected by the language commonly surrounding it. The medicalisation of disability is reflected by the fact that disabled people are often collectively grouped in depersonalised terms by their impairment; 'the deaf' and 'the spinal injured'. The influence of the personal tragedy model is illustrated by such phrases as 'suffering from', 'afflicted by', 'a victim of' and 'struck down by'. Disabled people are also spoken of as 'bound' to their wheelchairs or 'confined to their homes' by their individual impairments in way that neglects the restrictions imposed by the built environment.

The implications of this analysis for improving employment opportunities are important because it supports the need for a shift away from defining individual disabled people as being the root cause of the problem. An alternative strategy is required which values the contribution disabled people can make and questions the way that social barriers limit opportunities: the social model. When this model is applied to the disadvantages experienced by disabled people in work, alternative solutions can be developed. The explanatory power of the social model is revealed in the next section when it is used to demonstrate an alternative explanation for the failure of the quota system.

Applying the social model

The analysis offered by the social model provides a compelling explanation for the failure of the quota system. It was quite simply a maverick policy. The quota, by recognising, even in a compromised way (Bolderson, 1980) disabled peoples' rights, was incompatible with a whole range of other post-war policies which emphasised need and dependency and which largely determined the societal approach to disabled people.

The quota system recognised the employment rights of disabled people, but did so within a social environment which effectively restricted their access to exercise that right. The scheme did not take account of the institutional discrimination experienced by disabled people in all other areas of public provision: education, training, transport, environmental planning, housing, etc. This meant that disabled people were generally less well educated, less able to have access to transport, less geographically mobile and even less likely to be able to enter the very work places where the jobs, that they were supposed to have a sanctioned and assured right to, existed.

Instead of recognising the need to address the social restrictions faced by disabled people, other parts of the 1944 legislation placed a reliance on the rehabilitation profession to 'adjust' the individual disabled person to compete equally in the labour market. Emphasis on individual adjustment was, itself, consistent with the individualisation and medicalisation of disability.

The emphasis has subsequently been criticised both theoretically (Finkelstein, 1980) and empirically (Silver & Wortman, 1980). Bolderson's (1980) point about over-optimistic expectations of the rehabilitation professions is really therefore a point about the limits of individual adjustment as a means of accessing equal rights.

The result of this was that when presented with an unqualified and socially inexperienced disabled school leaver or a disabled applicant unable to move freely around the work place or use the existing office equipment, employers could simply refuse to recognise disabled applicants as suitable or fully rehabilitated or capable of competing on equal terms in their interpretation of the quota. That they were furthermore not required to do so was ensured by the prevailing political discourse, which defined disability in terms of personal deficiency, and which resulted in the passive implementation of the scheme.

Re-defining disability

The on-going development of a discourse which employs a social model of disability by both sociologists and disability rights activists has led to the attempt to re-define key concepts:

> **Disability** is the loss or limitation of opportunities to take part in the normal life of the community on an equal level with others due to physical and social barriers.
>
> With an accompanying definition of:
>
> **Impairment** is the functional limitation within the individual caused by physical, mental or sensory impairment.
> *(Barnes, 1991: 2).*

In other words people who have impairments are disabled by the society in which they live. It can be argued, therefore, that once all the disabling barriers to employment are removed disabled people will enjoy equality of opportunity in work. This situation will only ever be achieved if the social model is robust enough to provide all the solutions, which still remain open to question.

In beginning to develop a social model of disability, sociologists who are themselves disabled are linking the understanding of disability with developments in social theory in other areas. The dependency and personal tragedy models of disability may be compared with other 'victim blaming' social theories (Ryan, 1971) such as individualistic explanations based on the character weakness of the poor and unemployed and the 'sickness' of the criminal, lesbian or gay man. Alternative models incorporating social and economic factors have been constructed. In the social model definition the causation of disability is shifted from the individual's biological pathology and directed towards society and social organisation.

Social approaches argue that those who seek to address the disadvantage experienced by disabled people in society, by changing public attitudes or the attitudes of specific groups towards them are focusing on the manifestations and not on the root causes of disadvantage. The majority of the mechanisms revealed by the attitude theorists, based on ambivalence, guilt or fear of difference, are apparently supported by polls such as the recent Harris findings (Harris, 1991). These identified admiration, embarrassment, pity and fear as the predominant ways in which disabled people are viewed. Such views are likely to result from social organisation including segregating practices and the ideological construction of disability.

Some researchers (Stubbins, 1980; Siller, 1984), who write from an attitude research perspective, have expressed concern about the general orientation of their discipline to disability. For, by failing to look beyond the idea that only individuals develop attitudes and neglecting to examine the institutionalised patterns of behaviour and definitions of situations within the structural framework of the society that affect the disabled person (Atlman, 1981; Siller, 1984), they have realised that they are neglecting the most major variable of all, social organisation, which is not susceptible to analysis at the level of the individual.

In addition, researchers into attitudes towards disabled people, being part of society and part of the body of people who write about or do things to disabled people, are themselves influenced by prevailing ideological approaches and approaches that individualise and medicalise disability (Oliver, 1990). This happens both at a general level and at the more specific level of the discursive effect of these models on their particular disciplines.

This process by which a blend of science and culture constitutes the wisdom of a particular applied social science was discussed by Foucault (1965), although other writers have since recognised the need to be aware of the role of forces current in the larger society in shaping the evolution of a discipline (Kuhn, 1971). In other words, however well-intentioned the basic approach of attitude research, with its focus on the disabled individual, is both informed by and a manifestation of social organisation which itself causes the devaluation of disabled people. This implies a further problem with the attitude research approach. It appears to involve a degree of circularity, because it relies on a definition of disability that is created and sustained partly through the researchers' own activities.

The individual and social models

It has been suggested earlier that no one model can provide all the answers to a particular problem. A model is simply a set of ideas that have been developed to explain a particular situation. They can only ever be used to approximate to the true picture. It is argued here that the individual model of disability and the social model represent the opposite poles of a continuum. This spectrum is considered next to determine the most effective approach currently available to tackle employment discrimination against disabled people.

Historically, the individual model has been far more influential by presenting the impairment as the principal focus for intervention. Despite this, medical model practitioners have also recognised the existence of 'disabling barriers' which they often refer to as the 'handicapping' effects of disability. The derivation of this relationship is important because if, under medical definitions, the handicap results from the disability which in turn results from the impairment then logic would dictate that resource allocation and research effort should be directed primarily at ameliorating the impairment. This imperative is reflected by the dominance of impairment-centred research as reported in the majority of 'disability' journals, magazines and books.

Proponents of the social model take the opposite view. Their arguments lead to the conclusion that:

> It is in fact the posture of society at large that constitutes the most disabling parts of being disabled, not the physical effects of whatever condition one happens to have, unless it leaves the individual utterly bedridden or completely fatigued. On the whole, it is the organisation of society, its material construction and the attitudes of individuals within it, that result in certain people being disabled.
> *(Brisenden, 1986: 175).*

Despite stressing the organisation of society, Brisenden also recognised the importance of impairment: 'unless it leaves the individual utterly bedridden or completely fatigued'. It is important to note he has acknowledged that some features of a disabled person's experience are not socially defined. Indeed, the most recently refined definitions, as reported above (Barnes, 1991), refer to both disability and impairment.

In practice, however, the importance of the experience of impairment to individuals and the way in which they function with respect to others has not received the same degree of attention, nor has their been much campaigning on this aspect. This has happened for a variety of reasons.

Firstly, academics in disability research who are aligned to the social model have sought to redress the major imbalance resulting from medically-dominated ideas relating to 'disability'. Secondly, individual disabled people have not tended to go against the latest ideological emphasis on the social model by discussing personal concerns about pain or progressive impairment for fear of being thought of as not 'politically correct' enough to be part of the movement. Finally, the disability movement does not represent the views of all disabled people.

The differences of opinion over the most appropriate model to employ in disability research have emerged in a recent unpublished report presented to the Commissioning Group on Physical and Complex Disabilities (NHS R&D Programme, South and West Regional Health Authority, 1993). A sample of disabled people gave a higher priority to research on reducing impairments than they gave to questions based on the social model.

It is a fact that the majority of disabled people are over the age of 65 years (Martin & White, 1988). If the social model is to gain greater acceptance then the concerns of this group, and many other disabled people, who are still impairment-focused need to be considered. Continuing with an extreme polarisation of views might inhibit a broader acceptance of the social model and may result in a large number of disabled people adhering to the individual model. Partnerships are needed to gain a consensus perspective which represents the broader views of a larger number of disabled people about the balance between the individual and social models.

To achieve this, moderation may require shifting from a constraining adherence to a model that presents one particular pole of a spectrum of experiences. That is not to say that the social model or the individual model are wrong, each simply contains part of the true picture. This implies that there is a need for proponents of the social model to address the concerns of disabled people who focus on their impairment. Shakespeare has argued that:

> in order to reach out and foster collective identity, the disabled people's movement will have to work out new ways of dealing with the issue of impairment, and of developing conscienticization among the wide majority of disabled people.
> *(Shakespeare, 1993: 257)*

This development is needed not only to help those disabled people who view the social model as an anathema but also for professionals in the non-disabled field who feel threatened by recent developments. Avoiding the issue could lead to many important views being dismissed as belonging to a 'non-representative' minority. Professionals in the disability field are still, in the main, the gatekeepers of scarce resources which disabled people need to develop the application of different solutions. The USA experience suggests that significant progress can only be made when positive partnerships are developed between the disabled people's movement and employers, politicians, journalists, broadcasters, lawyers, rehabilitationists, academics, service providers, educators and other key social actors (Lunt & Thornton, 1993).

The latest demands from academics in disability research have been in favour of developing the concept of research based on an emancipatory model that strictly adheres to a method in which the research question, methodology, analysis and distribution of reports should be developed and conducted by disabled people and their representative bodies (Oliver, 1992). Shakespeare (1993) has questioned this concept of 'disabled people only' doing research. History is full of examples of the danger of any group within society believing that they are the only custodians of the truth.

A change in emphasis, however, is now required to start raising the priority of social model research. In addition, social model fundamentalists need to move from simply acknowledging that impairments exist towards developing a new way of thinking about the experience of being impaired which is a balance between the individual and social model. The experience of pain, even if the individual does not 'suffer' from it, needs to be considered in relation to productivity at work and general quality of life. The psychological impact of recurrent remissions for people with progressive impairments and the experience of people with expressive dysphasia are two further examples of many that require more thought. Although many of these issues can be illuminated by the social model the impact of the individual experience of impairment is important both to the employee and the employer.

This balance point in the spectrum of disability has yet to be reached. Despite this, and the relative explanatory powers of the social and individual models in our understanding of disability and impairment, there is still a concentration on the individual model by most employers. They still tend to favour medical retirement when an employee becomes disabled or justify not recruiting disabled applicants because of assumed sickness and low productivity. In research about disability, there is additional evidence of a bias towards the medical model. This is illustrated by considering the pain experienced by someone with juvenile onset arthritis. Research describes the development of treatments, therapies and drugs to limit the individual experience of pain but much less appears to have been done to explore the social model component. Research on the impact of the different height of seats, the benefits of using a wheelchair, the application of voice-activated computers, self-medication, unemployment, the height of the step on to a bus, the thickness of pens, the design of door knobs, social isolation or the distance required to walk to the shops are much more difficult to obtain, despite the importance of these considerations.

The social model is also helpful in understanding assumptions about dependency. The model proceeds from the *a priori* assumption that all human beings are dependent on each other. The presumed independence of non-disabled people is accompanied by a tendency to underestimate the interdependent nature of social existence. A routine flick of a switch to turn a light on actually engages the interrelated input of many thousands of people. The social apparatus is dependent on many such groups and activities, no matter how unremarkable and normalised the activity. These considerations put into context the view that certain people are dependent.

Oliver (1986) argued that the underlying ideology and associated concepts of individualism have made a large contribution to this emphasis on the individual model. Stone (1984) has added that there can be significant legal, medical, individual, political and economic pressure to change the number of people defined as 'disabled'. She argues that the flexible nature of the 'disability category' is important in times of either high or low unemployment. In other words, definitions based on the individual model can be deployed for ulterior motives.

In conclusion, it has been argued above that although the social model of disability is a useful way of examining the problems experienced by disabled people, the individual model may also be of value in considering the needs of newly disabled people, those with rapidly progressive impairments and those where medical intervention can improve function as is the situation for some people with mental health problems. In this chapter it has been necessary to consider the appropriateness, or otherwise, of the two models with respect to the cause of employment discrimination and measures taken to address it. While recognising the impact of particular impairments on productivity, an approach based on the social model has been selected as being more relevant and more effective. The social model can also be applied to the reduced productivity of people who experience pain or progressive impairments by providing solutions such as part-time work, job sharing, disability leave (like maternity leave) and flexible working hours. To date the individual model approach has led to a focus on attempts to rehabilitate people to fit them back into current work patterns with limited success. It has also been used to sanction early retirement on medical grounds and to segregate significantly disabled people into institutionalised employment. Social model solutions offer great utility and may be more appropriate when used to tackle employment discrimination.

The social model and discrimination

The conclusion that the social model has considerably more power than the individual model to explain the disadvantage experienced by disabled people in employment has several important implications. Duckworth (1995) has demonstrated that an approach attempting to change negative employer attitudes has definite limitations. The social model, however, presents a variety of solutions to the problems experienced by disabled people at work which otherwise would not be available.

Once it is recognised that discrimination is not a function merely of employer attitudes directed at individuals' impairments, but of social policy and practice, the focus of attention for challenging discrimination should be widened to include these factors.

Combating race and gender discrimination

In two areas where institutionalised discrimination has been recognised in the UK, namely sexism and racism, legislation has been employed in the Sex

Discrimination Act (1975) and the Race Relations Act (1976) to establish the illegality of discriminatory practice. That the Acts, in themselves, have not been completely successful in eradicating sexism and racism in the UK (Gregory, 1987) is indicative that the mere existence of anti-discrimination legislation does not provide a total solution to the problem of institutionalised discrimination. It has been suggested that legislation will only work effectively as part of an integrated approach comprising an independent structure for implementation, freedom of information and adequate funding for representative bodies to provide mechanisms for redress (Barnes, 1991).

Legislation, however, is an important first step. In addition to providing a framework for the enforcement of anti-discriminatory measures, it provides public confirmation that citizens from disadvantaged groups should enjoy the same rights and freedoms as other citizens and should not be subject to discrimination. In the terms of earlier discussion, anti-discrimination legislation for disabled people should reflect a change in ideological and political emphasis from individual needs to social rights.

The concepts of basic social rights and freedoms of citizens have increasingly become synonymous in international law and the national laws of some states with human and civil rights. These rights are not envisaged as divisible, and so legislation confirming civil rights is usually framed to be comprehensive. In the context of civil rights, therefore, another view of the 'failure' of the 1944 quota legislation is to recognise its partial nature as rights legislation.

Although there is no written constitution in the UK embodying the fundamental rights and freedom of citizens, successive governments have signalled a conceptual recognition of human rights, both through criticism of the human rights records of other nations and through subscribing to a number of relevant international Declarations and Conventions. These include the Universal Declaration of Human Rights (1948) and the particularly relevant United Nations Declaration on the Rights of Disabled Persons (1975) which specifically includes the right to freedom from discrimination.

The inclusion of disabled people in the concept of human rights was explicitly recognised in the United Nations Programme of Action (UN, 1988) which in outlining a global strategy for preventing disability and realising the full potential of disabled people also recognised the right of all human beings to equal opportunities.

None of the instruments mentioned above have been formally incorporated into the British legal system but the concept of civil rights has influenced the context of campaigns against racism and sexism. In the same way, organisations of disabled people in the UK, campaigning against institutionalised discrimination, have directed their campaigns towards asserting the human rights of disabled people and to obtaining equal civil rights in the community.

As there is no existing constitutional definition of individual rights, enforceable measures to prohibit or redress the effects of discrimination must be by statute. There has therefore been a growing campaign among UK disability organisation during the last 15 years for comprehensive anti-discrimination legislation in the field of disability.

The UK campaign for comprehensive anti-discrimination legislation

As early as 1978 MIND (an organisation seeking to help people with mental health problems) called for the introduction of equal opportunities legislation to counter the discrimination encountered by people with current or previous mental health problems in employment.

In 1982, CORAD, which had been set up by the Labour government in 1979, (following the recommendation of the Silver Jubilee Committee on Improving Access for Disabled People), surveyed the extent of architectural and social barriers facing physically impaired people and concluded that, while not being a universal panacea, legislation does have an extremely important part to play in combating discrimination and in providing a framework on which to base an integrated society.

The Conservative governments which have been in power since 1979 have, until 1995, not accepted the arguments for such legislation and have, as has been seen in employment policy, preferred measures that emphasised the need for persuasion and encouragement. This is entirely consistent with their other policies of minimalist intervention although this is usually held to be within a regulatory framework of law.

In a letter to Peter Large of the Association of Disabled Professionals the Prime Minister wrote:

> Many acts of apparent discrimination arise through thoughtlessness or ignorance of the special needs and the abilities disabled people, and we will carry on working to bring about the changes in attitudes and improved awareness among the general public, which are an essential step in removing barriers to full integration.
> *(Major, 1993: 6)*

Major's chosen language revealed the type of assumptions he made about disability, change mechanisms and ultimate goals. This statement indicated a commitment to address individual attitudes despite the evidence which points toward the need for more effective approaches to challenge institutional behaviours. Moreover, the mention of integration as the goal suggests that the norm is a non-disabled society into which disabled people must somehow fit.

Many opposition attempts to introduce comprehensive Anti-discrimination Legislation have failed. The Government's stated position of benevolent neutrality on this issue has been exposed to considerable question. As a result, mounting pressure from a variety of sources mean that the government had to reconsider its options.

In other countries the drive towards gaining recognition of disabled people's human and civil rights has met with varied responses. Substantial progress has been made in America on a civil rights act for disabled people that has provided a model for disabled activists elsewhere. It is interesting to note that in the country which has lead the world in attitude research and techniques to bring about attitude change there has been a realisation that anti-discrimination legislation, consistent with the social model of disability, is required.

In the UK this has resulted in the Disability Discrimination Act 1995 which has been criticised by many commentators as being weak and not comprehensive. The reason being that this new Act, like the failed 1944 Disabled Persons Employment Act, is based on partial rights legislation. Disabled people and others are already campaigning for a more comprehensive approach.

International responses

The Americans with Disabilities Act (ADA) came into force at the beginning of January 1992. On signing it President Bush declared, 'let the shameful wall of exclusion come tumbling down', while Senator Edward Kennedy referred to it as 'a bill of rights for the disabled' (IHT, 1989). These do not seem to be unduly extravagant claims for such an inclusive, comprehensive and prescriptive measure. It should be noted that the contrast between the language of the Conservative John Major and these Republican and Democrat politicians is quite marked. The ADA introduced detailed provisions to prevent discrimination in four main areas: employment, public services (including transport), private sector services and telecommunications.

Although it is as yet too early to judge the effect of the Act, disability rights campaigners are optimistic that it will make a major difference by removing institutionalised discrimination. Sufficient resources have to be available in both public and private sectors if changes are to be made without widespread invocation of the 'undue financial burden' defence.

Although the ADA is unique in that it is the first example of a unified piece of rights-based anti-discrimination legislation in respect of disability, similar law has also been developed in Canada and in some states of Australia as a result of case law developed from complaints under the human rights charters adopted by these countries and states.

On the basis of these developments some disability rights campaigners have looked to the Europe Union (EU) as a potential source of pressure on UK domestic policy. It would seem that the EU is unlikely to effect substantially British domestic policy towards disability, at least in the short term. Promotion of the social and economic integration of disabled people does not fit easily into the pattern of EU powers which were originally viewed as solely economic in nature. Certainly, it is not presently even within the powers of the Union, as defined by the Treaties which establish them, to introduce EU wide anti-discrimination legislation.

Conceivably, the EU could recommend that members states adopt comprehensive anti-discrimination legislation and provide a model act, but in practice such a Recommendation is likely to have little impact. Daunt (1991) notes that there is little significant commitment among national authorities to the idea of a European policy on disability. He believes that this stems from the tendency for national policies towards disability to have been developed in a largely *ad hoc* way.

Even if political will did exist for such an EU policy, there are numerous problems of subsidiarity that would need to be overcome before such a measure could be effective. For example, agreed definitions of disability and discrimination would be required in all EU languages. Yet Denmark, as a matter of policy, does not have an official definition of disability. There would also be considerable problems in the harmonisation of existing national provisions.

No European country has yet adopted comprehensive anti-discrimination legislation to protect the rights of disabled people.

Methods to challenge discrimination

Disabled people face discrimination in our society regardless of the model used to describe it. Discrimination contravenes conceptions of social justice but, in the field of employment, existing evidence seems to indicate that discrimination may also be unwarranted on pragmatic grounds. There is evidence to show that employed disabled people perform at least as well as non-disabled people across a broad selection of criteria.

In terms of British government employment policy, discrimination has been defined as a function of individual attitudes and anti-discrimination policy has been principally confined to trying to change these attitudes through information and persuasion. The force of law has only been adopted recently and in a way that is far from comprehensive and therefore destined to fail. This policy stance contrasts dramatically with the approach adopted to address racism and the unequal treatment of women. Although the current employment approach does not use an explicit definition of attitude, it shares the central assumptions found in attitude research literature in which attitudes are seen as abstract individualistic concepts, whose existence is assumed to explain regularities in behavioural responses. Although group attitudes may be studied, as in employer attitudes or peer attitudes, such studies merely provide an aggregation of the individual's attitudes within these groups to a more generalised level.

Attitude research has revealed a plethora of determinants and variables that are thought to determine attitude formation towards disabled people. The excessively varied and complex nature of its findings and lack of success in evolving modification techniques based on them is partly the result of methodological problems. Primarily, however, it is because this approach does not consider the effect of the prevailing ideological framework on individual attitude formation and on the very definition of the disability itself. By concentrating on the individual manifestations of institutionalised discrimination such research does not acknowledge the existence of institutionalised discrimination.

In an examination of the ideology relating to disability in our society, disability emerged as a category that is both socially constructed and socially created. This calls for a re-interpretation of the discrimination experienced by disabled people, away from the view that discrimination is a function of individual attitudes and toward the view that discrimination is a process which is institutionalised throughout our society in policy, ideology and social practice.

On this account, attitude change programmes, by accepting prevailing individualist definitions of disability and discrimination, and by identifying the disabled individual as the focus, can be seen as participating in the larger process of discrimination. Approaches based on the same assumptions, i.e. those which rely on changing the attitudes of individuals towards disabled people as a means of obtaining their equality of opportunity share the same conceptual and practical limitations, and are subject to the same criticism. This applies as much to attitude studies focusing on disabled people which are designed to accompany social change as to approaches that rely on attitude modification to produce change.

This carries the debate over individual attitudes and institutional behaviour one stage further. It has been argued that approaches using persuasion and education, which adopt the individual model of disability and aim to change the attitudes of individuals towards disabled people, will never result in substantial improvements in employment opportunities (Duckworth, 1995).

In other areas where institutional discrimination has been identified in the UK (i.e. with respect to race and gender), anti-discrimination legislation has been adopted as a primary form of redress. Internationally there are precedents for a similar approach to disability. In the UK, however, institutionalised discrimination against disabled people has become so deeply entrenched that neither traditional political activity nor the direct action employed by populist groups of disabled people has so far resulted in comprehensive legislation. The Disability Discrimination Act 1995, based as it is on partial rights, appears to be nothing more than a cosmetic exercise.

In the absence of comprehensive anti-discrimination legislation other approaches are required. This has led to the development of complementary strategies for change. Disability Equality Training (DET) is one such development. DET has been designed to enhance the case for the adoption of the social model of disability. It is based on an approach to training which is founded on the principles of the social model of disability and aims to challenge employment discrimination within an institutional framework.

Disability equality training and disability politics

The development of DET has been a natural progression from the growing sense of empowerment felt by many disabled people that has stemmed from the process of political emancipation enjoyed by an increasing number of disabled people throughout the world. The work of sociologists on disability in developing a social theory of disability has provided a theoretical basis for the pioneering work of disabled activists associated with the disability movement. The influence of both have enabled the emergence of a disabled identity based on the common experience of oppression by people with different impairments.

This new identity is one that disabled people can be proud of in a similar fashion to the way that other minority groups have declared that there is 'Strength in Sisterhood', 'Black is Beautiful' or that they are 'Glad to be Gay'. This has begun to challenge the historical divides created by the medical model among people with different impairments and identified contemporary social organisation, characterised by institutionalised discrimination against disabled people, as the alternative cause of limited opportunities.

The political agenda also began to change since the gradual theoretical transition from the individual model to the social model. Anti-discrimination Legislation, as the first line in removing institutionalised discrimination, came to be seen as the principal political objective of the newly emerged organisations of disabled people. It also came to be adopted by many of the traditional organisations for disabled people as the logic of the social model proved to be a catalyst for change. The emphasis on legislation as a primary requirement to combat institutionalised discrimination was reinforced by national precedents in the fields of race and gender and international examples of Anti-discrimination Legislation being incorporated into the statute books in respect of disability.

Various strategies have been developed among disability groups to maintain political pressure on the government or to press for change through other routes. These range from parliamentary lobbying through new alignments of disability groups (VOADL) and attempts to understand and redress the under-representation of disabled people in mainstream political activity (Fry, 1987), to direct action against particular manifestations of institutionalised discrimination (Disability Now, June 1990). All such strategies have in common a shared theoretical basis in the social model of disability and a shared concept of discrimination as an institutionalised process.

DET is a further strategy for change that has been developed by disabled people. It is underpinned by the same theoretical models of disability and discrimination as the more overtly political strategies outlined above. It also recognises that the achievement of Anti-discrimination Legislation is an essential step in eradicating institutional discrimination. In the presence of limited political progress in this area, however, DET is primarily conceived as a practical tool for tackling employment discrimination within current service provision and the employment policies and practices of organisations.

The first formalised and structured approach to training around disability, using the new theoretical model, was developed under the auspices of the London Boroughs Disability Resources Team (LBDRT). The new Training Forum outlined their view of the purpose of DET as follows:

> A Disability Equality Training Course will enable participants to identify and address discriminatory forms of practice towards disabled people. Through training they will find a way to challenge the organisational behaviour which reinforces negative myths and values which prevent disabled people from gaining equality and achieving full participation in society.
> *(LBDRT, 1991: 3)*

DET is therefore designed to spread acceptance of the social model of disability and demonstrate to different organisations their role in the model by showing how common organisational policies and practices may discriminate against disabled people. These policies may be shown not only to infringe the human rights of disabled people but also to be against the interests of the discriminating organisation.

DET is thus an essentially complementary activity to the political activities of the developing disabled peoples' movement. Within the present context it may be expected to achieve, if in a somewhat piecemeal fashion, some reduction of built-in discrimination within organisational policy and practice.

Various DET packages are now available from different training organisations and companies. There is debate within the disability movement about the appropriate use of training, as happens with all new movements. The debate focuses on degrees of conciliation, appropriateness of confrontation and even questions as to who should or should not benefit from training. As a consequence, training packages may vary accordingly, although all are based on the same basic principles.

An important element of all DET is that it should be delivered only by disabled trainers. This does not mean that trainers are able to claim to represent all disabled people. Trainers can only claim to be expert about their own experiences of discrimination. Even though these experiences may be unique there are many parallels that can be drawn. Although there are many variations and differences between disabled individuals and many groups within what appears as one category, there is an ideological framework that is discernible. Above all it is important that the trainer has some direct experience of this particular form of social oppression otherwise the message will become weaker. In addition, the very presence of disabled trainers adds an experiential component to the seminars.

DET is usually divided into two parts. The first part of the seminar is designed to familiarise participants with the social model of disability and the concept of institutionalised discrimination. The second part of the course is designed to address, in a practical way, measures and improvements that organisations may take to identify and redress employment discrimination within their own policies and procedures.

The social model and attitude

The social model is introduced to delegates by a series of exercises designed to show how people are disabled by the arrangement of the physical environment and transport, by segregative social policies and by prevalent negative images and false assumptions. In short, they are asked to identify the many and varied social barriers and attitudes while exploring how they have been generated in order to understand that they result from social organisation and practices rather than from people's impairments.

This transition by delegates away from viewing individual attitudes as the cause of employment discrimination towards regarding the institutional barriers as the main problem is essential. The first part of DET may superficially appear to have some similarity to the attitude modification model rejected earlier in this chapter. This is because of the inevitable discussion about attitudes. There are two important differences, however, between the attitude research approach rejected as being not only ineffective but also inappropriate and DET. The first is that, although DET is addressed to individuals as a first line, these individuals are intended to experience it within the context of their organisational roles. DET is thus targeted at a level between the individual and the state, recognising that organisations are both important political factors and major practitioners of institutional discrimination.

The second crucial difference is that DET and the attitude research approach are underpinned by radically different models of disability. Attitude research, in line with the medical and personal tragedy models, views disability as a problem of individual pathology. In line with this model, attitude research is directed toward modifying attitudes concerning disabled people as a means to removing discrimination. In contrast, DET views disability as being primarily caused by social organisation. Accordingly, it rejects the uncritical acceptance of a view which argues that employment discrimination, or prejudice, results from negative attitudes in favour of considering social organisation, and the underlying ideology, as the critical factors to be challenged in an attempt to remove employment discrimination.

A major difference in focus has been noted between the attitude or persuasion approaches and the approach used by DET that is based on the social model. While it is true that both approaches concern attitudes, DET recognises that the attitudes of individuals within society are conditioned by prevailing misconceptions and the underlying ideology. It is these factors that are oppressive to disabled people and inevitably result in the disadvantaged position that disabled people experience and the negative perceptions about them.

By introducing the social model, therefore, trainers are asking delegates to identify attitudes and redirect their understanding away from viewing the individual's impairment as the problem towards considering how contemporary social organisation, and the underlying ideology encapsulated by individualism, is responsible for creating the many disabling barriers. In many ways this approach requires delegates to adopt a new paradigm.

Synopsis of the research study

In summary, the research evaluated six two-day DET seminars designed by the researcher to challenge employment discrimination. The training was supported by comprehensive training notes provided for each delegate. The modular training seminar introduced the social model and gradually progressed to present information to delegates about the behavioural changes required within their organisations to reduce or eliminate employment discrimination.

The research study focused on the participation of 66 delegates from large employers who attended one of a series of six two-day seminars. To attract the eight to 16 delegates required by the seminar design, a data base of 2150 personnel managers was constructed using The Personnel Managers Year Book (Kaminsky, 1989) of 5300 Members of the Institute of Personnel Managers in London and the South East of England. Seminar publicity was then mailed to publicise the seminars. As a result, 66 delegates self-selected to attend the six scheduled seminars.

Next, the evaluation tools selected for the purpose of this research project were critically assessed. Four principal methods were selected to evaluate DET. The first involved an immediate post-seminar evaluation that is used by many training providers and is an evaluation tool often described as a 'happy-chart'. It provided an opportunity for delegates to give their initial response to the seminar content, intensity, style and delivery. The second approach involved an investigation into the effectiveness of the implementation of an action plan developed by the delegate during the last day of the seminar. Delegates were required to complete an action plan form, a copy of which was retained by the researcher. After 12 months a questionnaire was sent to delegates in order to evaluate how much of their action plan each had managed to complete. The final evaluation tool was a longer term (two to three year) follow-up of four selected organisations to identify what further action had been taken to improve opportunities for disabled employees and applicants. These evaluation tools were critically analysed and it was concluded that despite significant problems with their application they were the best tools available.

The results indicated a positive response to the immediate post-seminar questionnaire and that delegates' action plans were based on the social model of disability. They also provided good evidence that demonstrated that DET proves to be a potent tool in effecting change. On considering the limitations of these seminars, however, it was revealed that the success of DET in challenging institutionalised discrimination throughout the employment market is contingent on the introduction of comprehensive and effective Anti-discrimination Legislation.

References

Abberley, P. (1987). The concept of oppression and the development of a social theory of disability. *Disability, Handicap and Society*, **2**, 5–19.

Altman, B. M. (1981). Studies of attitudes toward the handicapped: the need for a new direction. *Social Problems*, **28**, 321–37.

Barnes, C. (1991). *Disabled People in Britain and Discrimination: A Case for Anti-Discrimination Legislation*. London: Hurst.

Bolderson, H. (1980). The origins of disabled persons employment quota and its symbolic significance. *Journal of Social Policy*, **9**, 169–86.

Bowe, F. G. (1980). *Rehabilitating America: Toward Independence for Disabled and Elderly People*. New York: Harper & Rowe.

Brisenden, S. J. (1986). Independent living and the medical model of disability. *Disability, Handicap and Society*, **1**, 173–8.

BRU. (1990). *Images of Disability on Television*. London: Broadcasting Research Unit.

Campbell, J. (1990). *Developing our Image – Who's in Control?* Paper presented to the Cap in Hand Conference, London, February.

Cornes, P. (1984). *The Future of Work for People with Disabilities: A View from Great Britain*. New York: World Rehabilitation Fund.

Daunt, P. (1991). *Meeting Disability – A European Response*. London: Cassell Education.

Duckworth, S. C. (1995). *Disability and equality in employment: the imperative for a new approach*. PhD Thesis, University of Southampton, UK.

Finkelstein, V. (1980). *Attitudes and Disabled People: Issues for Discussion*. New York: World Rehabilitation Fund.

Foucault, M. (1965). *Madness and Civilisation*. London: Tavistock.

Freud, S. (1961). The Ego and the Id. In *The Standard Edition of the Complete Works of Sigmund Freud*, ed. and trans J. Strachey, vol. 19, pp. 3–66. London: Hogarth press (Original work published in 1923).

Fry, E. (1987). *Disabled People and the 1987 General Election*. London: The Spastics Society.

Gramsci, A. (1971). *Selections from the Prison Notebooks*. London: Lawrence & Wishart.

Gregory, J. (1987). *Sex, Race and the Law*, London: Sage.

Hanks, J. R. & Hanks Jr, L. M. (1980). The physically handicapped in certain non-occidental societies. In *Social Scientists and the Physically Handicapped* ed. W. Philips & J. Rosenberg. London: Arno Press.

Harris, L. (1991). *Remarks of Chairman and Chief Executive Officer*. L. Harris, to Press Conference, National Press Club, 11 September, Washington, DC.

Ignatieff, M. (1983). Total institutions and the working classes: a review essay. *History Workshop Journal*, **15**, 63–7.

IHT. (1989). *International Herald Tribune*, 26 July, New York.

Kamainsky, A. (1989). *The Personnel Managers Yearbook*. London: AP Information Service.

Kent, D. (1987). Disabled women: portraits in fiction and drama. In *Images of the Disabled: Disabling Images* ed. A. Gartner & T. Joe. New York: Praeger.

Khun, T. S. (1971). The relations between history and the history of science. In *Interpretative Social Science: A Reader* ed. P. Rubinow & W. M. Sullivan.

Berkeley, CA: University of California Press.
LBDRT. (1991). *Disability Equality Training: A Trainer's Guide*. London: London Boroughs Disability Resource Team.
Longmore, P. (1987). Screening stereotypes: images of disabled people in television and motion picture. In *Images of the Disabled: Disabling Images* ed. A. Gartner & T. Joe. New York: Praeger.
Lunt, N. & Thornton, P. (1993). *Employment Policies for Disabled People: A Review of Legislation and Services in Fifteen Countries*. University of York: Social Policy Research Unit.
Major, J. (1993). Letter to Peter Large, *Association of Disabled Professionals Bulletin*, March, p.6.
Martin, J. & White, A. (1988). *The Financial Circumstances of Disabled Adults Living in Private Households*. London: HMSO.
Martin, J., Meltzer, H. & White, A. (1989). *Disabled Adults: Services, Transport and Employment*. London: HMSO.
Morris, J. (1989). *Able Lives; Women's Experience of Paralysis*, London: Women's Press.
Murray, B. & Kenny, S. (1990). Home-based telework opens up new employment opportunities. *Rehab Network*, City University, London, Autumn/Winter, pp. 3–5.
NHS R & D Programme (1993). South and West Regional Health Authority.
Oliver, M. (1986). Social policy and disability: some theoretical issues. *Disability, Handicap and Society*, **1**, 5–17.
Oliver, M. (1990). *The Politics of Disablement*. London: Macmillan.
Oliver, M. (1992). Changing social relations of research production? *Disability, Handicap and Society*, **7**, 101–14.
RADAR, (1994). *The Cost of Reasonable Accommodation: The Americans with Disabilities Act*. RADAR Bulletin, October, London: The Role Association for Disability and Rehabilitation.
Reiser, R. & Mason, M. (1990). *Disability Equality in the Classroom: a Human Rights Issue*. London: Inner London Education authority.
Rogers, M. (1991). The case for the amputee astronaut, *New Scientist*, February, 13–14.
Ryan, W. (1971). *Blaming the Victim*. Orbach and Chambers, US.
Schworles, T. R. (1983). The Person with disability and the benefits of the microcomputer revolution. *Rehabilitation Literature*, **44**, 322–30.
Shakespeare, T. (1993). Disabled people's self-organisation. *Disability, Handicap and Society*, **8**, 249–64.
Siller, J. (1984). Attitudes toward the physically disabled. In *Attitude and Attitude Change in Special Education: Theory and Practice* ed. R. L. Jones. Reston VA: Council for Exceptional Children.
Silver, R. & Wortman, C. (1980). Coping with undesirable life events. In *Human Helplessness: Theory and Applications* ed. J. Gerber & M. Seligman. London: Academic Press.
Stone, D. (1984). *The Disabled State*. Philadelphia: Temple University Press.
Stubbins, J. (1980). *A Critique of Vic Finkelstein's Changing Attitudes and Disabled People: Issues for Discussion*. New York: World Rehabilitation Fund 5.
Tackney, J. (1989). The pathway employment service. *Rehab Network*, Issue 14, pp. 14–16.
Thurer, S. (1980). Disability and monstrosity: a look at literary distortions of handicapping conditions. Special Article. *Rehab Literature*, **14**, 1–2.

4

Towards a therapeutic alliance model of rehabilitation

SANDRA HORN

In this chapter, the descriptor 'patient' is used rather than 'client'. This follows the convention adopted by Davis & Fallowfield (1990) when they speak of the inappropriate consumerist flavour of the word, and its derivation from 'cliens' meaning 'dependent, client, adherent, follower or vassal'. While 'patient' may not be ideal either, it does at least carry the connotations of perseverance, forbearance and endurance, all of which are valuable qualities in the field of rehabilitation.

In recent years, the patterns of disease and disorder in industrialised nations have changed, with the balance moving away from acute infective diseases and towards more chronic conditions, many of which have environmental and/or behavioural causal factors. Changes in the pattern of health care have therefore become necessary, with the emphasis on long-term management rather than on short-term medical intervention, and on coping, adjustment and management rather than cure in many cases.

These issues invite consideration of the psychosocial aspects of health care, and in particular the question of whether patients and health care professionals (HCPs) have a common language, a common way of understanding and dealing with the issues of health and illness, and common expectations of processes and outcomes. Where there are differences rather than commonalities, they invite a consideration of the status of patients' perspectives, and ways of dealing with fears and with unrealistic expectations of therapy. They invite a consideration of patients' and HCPs' coping strategies, and the conditions under which they are facilitated or break down. They invite a look at commitment to staying the same and commitment to change, for HCPs and patients alike. Finally, they invite a consideration of a clear contract between patients and HCP; one that identifies mutual goals, role expectations and responsibilities.

This 'new' approach, was foreshadowed by Szasz & Hollender (1956) when they wrote 'A contribution to the philosophy of medicine' in which three contrasting models of the relationship between patients and doctors were described:

1. *Activity–passivity*, or parent–infant, in which the patient is unable to respond because of anaesthesia, coma, etc., and so is the passive recipient of something the HCP does. This category will also include those unable to take an active part in decision-making on their own behalf. This relationship requires that the HCP 'disidentifies' with the patient. It is not an interaction, because the input is all one way, **from** the HCP **to** the patient.
2. *Guidance–cooperation*, or parent–child, in which the patient is suffering from, say, an acute infection and the expected behaviour is of cooperation with/obedience to the HCP, whose role is to tell the patient what to do. Again, the HCP does not identify completely with the patient, but rather sees her or him as something that can be moulded into a better shape.
3. *Mutual participation*, or adult–adult, in which the patient and HCP participate in a partnership, and the HCP's role is to facilitate self-help. The HCP alone does not and cannot know what is best for the patient. The search for what is best is the essence of the therapeutic relationship, and the patient's contribution is indispensable.

Szasz & Hollender went on to observe that in the mutual participation relationship, it is crucial that the participants have approximately equal power; that they are mutually interdependent (need each other) and that they engage in an activity which is satisfying to both of them in some way. The relationship is characterised by empathy and by identification; the HCP's inner needs and satisfactions 'form a complementary series with those of the patient'. The most obvious clinical application of this model is in rehabilitation and most chronic diseases, but it also has its place in a wide range of healthcare settings, including acute care.

Since Szasz & Hollender's paper, the mutual participation model of health care has reemerged from time to time as a cause of concern. Later still, Barofsky (1978) explored some of the issues in the evolution of the relationship between a patient and HCP into a therapeutic alliance in a study of self-care behaviours, and Brody (1980) presented an approach to encouraging patient participation in clinical decision-making. Brody quoted several studies which demonstrated the increased therapeutic effectiveness of regimens that involved active patient participation.

These papers were part of the groundswell that culminated in the modern concept of 'empowerment'. It is a principle to which many forward-thinking HCPs and some patients subscribe, but one that demands more than mission statements and patients' charters. It requires from HCPs an understanding of how patients make and carry out health-care decisions, and the influences which bear on that behaviour. It requires highly-developed communicative and interpersonal skills. It also requires an understanding of the place of health in the hierarchy of concerns of the patient. These are significant issues, and it is pertinent to ask to what extent they are being addressed in education and training. There are also wider implications for the health-care professions if the sharing of power and decision-making by negotiation are to become standard practice. The nature of clinical responsibility will be changed significantly; more of it will reside with the patient. How is that change to be signalled and implemented for staff and patients? What changes in staff contracts and job descriptions, in management procedures, in support systems, should be in place in order that HCPs may function confidently and effectively under the new regimen?

The new demands on HCPs if empowerment is to become a reality are mirrored by new demands on patients. The mutual participation model requires an understanding of what is and is not an offer from the HCP, a degree of knowledge about their condition and its treatment, and a willingness to take an active part in the transaction. Brody (1980: 721) commented that not all patients will have the desire or capability to participate in clinical decisions, nor will all physicians possess the time, interest, sensitivity and communication skills needed to foster enlightened patient participation. While it is true that some patients with certain conditions affecting cerebral functioning may not have the capability to take decisions for themselves, and others (not necessarily HCPs) may therefore need to speak for them, the unwillingness of patients and the lack of time, interest, sensitivity and skills of HCPs cannot be taken as given. They may be regarded as remediable conditions.

Kerr (1970) identified a number of areas in health care in which research was needed:

- the decision-making power of the patient and what can be done to increase it
- the nature of the staff–patient interaction, a clearer understanding of which should lead to the specification of the conditions under which such interactions can become more positive and growth-inducing
- the social structure of the general hospital or rehabilitation centre, so that barriers to patients' psychological progress inherent in these institutions can be identified
- the conditions under which staff facilitate the relearning of the mature and responsible adult role in patients who have accepted the patient role too well.

In the following pages, these and other issues will be explored by reference to the literature and case examples, together with some speculations about future directions.

The decision-making power and commitment of the patient

Much of the literature about decision-making on the part of the patient carries the implicit assumption that the goal is to match the patient's view to that of the HCP, i.e. the goal is compliance. Compliance is not an attractive word, carrying as it does the connotation of the submission of will of a less powerful individual to the will of a stronger one. Some writers have suggested 'adherence' as an alternative, but it is not much of an improvement. Barofsky (1978) has argued that compliance, adherence and negotiation make up a continuum, with others largely determining the patient's behaviour at one end, and the patient largely exercising self-determination at the other. This is an interesting idea, but it begs many questions about the relationship between self-determination and compliance or non-compliance.

So-called 'noncompliance' with advice and with treatment regimens is very common and takes a variety of forms, from failure to heed advice about disease prevention, failure to seek professional help appropriately and failure to keep appointments to failure to follow medication or other regimens. Non-compliance also describes the behaviour of the significant number of people who undertake programmes to enable them to make important behavioural changes (e.g. giving up smoking, learning pain-management techniques) and having completed the programme successfully, relapse.

In extreme cases, failures to comply with advice and treatment regimens may result in premature death. In one study of a series of 250 deaths in people under 50 years of age, Clarke & Whitfield (1978) found 98 cases of 'self-destruction'. Of the 98, eight died from deliberate self-poisoning and the others from a variety of causes to which alcohol abuse, smoking, obesity and a delay in seeking medical advice were implicated. Thirty-seven of the patients had refused admission to hospital, refused investigations, discharged themselves from hospital, defaulted from diabetic clinics or failed to cooperate in taking medication. Clarke & Whitfield were of the opinion that 'an anxious and nervous temperament was responsible in many instances but in others a lack of cooperation seemed to stem from fecklessness or a psychopathic attitude to life and to doctors in particular. There was little to indicate that lack of intelligence played any significant part'. The authors also state that the uncooperative attitudes were often encouraged by spouses. There is no reason to think that the sample was unrepresentative, and yet in a substantial proportion of the cases, terminally non-compliant behaviour was exhibited. The figure is too large to be attributed to fecklessness or nervous temperament without further enquiry. So far the search for the typical non-compliant patient has proved fruitless, and it is likely that a number of different factors are operating.

The extent to which these behaviours are the result of conscious decision-making (self-determination), or lack of commitment, or insufficient information or support, or a combination of these and other factors is unknown, although a number of studies have addressed the issues. Brannon & Feist (1992), for example, have reported on a number of predictors of 'compliance', among which are the severity of illness as perceived by the patient (HCP perception of severity has no effect), the patients' cultural beliefs (if they are congruent with the HCPs recommendations) and the personal qualities of the HCP, such as friendliness. Factors with a negative relationship to 'compliance' include delay in getting an appointment, delay in the waiting room and duration of treatment. Other factors involved in non-compliance have also been identified in research studies. Some, such as the complexity of the regimen and unpleasant side-effects of treatment, demand technical solutions, and the search for answers goes on. Others, such as the need to address 'silent' symptomatology in conditions such as hypertension, require imaginative and innovative effort in patient education as well.

Meichenbaum & Turk (1987) have identified a number of factors in non-compliance, some of which are matters of patient education, information and support:

patients do not know what to do
they do not have the skill or resources to carry out the treatment regimen
they do not believe that they have the ability to carry out the programme
they do not believe or feel that carrying out the treatment programme will make a difference
the treatment regimen is too demanding and patients do not believe that the potential benefits of adherence will outweigh the costs.

Some are matters of HCP education, information and support:

the quality of the relationship between the HCP and the patient is poor
there is no continuity of care
the clinic is not geared to facilitating adherence.

Some of these issues have been explored in further studies. They include the impact of the way information is presented (Ley *et al.*, 1973; Ley, 1972; Wilson, 1989) and such things as reminders, provider continuity and the modification of clinic procedures to allow for more personalised, convenient care (Becker & Rosenstock, 1984). Deyo & Inui (1980) have also noted the importance of the relationship between patient and HCP, arguing that successful interventions for broken appointments and drop-out rates have included time for discussion about the disease, the therapy and the importance of continuing the regimen, exploring and modifying health beliefs, and eliciting and discussing reasons for previously missed appointments.

A treatment regimen which is long term, difficult or associated with adverse side-effects, for example, can be dealt with by breaking down the regimen into a series of specific, achievable subgoals, and by the use of rewards for achievement in the goals; rewards, that is, not of a concrete nature, but intrinsic or internalised (self-satisfaction, self-esteem, realisation of self-competence and the ability to cope with one's environment) (Caplan *et al.*, 1976). Measures such as these inevitably involve discussions in which the patient plays an active, and often a leading, part. They are able to be in control *and* to participate in their own care, as opposed to taking control by opting out of an uncomfortable situation in which the rules are imposed on them.

Individual differences are also an important factor in determining the direction and strength of decision-making and commitment in patients. Among the cognitive variables patients bring to encounters with HCPs are their expectations, beliefs, attitudes and attributions: the things we have learned to know, believe and hope for. Beliefs about the causes of illness may cause problems with acceptance and adjustment, especially if they are associated with 'dirtiness' or moral laxity. Leprosy has been associated with uncleanness, for example, leading to a sense of shame and guilt on the part of many sufferers, and to ostracism by the social group. Incorrect beliefs about infectiousness or heredity in illness and disability may have similar consequences. While many health education programmes have had some success in combatting superstitious beliefs ('Head lice like *clean* hair', 'You can't catch it (AIDS) from a toilet seat') other campaigns designed to combat conditions where there is a causal component linked to the behaviour of the victims have been relatively ineffective. There have been a number of attempts to identify key personal beliefs and attitudes in health-related behaviour. Some of the clusters of beliefs, attitudes, etc. which have been studied are self-referent/self-efficacy (Bandura, 1977) for example, and the locus of control (Rotter, 1966). Others take into account the perception of external factors such as the assessment of threat or beliefs about the opinions of others. These perceptions have both emotional and cognitive components.

Breakwell (1986) has illuminated some emotional factors in writing about the importance of a sense of self in human behaviour, and about the causes and consequences of a perceived threat to one's identity. Threat is experienced when deep-rooted needs are prevented from being fulfilled. These include a need for autonomy, for continuity in self-definition, for distinctiveness and for self-esteem. Those who come into contact with the rehabilitation services as patients will be in the process of attempting to adjust to significant life changes.

The disease or disability causing those changes may bring pain, disfigurement, increasing limitation of movement, increasing physical dependence and decreasing choices in many areas of life. In Breakwell's terms, the lack of control over changes being imposed on the person by the disease process or disability constitutes a threat to identity by affecting self-esteem and disrupting the continuing sense of self-definition. A further threat may come if there is a need for institutional care of a kind that undermines a sense of distinctiveness ('It's the rheumatoid in bed 8 . . .') and the drive for autonomy. The person who must add 'patient' to the list of roles by which he or she is identified is therefore engaged in a struggle at many levels, from dealing with the outer and obvious manifestations of the problem and its management, to inter- and intrapersonal adjustments, many of which will be difficult and painful. There is an obvious need for these concerns to be addressed.

The cognitive aspects of coping with health concerns have been addressed by models such as the Health Belief Model (Rosenstock, 1966; Becker, 1979) and the Theory of Reasoned Action (Azjen & Fishbein, 1980). However, these models of the impact of beliefs tend to be weak predictors of behaviour on their own, and Ingham (1994) has suggested that it is because the information to support them is typically collected by questionnaire, thus forcing responses into predetermined categories and ignoring other powerful variables such as contextual factors. Other writers have looked beyond these cognitive or rational models of human behaviour and concerned themselves with the symbolic meanings of illness. Barnlund (1978) for example, typified the apparent vagaries of human behaviour when it comes to ill health in the following words:

> No animal talks itself into becoming sick, suppresses its symptoms because it fears a diagnosis, prolongs recovery because of the symbolic pay-off it receives or spontaneously recovers because it has redefined its situation. Yet human beings do all of these things. They avoid critical examinations that might save their lives. They seek unnecessary treatments and disregard essential ones. They often suffer more in the name of their illness than the physical discomfort it produces. They suppress some symptoms and disregard others. They convert discomfort into excruciating pain and transform extreme suffering into tolerable discomfort. They can go into shock without physical justification and accept a painful death with serenity.
> *(Barnlund, 1978; 717)*

Barnlund argues that the meaning we place on events, including illness and disability, governs our response to them, and that health-care professionals must acknowledge and understand these meanings to be effective agents in therapy.

Some of these personal and subjective aspects of illness have been further explored by Lipowski (1970), and Schüssler (1992). Lipowski described eight individual personal meanings of illness: illness experienced as a challenge (constructive acceptance), as an enemy, as a punishment, as a weakness, as a relief, as a strategy, as loss or damage, and as a value. Lipowski's illness concepts were derived from clinical experience, and he related them to characteristic emotional reactions and coping strategies.

Schüssler (1992) attempted to investigate these clinically-derived concepts and their relationships to coping strategies in chronic patients. He added 'controllability' to Lipowski's original eight concepts. His study involved a series of 205 patients with chronic physical disease: 50 with rheumatoid arthritis, 59 with coxarthrosis and 44 with sarcoidosis, first examined at least six months after diagnosis. He used a variety of assessment tools, some carried out by investigators, such as the Bernese Coping Modes, a psychoanalytic defense rating, a biographical case history and evaluation of the illness concepts. Patients also completed self-rating scales of personality traits and the Ways of Coping Checklist. Six months after the initial ratings, patients were asked about their well-being and the course of their illness. Schüssler found relationships between the concepts 'illness as challenge/acceptance', 'illness as value' and 'internal control', and the positive coping strategies cognitive reconstructing (positive reappraisal), valorisation, constructive activity, giving meaning, relativising, optimism and compensation, and to emotional stability. On the other hand, the concepts 'illness as enemy', illness as punishment' and 'illness as relief' were related to negative emotional coping such as wishful thinking, and symptoms such as anxiety and depression and emotional instability. Those who saw illness as an enemy or as punishment or damage tended to use emotion-related coping strategies, and to exhibit social withdrawal and passive dependence, whereas those who accepted the illness or believed they could control it tended to use problem-solving coping strategies.

It is clear that a consideration of individual responses such as those identified by Schüssler and Lipowski is important in any situation where the patient's coping skills are a major contributing factor in successful management.

Another important area of health care identified by Kerr (1970) is the nature of staff–patient interaction. She suggests that before problems such as dependence and over-demandingness are attributed to a personal defect on the patient's part, the following questions should be addressed:

> does the patient have reason to believe that he/she can succeed in the task required?
> is the patient afraid?

is the patient assured of social contact and the right kind of attention if he/she develops self-care skills?
is the patient angry with anyone?

These questions set the patient's personal meanings into the social context of the hospital or treatment centre and invite a look at the relationships therein.

The nature of the staff–patient interaction

There is a growing body of literature that suggests that the quality of interpersonal relationships in health care is highly valued by patients; often, the 'human' characteristics of doctors are felt to be more important than their technical skills. For example, Reader *et al.* (1957) found that 50% of out-patients they surveyed listed 'kindness, understanding, sympathy, interest and encouragement' as the most important aspects of a physician, and only 26% rated the physician's ability to treat their illness effectively as most important. Ware & Snyder (1975) surveyed 560 households and found that many people could not distinguish between the caring and curing functions of physicians. Koos (1955) in a sample of 1000 patients found that 64% criticised their doctors for lack of warmth and too much emphasis on such technological aspects of care as tests, diagnosis and drugs. Korsch *et al.* (1968) found that communication was adversely affected by the lack of warmth and friendliness on the doctor's part. There is little or no evidence that things have changed significantly since these studies were carried out.

Communication

The need for a shift in the balance of responsibility for health care must be addressed as it moves towards a collaborative endeavour with shared decision-making and goal-setting. Although the HCP will need to pass on information to the patient as part of the collaboration, the educative process cannot be one way. It will not be sufficient for the patient to give a list of symptoms; collaboration demands a deeper level of understanding than that provided by a catalogue of the manifestations of disease. It requires the collaborators to learn from each other about the hierarchy of concerns each has, the skills each can bring to the problems, the limits of their skills and knowledge, the barriers there might be in attaining the goals they have identified and agreed, and what they need and expect from each other.

Barnlund (1978) argues that interpersonal communication, the process of sharing meanings, is the key issue in health care. Barnlund talks about 'communicative negligence': the failure to listen, the failure to comprehend, the failure to respect and collaborate, as a cause of suffering in health that needs a vigorous effort to remedy it. These may seem like self-evident truths, but they have wide-ranging implications for service delivery, from the planning of entire health-care systems to individual therapeutic interventions, and they beg many questions. For example, if the patient's perspective is crucial, what mechanisms are in place to ensure that it is understood and acted on? What do we know about how patients and their families make decisions about important issues in their daily lives, or manage those issues, or communicate about them to others?

Trieschmann (1974) has pointed out that while we (HCPs) may know how to set goals for rehabilitation patients, we may not know about the relationship between our goals and theirs. We tend to focus on what disabled people *can* do, but what they *do* do or *will* do is equally important. These issues highlight the need for HCPs to build relationships with patients in which the free exchange of information is facilitated, and where there are difficulties, to consider the effect they and their institution are having on their patients. It is legitimate to ask how we as individual HCPs address these questions in training and in professional work, and how they are acknowledged and addressed by the organisations in which we work, as they are basic questions about therapeutic effectiveness. There are important issues around the delicate relationship between all those involved in health care, and the barriers to forming effective therapeutic alliances. The issues will be addressed under the following headings:

becoming a patient: some determinants of behaviour
power in health care relationships
communication and information
the need for new initiatives in education, training and management.

Becoming a patient: some determinants of behaviour

In his phrase '. . . the Christlike and the querulous', Hodgins (1977) identifies the two stereotypes for invalids, found in drama and literature. He goes on to suggest that querulous demanding behaviour may be not so much a personal attribute as a response to the kind and quality of health care the patient receives. Users of the health-care system are often vulnerable, and are entering into relationships with HCPs that are unusual in many respects. The HCP may be a stranger, and yet may be empowered to ask intimate questions and encroach on personal space in a way that would be intolerable in almost any other social situation. HCPs are further empowered by being integral parts of the system, which is often located in their workplace. Users must find ways of dealing with the discomfort of being in a place they would rather not be in, and in which they do not seem to belong, and an important aspect of the HCPs role is to minimise that discomfort, to be, at the very least, a considerate host or hostess. Failure to address the problem may be one of the antecedents of passive compliance (learned helplessness) or alternatively, of 'non-adherence', i.e. the users removing themselves from the uncomfortable situation in one way or another. Consider the following example of 'host' behaviours described by journalist Sandra Barwick in extracts from 'One of the waiting room herd' (*The Independent*, Saturday 10 October 1992: 15). This encounter with the hospital system took place more than six months after the Patient's Charter was published.

Sandra Barwick arrived early for her 1.30pm outpatient appointment, and having checked in at the reception desk, settled down to read 'A Charter for Patients – Our Aims', sent by the hospital with her appointment letter. The brochure announced that outpatients would be seen within 30 minutes of their appointment time, and that all staff would wear name badges, so that patients and visitors know who they are.

> it was difficult to check this one, since no staff were present, The group waiting dumbly by the reception desk (now empty) had now grown to about a dozen, mainly elderly people, who were standing holding their letters towards an empty space with expressions of hopefulness and resignation, as though waiting was something to which they had long become accustomed. . .
>
> 'Sit down! Over there! Until the receptionist comes!' The order came from a person in a green overall walking briskly across the room. There was no name badge. . .
>
> The group by the desk shuffled obediently and silently to various seats and began to gaze at the walls. 'Sit down!' commanded the green-overalled one to the few who had not yet yielded. I searched my optimistic pamphlet to see any plans for future provision in the Patient's Charter of the words 'Please' or 'I am sorry there is no one here to help you yet', or even 'Do sit down, sir, we will be with you shortly', but the pamphlet, like the patients, was dumb.
>
> If the appointment was not to be kept within 30 minutes, 'patients will receive an explanation and an indication of how long they will have to wait'. No explanation came to any of us. An hour after my appointment time, I asked the receptionist for one. With an air of faint surprise he checked, and said he thought the consultant would be coming soon. . .
>
> What were we, this small bundle of worried people, being given orders rather than service, condescension rather than courtesy?. . . I had begun to feel remarkably like a cow waiting hopefully with its herd to be milked. We had become objects. . .

> I wondered how single parents managed, those with dependent relatives, demanding employers. Still there was no word of explanation, let alone apology.
>
> On my way out, past the rows of those still waiting, patient as monuments, I asked a green-overalled figure whether it was usual for appointments to run an hour and a half late. She looked at me with great reproof. 'He has been operating', she said. It was, of course, no answer.
>
> No resources are necessary for courtesy or explanations. These are small things which would have transformed that anxious waiting room.

We do not know why courtesy and explanations were absent in this case, and it may be that shortness of staff and other resources were in part to blame, but questions about staff training and support must be asked. What understanding of their jobs and roles did the staff have? What status did the patients have? Was 'good' behaviour on the part of the patients equal to dumb submissiveness? Why?

One of the problems in knowing how to be a good patient is that the rules of the game may not be made explicit, and by the time you have worked them out, they may have changed. At one point in your career as a patient, you may be smiled on for being passive, uncomplaining and unquestioning; indeed, there are times when loss of consciousness is a distinct advantage. At other times, however, passivity will be frowned on, and failure to ask appropriate questions will attract blame. If it is hard for outpatients, the lot of the inpatient is infinitely more difficult. You are in hospital, in someone else's house, as it were. Who decides when you may bathe or wash your hair? Is it you, as it has been all your adult life, or must you wait for your host/ess to give you permission? Are you more of a nuisance when you ask, or when you don't? Some people, from sheer good manners, try to behave according to the rules of the house as they perceive them. Others behave as they always have in their own homes. This may be a nuisance when it does not fit the ward routine, but it will be praiseworthy at discharge time when they must resume their normal lives. The failure to make the 'rules' explicit, and to identify those things which are open to negotiation (e.g. bathtimes), may be a cause of much discomfort and discontent, which may in turn lead to 'difficult' behaviour.

Power in health-care relationships

Barofsky (1978) has argued that the relationship between the patient and the HCP almost always starts as unequal, with differences between them which make one more in control than the other. The HCP, for example, is familiar with the geography of the hospital or unit, is part of its working structure, shares a common language with colleagues, is accorded a certain status; none of those things may apply to the patient, who may also be feeling anxious and vulnerable. Initially and legitimately, patients are directed as to what to do, or told what is expected, although with time and continued interaction, they may become active in the therapeutic decisions being made, and develop self-care behaviours. Where the HCP–patient relationship not only starts but remains unequal, it is because the patient has little or no influence over the HCP's behaviour, and the distribution of power between them is a barrier to the initiation and maintenance of self-care behaviour. French & Raven (1968) have identified a variety of power bases HCPs may use to influence patients' behaviour: expert, legitimate, referent, coercive and reward. If the HCP is perceived as an expert, patients are more likely to accept his advice. If patients adopt the sick role, they may decide that the HCP has a legitimate role to prescribe a particular path towards a goal; acceptance of 'the doctor's orders' makes sense when the HCP has technical competence and the patient has need for direction and guidance. The knowledge, beliefs, attitudes and expectations of the patient, however, are still operating on the encounter.

The referent power base operates when the patients like the HCPs and identify with them, and will therefore do what they say (the converse is also true). Coleman (1985) has identified components of HCP behaviour that have an impact on patient behaviour; among them are compassion, communication and an attitude of concern, with hope and interest in the patients' future wellbeing. Coercive power, on the other hand, is in use when patients receive the message 'do this or else...' It tends to lead to the production of quotas (if it works at all), i.e. they will do precisely what they are instructed to and not an atom more. Furthermore, when someone uses coercive power, the required behaviour is often only performed in their presence or when they are likely to find out about it. Finally, coercion and coercive people are often disliked, so referent power works against cooperation.

The model of mutual participation described by Szasz & Hollender (1956) implies not so much a loss of power and status on the part of the HCP as a different way of obtaining gratification; satisfaction comes not from exerting control over another person but from a different kind of mastery, arising from mutuality and cooperation. They suggest that these attributes are deep human sources of gratification, as strong or stronger than the need for power and control, given the right circumstances. The identification of those circumstances has yet to be undertaken.

Communication and information

> 'When I use a word', Humpty Dumpty said, in a rather scornful tone, 'it means just what I choose it to mean – neither more nor less'. 'The question is', said Alice, 'whether you can make words mean so many different things'. *(Carroll, 1871).*

Blaxter (1976) has pointed out that the perspectives of providers and patients may differ on both the definition and treatment of illness. A study of the literature reveals that they may also be using words differently. It is not just that patients misunderstand technical words or HCPs do not get to grips with vernacular terms. The report of the National Fitness Survey (Allied Dunbar, 1992), which surveyed 6000 adults selected at random throughout the country, showed that apparently simple, everyday words like 'fitness' and 'health' meant different things to the surveyors and surveyees. Health-related behaviours, attitudes and beliefs were assessed during interviews conducted in people's homes. The interviews included questions about current health status, level of participation in sport and active recreation, physical activity at work and at home (housework, DIY, gardening, stair climbing, etc.) and psychological variables including wellbeing, social support, stress and anxiety. In addition, physical appraisal measures were taken in a mobile laboratory, including body measurements, blood pressure, muscle functions (strength), flexibility and aerobic fitness.

Participants' responses indicated that 80% of both men and women of all ages believed themselves to be fit, and the majority believed that they did enough exercise to keep fit. Eighty per cent also expressed a strong belief in the value of exercise in health and fitness. Only a tiny minority actually engaged in regular physical activity of a moderate or vigorous intensity. In contrast, the researchers estimated that nearly one-third of men and two-thirds of women would find it difficult to sustain walking at a reasonable pace (3 miles per hour) up a 1 in 20 slope.

There are a number of ways of interpreting these findings; a particularly interesting one is that the participants and researchers are using words in completely different ways. The participants seem to regard 'fit' as meaning 'not actually feeling ill at present, and able to carry out my normal daily routine comfortably'. The researchers, on the other hand, are thinking in terms of aerobic fitness, and the ability to walk up a slope without breathlessness and discomfort. It is not that one is right and the other wrong; they are simply using the same word to mean different things: one referring to everyday subjective experience, the other to a precisely-defined piece of technical information.

'Exercise' also appears to be a Humpty Dumpty word. If most people in the survey thought they did enough exercise to keep fit, but only a very small number engaged in moderate or vigorous physical activity on a regular basis, it is likely that most people were talking about the exercise inherent in their daily activities (walking, housework, shopping, work) rather than actually attending aerobics classes or jogging or playing at sports. The mismatch is reinforced by the perceived inappropriateness and unattractiveness of many 'healthy' forms of exercise, and the fact that most people do not identify with those who attempt to sell exercise by displaying bodies which are often seriously underweight or grossly overmuscled.

'Improvement' is another deceptively simple word in health care, but there is evidence that it too can have different meanings when used by different groups of people. For example, Jachuck *et al.* (1982) report on a study in which quality of life after antihypertensive therapy was assessed in 75 patients with controlled hypertension using questionnaires given to patients, close companions and doctors. The overall assessments of the three groups differed widely. The doctors registered 100% improvement in patients because their blood pressure was adequately controlled, there had been no clinical deterioration and the patients had not complained about the effects of the treatment to the doctors. Only 48% of patients felt improved after treatments, however, and 8% felt worse. They were reporting subjective feelings, not clinical changes. The relatives reported only two patients as improved and 25% to be negligibly or mildly worse, 45% to be moderately worse and 30% to be severely worse. The adverse changes they were concerned to report included affect, outspokenness, tearfulness, tact and dependence: all attributes that would tend to create problems with relationships. Each group was responding to the most obvious interpretation of 'better' or 'worse' as they saw it, but they each meant something entirely different.

Similarly, Doolittle (1991), in a study of personal experiences of stroke, demonstrated differences in ideas of what constitutes recovery between patients and rehabilitation staff. The staff described recovery in terms of task performance, improved mobility and independence in self-care. Patients, on the other hand, saw recovery as a return to previously-valued activities in life. They saw independence in self-care as an improvement in their condition, but their major point of reference was their prestroke life. The health care team could, of course, adopt the approach of educating patients to share the team's perspectives and use of language, and to some extent that may be valuable. After all, the HCPs have technical knowledge that patients may need. On the other hand, patients have crucial information too, which must be acknowledged and used if they are to be active agents in the management of illness or disability. A vivid example of missed opportunities in two-way communication is given in a study by Brody (1980) in which 235 patients were interviewed after being prescribed medication, or having changes in their medication or were given advice about ancillary health matters. Twenty-six per cent of those who had medication changes had failed to understand them, 54% had tried but not been successful at following advice for ancillary health measures, 8% had not tried, 36% had underconsumed their regular prescribed medication in the preceding week and 13% had overconsumed it. The surprising result of Brody's study, however, came when the results of the first interviews were fed back to the prescribing doctors between the first and second visits. The feedback had *no effect* on detection rates at second visit. Doctors failed to identify underconsumption of medication in 70% of cases at first interview but this *increased* to 82% at the second interview. Doctors were also asked about psychological problems and stressful life events in their patients at first and second interviews. Again, they failed to detect 36% of psychological problems at first interview and 35% after feedback, and also failed to detect 82% of stressful life events at first interview and 73% after feedback. Thus, significant numbers of these HCP/patient encounters resulted in failed communication on *both* sides.

The need for new initiatives in education, training and management

Craddock & Reid (1993) described a bold, all-or-nothing experiment in which a Well Woman Centre in Glasgow was remodelled so as to facilitate responsibility and decision-making by the users. The changes were wide-ranging, and included creating a homely informal setting in which services were easily accessible. For example, the appointment system was abandoned, and instead women were invited to fill in a 'service sheet' when they arrived, indicating which of the services they wanted. They held their case records for the duration of their visit. Attendance at the centre increased fourfold during the experiment, good use was made of the counselling service, and nine self-help groups were set up. They included particularly successful Healthy Eating and Agoraphobia groups. The project was not without its difficulties, however, including the extra work for the staff caused by long extended hours (a consequence of appointment-free clinics), and by their professional roles and responsibilities being rapidly and radically changed and sometimes blurred. The study highlights the need for careful consideration to be given to staff training, management and support if changes are to take place with the minimum of difficulty and distress, and for the issues noted by Kerr to be addressed systematically.

The changes in the pattern of diseases, and changes in the delivery of health care, offer exciting possibilities for the future. Greater participation for patients in decisions about their treatment is surely to be welcomed. If the new challenges engendered by the changes are to be met, however, new initiatives in staff training and support must be in place, or the HCPs will be in danger of becoming demoralised as their old role expectations are no longer valid. New ways of conducting the business of health care may be evolved slowly and painfully through trial and error, or smoothly and efficiently through training programmes that facilitate personal growth and responsibility. Innovative techniques pioneered by McMaster University in Canada use interactive learning in workshop and role-play formats to teach a variety of skills in health care, and have been adapted and extended here by trainers such as Fallowfield (1993) in areas of health work demanding a high degree of interpersonal sensitivity, such as breaking bad news. Listening and communication skills, goal-setting, problem-solving approaches, are examples of other skills that are readily learned through interactive programmes, and which engender confidence in the HCPs who deal daily with vulnerable people. It is also crucially important to give HCPs the wherewithal to deal with the problematic side of decision-sharing with patients. For example, what about the patient who refuses vital treatment? Or the patient who 'wants to know the truth' but has difficulty in accepting it? Or the anxious relative who 'doesn't want mother told?' No HCP should shoulder these burdens alone; an explicit support system *which is independent of job appraisal and line management* should be in place for all care staff if the new demands are to be met with skill and confidence rather than confusion and despair. New jobs need new tools.

References

Allied Dunbar National Fitness Survey. (1992). Sports Council Health Education authority. London: HMSO.

Azjen, I. & Fishbein, M.(1980) Understanding attitudes and predicting social behaviour, Englewood Cliffs, NJ: Prentice-Hall.

Bandura, A. (1977). Self-efficacy: toward a unifying theory of behavioural change. *Psychological Review*, **84**, 191–215.

Barnlund, D. C. (1978). The mystification of meaning: doctor–patient encounters. *Journal of Medical Education*, **51**, 716–25.

Barofsky, I. (1978). Compliance, adherence and the therapeutic alliance: steps in the development of self-care. *Social Science and Medicine,* **12**, 369–76.

Barwick, S. (1992). One of the waiting room herd. *The Independent*, Saturday 10 October, p.15.

Becker, M. H. (1979). Understanding patient compliance: the contribution of attitudes and other social factors. In *New Directions in Patient Compliance* ed.

S. J. Cohen Lexington, MA: Lexington Books.
Becker, M. H. & Rosenstock, I. M. (1984). Compliance with medical advice. In *Health Care and Human Behaviour*. London: Academic Press.
Blaxter, M. (1976). *The Meaning of Disability*. London: Heinemann educational Books.
Brannon, L. & Feist, J. (1992). *Health Psychology: an Introduction to Behaviour and Health*. Belmont CA: Wadsworth Publishing.
Breakwell, G. (1986). *Coping with Threatened Identities*. London: Methuen.
Brody, D. S. (1980). The patient's role in clinical decision-making. *Annals of Internal Medicine*. **93**, 718–22.
Caplan, R. D., Robinson, E. A. R., French, J. R. P., Caldwell, J. R. & Shinn, M. (1976). *Adhering to Medical Regimens: Pilot Experiments in Patient Education and Social Support*. Ann Arbor, MI: Institute for Social Research, University of Michigan, pp. 22–7.
Carroll, L. (1871). *Through the Looking Glass, and What Alice Found There*. London: Macmillan.
Clarke, C. & Whitfield, A. G. (1978). Deaths under 50. *British Medical Journal*, **2**, 1061–2.
Coleman, V. R. (1985). Physician behaviour and compliance. *Journal of Hypertension*, **3**, 69–71.
Craddock, C. & Reid, M. (1993). Structure and struggle: implementing a social model of a well-woman clinic in Glasgow. *Social Science Medicine*, **36**, 67–76.
Davis, H. & Fallowfield, L. (1990). *Counselling and Communication in Health Care*. Chichester: John Wiley.
Deyo, R. A. & Inui, S. (1980). Drop-outs and broken appointments: a literature review and agenda for future research. *Medical Care*, **18**, 1146–57.
Doolittle, N. D. (1991). Clinical ethnography of lacunar stroke: implications for acute care. *Journal of Neuroscience Nursing*, **23**, 235–9.
Fallowfield, L. (1993). Invited paper presented to the Medical Education Seminar. University of Southampton, 5 July.
French, J. R. P. & Raven, B. (1968). The bases of social power. In *Group Dynamics*, ed. D. Cartwright & A. Zander, 3rd edn. New York: Harper and Row.
Hodgins, E. (1977). Listen: the patient. In *Social and Psychological Aspects of Disability: a Handbook for Practitioners*. ed. J. Stubbins Austin, TX, Pro-Ed.
Ingham, R. (1994). Some speculations on the concept of rationality. In *Advances in Medical Sociology*, ed. G. L. Albrechet, vol. *iv*, pp. 89–111. Greenwich, CN: JAI Press.
Jachuck, S. J., Brierley, H., Jachuck, S. & Willcox, P. M. (1982). The effect of hypotensive drugs on the quality of life. *Journal of the Royal College of General Practitioners*. **32**, 103–5.
Kerr, N. (1970). Staff expectations for disabled persons: helpful or harmful. *Rehabilitation Counselling Bulletin*, **14**, 85–94.
Koos, E. L. (1955). 'Metropolis' : what city people think of their medical services. *American Journal of Public Health*, **45**, 1551.
Korsch, B. M., Gozzi, E. K. & Francis, V. (1968). Gaps in doctor–patient communication: 1. Doctor–patient interaction and patient satisfaction. *Paediatrics*, **42**, 855–71.
Ley, P. (1972). Comprehension, memory and the success of communications with the patient. *Journal of the Institute of Health Education*, **10**, 23–9.

Ley, P., Bradshaw, P. W., Eaves, D. E. & Walker, C. M. (1973). A method for increasing patients' recall of information presented to them. *Psychological Medicine*, **3**, 217–20.
Lipowski, Z. J. (1970). Physical illness, the individual and the coping process. *Psychiatric Medicine*, **1**, 91–102.
Meichenbaum, D. & Turk, D. C. (1987). *Facilitating Treatment Adherence: a Practitioner's Guidebook*, Plenum press, New York.
Reader, G. G., Pratt, L. & Mudd, M. C. (1957). What patients expect from their doctors. *Modern Hospital*, **89**, 88.
Rosenstock, I. M. (1966). Why people use health services. *Millbank Memorial Fund Quarterly*, **44**, 94–127.
Rosenstock, I. M. (1974). Historical origins of the Health Belief Model. *Health Education Monographs*, **2**, 328–35.
Rotter, J. B. (1966). Generalised expectancies for internal versus external control of reinforcement. *Psychological Monographs*, **80**, 1–28.
Schüssler, G. (1992). Coping strategies and individual meanings of illness. *Social Science and Medicine*, **34**, 427–32.
Szasz, T. S. & Hollender, M. H. (1956). A contribution to the philosophy of medicine. *AMA Archives of Internal Medicine*, **97**, 585.
Trieschman, R. B. (1974). Coping with disability: a sliding scale of goals. *Archives of Physical and Medical Rehabilitation*,**55**, 556–60.
Ware, J. W. & Snyder, M. K. (1975). Dimensions of patient attitudes regarding doctors and medical care services. *Medical Care*, **13**, 669–82.
Wilson, B. (1989). Improving recall of health service information. *Clinical Rehabilitation*, **3**, 275–9.

5

Rehabilitation education: a learner-centred approach

COLIN COLES

Introduction

This chapter focuses on rehabilitation education and explores the application to it of learner-centred principles. It is primarily directed towards people engaged in the education of health professionals about rehabilitation both in their preregistration or postregistration training. It is hoped too that the concepts outlined here could also be applied to the education of people with disability, their relatives and their non-professional carers. The essential message being conveyed is that the principles of learner-centred education are generalisable.

Learner-centred and teacher-centred education

Studies in which the behaviour of teachers and learners were carefully observed have provided valuable insights into the process of education. Learner-centred education occurs when a teacher helps a learner achieve some educational objectives agreed between them which address both the teacher's and the learner's agendas. Teacher-centred education on the other hand occurs when teachers merely inform learners about what they think they ought to know. The most fundamental way in which these two educational approaches differ then is this: in learner-centred education the teacher helps the learner to learn, whereas in teacher-centred education teachers pass on what they know to learners. Learner-centred education involves learners identifying for themselves the gaps in their knowledge, whereas teacher-centred education assumes gaps are there, and sets out to fill them. In learner-centred education the learner is active. In teacher-centred education the learner is passive. Learner-centred education is concerned with helping learners direct their own learning. Teacher-centred eduction, on the other hand, is concerned with directing what learners should learn, and often how they should learn it. In learner-centred education the learners are encouraged to evaluate their own performance, whereas in teacher-centred education the teacher is the learner's assessor. What is wrong, then, with teacher-centred education? Why is it a problem? The evidence comes from both pre- and postregistration education, and from patient education.

Preregistration students experiencing teacher-centred education have been shown to feel overloaded with content, lose their motivation to learn, become cynical about what they are doing, find difficulty in seeing the relevance of much of what they are learning, commit large amounts of information to memory and find it difficult to retrieve and use this information in a practical setting (Becker *et al.*, 1961; Simpson, 1972; Maddison, 1978). Rather than trying to understand what they learn, they adopt a 'surface' approach to learning, and their study habits quickly deteriorate (Coles, 1985*a*). In learner-centred education, on the other hand, students have been found to develop much more appropriate ways of studying (De Volder & De Grave, 1989). No longer do they see courses and subjects as separated from one another and isolated, but they actively seek the links between them. Theory and practice, which often are separated in teacher-centred courses, are now seen to be related and relevant to one another. They experience 'things fitting together', and are more able to remember and apply what they have learnt in a practical setting (Coles, 1990*a*). These students have a greater sense of achievement, and enjoy their learning. They **elaborate** their knowledge, i.e. they build up more and more complex interconnections between the things they are learning. They develop a network of knowledge rather than a collection of isolated, independent facts.

In postregistration education, the main problem is not so much poor education but a lack of it. Medical trainees in particular complain that their education is displaced by the demands of a heavy clinical workload, and that they receive little feedback from their seniors on their performance. Junior staff can become disillusioned, and feel stressed and unsupported. They often complain of a lack of any clear idea as to what they are expected to have achieved by the end of their training. Perhaps even more worryingly, there is a disparity between the perceptions of the junior staff and their educational supervisors regarding the amount and quality of education being given and received. (Grant *et al.*, 1989; Allen, 1988; Biggs, 1989; Dudley, 1990; Dowling & Barrett, 1991; Hunter, 1991; Royal College of Physicians, 1991).

The problems of patient education are remarkably similar to those experienced by health professionals. Patients complain about their needs not being addressed. The health professionals say their patients forget what they have been told, and fail to comply with clinical management plans (Ley, 1988). Patients are often given a welter of information about their condition but much of it seems to be unconnected with the problem of coping with their daily routines.

The theoretical basis of learner-centred education

Learner-centred education has it origins in two sources: cognitive learning theory and humanistic learning theory.

Cognitive learning theory

A reasonable analogy of learning is a library (Broadbent, 1975). Newly-acquired books are accessioned by a librarian using an agreed classification and storage system. A library user wishing to retrieve a particular book but knowing only part of the title or the topic first goes to the appropriate index, and thereby finds out where the book is located within the library. Effective retrieval requires having 'multiple routes of access' to the information that has already been stored.

Similarly, learning can be thought of as 'information processing'. Ausubel *et al.*, (1978) suggested that learning is aided by an 'advanced organiser' which is some prior knowledge or experience that helps us process new information. Educationally this means ensuring that learners are 'prepared' in some way for the information being presented to them. Kolb (1984) argues that learning should start with some kind of experience. The learner then reflects on that experience in some significant way, constructs some abstract principles concerning it, and applies those principles to practical situations, thus providing a new experience on which to reflect. So the experiential learning cycle proceeds as follows: experience - reflection - abstraction - experimentation - experience - reflection - abstraction - etc.

Schon (1983) suggests too that professional learning is a reflective process. He argues that professional practice is based on often unstated principles that involve the practitioner in a process he calls 'reflection in action'. In the course of their daily work, professionals hold a kind of dialogue with themselves in order to define the problems they face and then begin to solve them. They hold 'theories of practice' which guide their actions, and they carry out 'on the spot experimentation' that subtly modifies their approach in ways that are untried and untested before they meet the unique demands of each new situation. He suggests, also, that professionals can best be educated by being helped to develop the capacity to reflect on their practice, and so derive general principles concerning it to guide their work and further extend their theories of practice (Schon, 1987).

Polyani also suggested that much professional knowledge is implicit and personal (1958). Any two professionals may practice in similar ways yet their knowledge base is likely to be quite different. This suggests it would be quite wrong to assume that there is some core knowledge underpinning practice that can be transmitted through professional education. Rather professionals should be allowed to create for themselves their own personal knowledge through the opportunities afforded by professional education.

Cognitive learning theory suggests, then, that professional learning is more than merely giving people information. It is concerned with the processing of information, and is highly dependent on what the learner is experiencing. The knowledge-getting process is unique to each individual. Learning is a personal adventure : an individual journey. The teacher cannot learn *for* the learner. Learners have to do it for themselves.

Humanistic learning theory

Humanistic learning theory originated in the work of occupational psychologists in industrial and commercial processes, particularly with the introduction of automated work practices and repetitive business routines (Munn, 1956). Employees were observed carrying out everyday tasks in the workplace itself. Employment was seen from the point of view of the employee. Initially, these studies were carried out with the aim of improving worker efficiency but it soon became apparent that the analysis of job performance also helped employee training. Once skills has been observed and recorded, they could be broken down into their constituent parts, which could form the basis for training programmes. It became clear too that the working environment affected how people performed. Employees subjected to excessive noise, heat, fumes, fatigue, etc performed less well than those who were not. The morale of the workforce was also influential. Deliberately altering the environmental conditions led to increased efficiency because the group being studied felt valued. As their self-esteem and motivation improved so too did their performance. Giving employees constructive feedback on their work also increased their efficiency. Successful working practices that were praised led to enhanced performance, and poor working practices could be rectified. It was found, though, that critical appraisal should be constructive and allow employees to see for themselves the nature of their errors. They improved when they had the opportunity to observe the results of their efforts and discover where they could make changes. What was more, it was shown that even higher levels of proficiency and more effective work practices could quickly be gained by trainees who were taught by people who themselves had been trained as trainers.

It was recognised many years ago, then, that work efficiency in an industrial setting was directly connected with the employees' state of mind but it was not until the 1960s and 1970s that these concepts began to be applied to education. Rogers (1969) argued that the learner was the most significant focus for education, and that the teacher's role was to provide support for learning to occur. Learning he said was a 'self actualising tendency'. If learners were faced with the task of solving problems relevant to them they would learn automatically. The teacher's role was to provide a supportive environment in which this could happen, i.e. to facilitate learning.

Knowles further developed these ideas in relation to adult education (Knowles, 1970, 1986). He introduced the term 'self-directed learning' to describe situations where learners are encouraged to set their own learning objectives and seek their own solutions to their problems.

Cognitive and humanistic learning theories, then, provide two strands which together contribute towards the concept of learner-centred education. One sees learning as the processing of information that is unique to the individual, and the other looks at the learner's context, i.e. the circumstances in which the learning takes place. Taken together, these two views show that education should be concerned not just with ensuring that somebody is *able* to work well, but also that the person *wants* to work well. The first view is concerned with the learner's competence. It is about making sure that the person *can* do the job. The second, which is equally important, concerns the person's motivational state, their desire to do the job to the best of their ability. Educators should be asking whether someone, as a result of educating them, is prepared to do the job in the sense not just of being competent but also willing to do it.

An example of learner-centred education : training medical teachers

The following example illustrates how learner-centred education works in practice. In the Wessex region of the UK general practitioners are being trained to teach in a way that provides a clear example of learner-centred education in practice. They attend a five-day residential educational workshop, bringing along a video recording of recent consultations with patients. In small groups with an experienced group leader they learn how to teach each other about general practice.

The procedure is as follows. Initially, two of the group engage in a piece of teaching. One of the pair shows his or her consultation video, following which the other (the teacher) carries out some teaching on it. The remainder of the group silently observe. Then, with a group leader facilitating discussion, the group gives feedback to the teacher on the teaching they observed (rather than the consultation) and they do so by using the protocol shown in Table 5.1. The teacher identifies what he or she believes went well in the teaching. The remainder of the group then say what they thought went well and the teacher makes a record on a flip chart of the points raised. The group leader then asks the teacher to identify the weaknesses in the teaching, and following this the remainder of the group identify the weaknesses in the teaching they observed.

On the basis of what has been said and written up, the teacher says what he or she would *want* to do differently next time. Again these points are listed. Following this, the group are asked to say what they think the teacher *needs* to do differently next time.

Clearly these two lists, the teacher's identification of his or her educational 'wants' and the corresponding list of what the group sees as the teacher's educational 'needs', can be different, and some negotiation may be needed. Through this the teacher is helped by the group to arrive at a set of learning objectives for the development of his or her own educational skills. These objectives are then dealt with there and then as far as possible. Next the teacher is asked to say what he or she has learnt as a result of the process and, finally, the group members have the opportunity to say what they believe the teacher should have learnt about his or her teaching.

Once this process has been completed another pair volunteers to demonstrate some teaching, again beginning with one of them showing a video of a consultation with the other then carrying out some teaching on it. Again the group will discuss the teaching they observed by using the protocol shown in Table 5.1.

When this procedure has been employed two or three times the group leader will ask the group to reflect on what this process has suggested about the nature of education. These points, too, will be listed on a flip chart and displayed around the walls. Following all subsequent discussions the group's attention will be focused back to the list of educational outcomes, which is extended or amended in the light of their growing insights.

By the end of the five-day workshop, participants will have derived their own list of educational principles and attributes of competent educators. A typical list is shown in Table 5.2. Follow-up evaluations of participants have shown that people's attitude towards teaching shifts significantly towards a learner-centred approach, and even their attitude to consultations becomes more

Table 5.1 *Protocol for reflecting on practice*

Begin with someone (the presenter) presenting to others some aspect of his or her practice	
1. What went well, and what was the presenter's contribution to this? (Presenter first)	2. What didn't go well, and what was the presenter's contribution to this? (Presenter first)
3. What does the presenter see as his or her wants?	4 What do others see as the presenter's needs?
5. Negotiate these wants and needs, and prioritise them.	6. List the agreed learning objectives, and deal with them
7. The presenter articulates what he or she has learnt.	8. Others say what they think the presenter should have learnt.

Table 5.2 *Educational principles derived by workshop participants*

Discussions are most useful when they begin with some shared concrete experience
The learner must be the focus of education
The learner must be given the first say
The learner holds the pen and writes up discussion points
Positive points must be heard before negative ones
The teacher is the group leader, and vice versa
The teacher acts as a facilitator, encouraging others to contribute
The learner's 'wants' can be different from the learner's 'needs'
Learning objectives emerge by negotiating wants and needs
Learners only achieve objectives (= learn) they have had a say in setting
Learning priorities must be set
Learning objectives can be dealt with often by the learner alone from his or her own resources
Knowledge emerges through the articulation of ideas
Learning occurs when outcomes are clarified
Assessment is best when it is facilitated self-appraisal that can involve peer review
The protocol (Table 5.1) sets the right conditions for learning to take place. It is positive without being collusive, challenging without being threatening, supportive not humiliating, and safe without being bland

patient-centred (Pitts, 1991). Informal feedback from participants indicates that the workshop has provided them with a unique opportunity, which very few have experienced previously in their own professional education, to develop new and exciting ways of providing high quality, learner-centred education for trainees in general practice.

Applications of the learner-centred model

Having now seen learner-centred education in action we could now apply this to a number of situations involving both informal and formal education, curriculum design and patient education.

Informal education

Most clinical learning occurs informally on-the-job. Learner-centred education can occur through everyday clinical situations such as when a trainee has to refer to his or her supervisor for help. What could the supervisor do to make these situations learner-centred as well as clinically sound?

First the trainees could be asked to describe the situation or situations giving concern, thus providing them with something concrete to discuss. The supervisor should ask questions only for clarification at this stage, and the questions themselves should be 'open' rather than 'closed', such as 'What did you do?' rather than 'Did you take a blood test?' The nature of the problem (whether clinical, educational, or both) should be left open at this stage. Then the trainee should be asked to say what he or she has done well so far, and the supervisor should reaffirm and reinforce good practice. After this the trainee should be asked to say what hasn't gone so well, and here the problems are likely to emerge. What does the trainee want to do about things at this stage? Quite often, the trainee will say precisely what the supervisor would have chosen, and has only not taken the decision because of being uncertain that this was right. The supervisor is doing two things: firstly, evaluating the trainee's competence, and secondly, allowing the trainee an opportunity to articulate his or her own thoughts, and thereby quite probably coming to see the problem and its solution more clearly. Only then, should the supervisor say what he or she believes needs to be done. This too might merely be a reaffirmation of what the trainee has already said but it might also show that they are not in agreement or there is a gap between what the trainee wants to do and what the supervisor believes the trainee needs to do. In short, there may be the need for some negotiation concerning what should happen. This should be handled constructively and out of it should come some objectives (whether for attending to the clinical situation or to the trainee's educational needs).

Although the trainee's educational needs and the necessary clinical provision to meet the patient's needs go hand in hand, care should be taken to distinguish between them. Clinical action will need to be taken, and so too will educational action. The supervisor should make sure that the necessary resources are available for both to be met, and should check the trainee's understanding of what should happen now. Clearly, too, at some future point, the supervisor will need to revisit the situation, both clinically and educationally, to see what progress has been made and what the outcomes are. The immediate interaction should be concluded with some positive statements on the part of the supervisor that motivate the trainee to deal with what needs to be done clinically and educationally.

Informal clinical education also occurs off-the-job as when trainees and supervisors meet privately away from the immediate demands of their clinical work to discuss progress. Learners need regular feedback but more importantly they must develop the skills of self-appraisal. This will be helped by the way the educational supervisor conducts these meetings, so how should they proceed?

Supervisor and trainee should meet regularly, if possible once a week. The timing should be agreed and the time available, which need be no longer than ten or 15 minutes, should be clear and adhered to. Punctuality and good time keeping are crucial for mutual respect. The environment in which these meetings occur is important too. While the meetings might take place in the supervisor's office, and therefore not on neutral territory, every attempt should be made to limit the effect of the hierarchical position one has over the other. Rather than talking across a desk, the seating arrangements might involve easy chairs around a coffee table. A cup of coffee or tea could be offered. Whatever the pressures of time on both parties, neither should give the impression they are eager to get away.

Next the agenda needs to be set, but whose agenda should it be? Initially, the trainee should be encouraged to say what he or she wants to talk about, what are his or her concerns and what is of pressing importance, using the protocol shown in Table 5.1. The supervisor may consider that other matters also need to be discussed. Clearly this has to be handled delicately. The supervisor might know of some knowledge areas in which the trainee has gaps, perhaps as a result of some routine clinical contract or on-the-job teaching in the course of their day-to-day work. The supervisor should first explore what the trainee already knows in the area, especially where he or she perceives knowledge gaps, and out of this discussion the trainee should be encouraged to identify and agree some educational objectives with the supervisor, again following the procedures just outlined.

Subsequent meetings to discuss progress could deal with 'matters arising' from the previous discussions, to follow-up what the trainee has been pursuing in the interim, and to look at what the learning outcomes have been. The supervisor needs to show interest in what the trainee has been able to achieve between meetings and to reinforce positive learning, while perhaps correcting any inaccuracies or misunderstandings. Some form of record keeping might prove valuable for both trainee and supervisor to know what has been agreed, and to provide an informal learning contract between them.

As a consequence of adopting this approach the trainee will be engaging in a fruitful educational programme directed at his or her own particular learning requirements that supplements the daily on-the-job teaching. In addition, and perhaps even more significantly, the trainee will be learning the art of self-appraisal and its necessary links with self-directed learning. He or she will develop ways of looking at his or her own progress, find out how to identify personal strengths and weaknesses, and through this to be more able to set self-learning objectives. Ultimately, the aim is for the trainee to be able to do this alone without the intervention of the supervisor.

A further way in which informal training can occur is through counselling, and this too can utilise a learner-centred approach. Very importantly, when a trainee enters a post for the first time, or comes to it from another post as part of a rotational scheme, the supervisor should welcome the trainee and provide some kind of positive induction to the unit, introducing the trainee to colleagues, explaining the way the unit works and any particular conditions and circumstances that the trainee should know about. Alongside this, supervisors should ensure that the trainee's domestic arrangements are satisfactory, and show some interest in the trainee's personal well-being as well as professional development. The two are closely interlinked. Importantly, too, the supervisor who in the general course of events takes the approach to learning-centred education described earlier will be laying an important foundation for a constructive working relationship with the trainee.

The development of active listening skills is perhaps the single most important attribute that supervisors can acquire. Even though their own schedule is extremely busy, supervisors should make time to hear the concerns that trainees express, and show what Rogers (1961) has called unconditional positive regard towards them, even though on occasions these concerns may appear trivial or unnecessary.

Trainees need also to know how to manage their own professional work. Time management is important, and trainees should be helped to acquire good habits. Managing their stress is equally important, and supervisors can help by taking some interest in their trainee's outside interests, and by getting to know them as individuals.

The skills needed here by supervisors are closely related to basic counselling (Murgatroyd, 1985), and include attentive listening, the use of open rather than closed questions, summarising, confrontation, etc. The protocol for reflecting on practice described earlier (Table 5.1) provides an ideal basis for this.

Formal education

Learner-centred education can occur in formal teaching situations too. Working in small groups (Walton, 1973) can be very effective, and is the basis on which workshops are organised (Woolf, 1987) as well as problem-based learning (Boud & Feletti, 1991). Often a group of learners can achieve educational goals that surpass what an individual can achieve alone. Largely because of group dynamics, ideas can be generated, explored, expanded and elaborated; however, these group dynamics need to be clearly understood and harnessed.

When a group first meets, people are very hesitant about what to say and how to say it. At this 'forming' stage they tend to 'play safe'. Often there is a high level of anxiety, and a strong dependence on the leader. People are uncertain of themselves, worry how others see them and can be quite defensive. Frequently they are confused about what they are supposed to be doing. Group leaders can help this 'forming' stage by ensuring that people get to know each other and that the group's task is as clear as possible.

The second stage of group development is sometimes called 'storming'. Group members begin to open up and express themselves more freely. Sometimes this can be a time of conflict, and even rebellion against the leader. There may be a polarisation of opinion, and subgroups may form. Often there is a resistance to control, and very typically opposition to the task itself. From a positive point of view, this means that the group members are starting to take this task seriously and to work out the implications for themselves of working in this particular way. The group leader needs to remain patient and be non-confrontational.

The third stage of group work, 'norming', occurs when group members start to develop a stronger sense of cohesion. The earlier resistance is overcome and conflicts resolved. The group now feels able to achieve the task. People are freer in expressing their thoughts and feelings, and offering their expertise to help solve the group's task. There is a feeling of cooperation and collaboration. The group leader can help by providing encouragement.

The fourth stage of group development is sometimes called 'performing': carrying out the task productively. Roles within the group become clearer, and particular people take on certain functions. Individuals feel more able to express differences of opinion, and to find compromises if necessary. There tends to be a great deal of energy available within the group for carrying out the task, even when new problems arise. The group leader is often used now as a resource.

Finally, the group process ends, hopefully with the completion of the task.

There can be a sense of great satisfaction and achievement if this happens, but equally a sense of frustration and disappointment if it doesn't. There can too be sadness at separating. The group leader may need to be quite supportive at this stage.

The group leader can therefore be instrumental in enabling people to learn by the way the group is handled. Again, the principles of learner-centred education outlined earlier can be applied, with the group leader helping individuals to achieve their learning objectives.

A principle feature of learner-centred education is that teachers and learners negotiate the learning objectives. Right at the start the teacher can ask the group what it wants to get out of the session, and then discuss the points he or she feels they need to know. The teacher may possibly have to modify what had been prepared in advance. Teachers who teach in a learner-centred way have to be ready to be flexible about what they feel they should be teaching. In small group learning, the class should be actively engaged. In a workshop approach (Woolf, 1987) the teacher provides some educationally appropriate task that is pertinent or relevant to the learner's situation. This could be a clinical problem carefully chosen by the teacher to provide an appropriate learning context for what he or she would like the group to learn. It might also be a problem or case brought along by the participants. This might require the provision of additional resource material where the group members' knowledge is inadequate for the solution of the problem or the completion of the task. At the end of the group-learning session the learners should be invited to state for themselves the outcomes of their learning, and what they need to do next on their own.

Problem-based learning is one variant of this workshop process (Boud & Feletti, 1991). Learners begin by analysing a clinical problem or situation, and out of this derive some learning objectives to enable them to solve that problem. They then seek out the necessary information, either through resources provided for them by their teachers, even through lectures (Gibbs *et al.*, 1989), or possibly by consulting materials in a library. They bring back information gathered in this way to their group, possibly then redefining the problem and the need for further information which is gathered prior to attempting to solve the problem. The teacher's role is to help the group through this process, to ensure that group members have adequately defined the problem, and that they are directed towards appropriate resource material. Misunderstandings and errors can be clarified by the teacher, whose role is not to tell them what to do or what they should know.

Lectures too can be learner-centred, although at first sight this may seem paradoxical. Many lectures are almost entirely teacher-centred. Lecturers often pursue their own objectives, and merely give information to students. At worse they are a monologue: the transmission of facts from the lecturer's notes to the students' without passing through the brains of either! Lectures can also be an extremely valuable learning experience. The challenge to lecturers is to create the necessary conditions for effective learning to occur (Gibbs *et al* ., 1989; Jenkins, 1992), and this can be achieved by applying the principles of the learner-centred educational model presented earlier.

Right from the outset the learner's mind must be actively engaged in the process of the lecture. Fundamentally the learner must have a sense of 'ownership' of the learning objectives. The learner must 'want' to know what the lecturer believes the audience 'needs' to know. How can this be achieved? Certainly not just by telling people what the lecture is about, or even by saying how important it is likely to be for them. One way to engage the learners in the process would be to pose some questions that would be answered in the course of the lecture. Another approach is to ask people to spend a few moments writing down what they hope to achieve from this particular lecture. Even better, the lecturer could show some example or illustration, perhaps in some vivid manner such as through a video recording or film, of a situation that is highly relevant to the content of the lecture (Coles, 1990*a*). Frequently, lecturers do indeed use examples to illustrate abstract points they are making, but often these come later on in the lecture, once the 'theory' has been presented. Theoretical principles are unlikely to 'engage' the audience, but practical examples and illustrations can.

Once the audience has been engaged in the lecture the lecturer can begin to present information. It is very important that this information is potentially relatable to the examples and illustrations given at the outset, and that this information relates to previously presented information if the lecture is part of a series. The information could also be related to other courses running concurrently, and certainly to lectures and courses that will run in the future. The lecturer should indicate these connections at the time the information is being presented, although this will mean knowing more than most lecturers do about the course as a whole.

A further feature of learner-centred education concerns the learner's role in handling the information appropriately. What activities can the lecture audience undertake? Some work could be carried out by the learner before the lecture occurs, although probably the most valuable previous activity is to reflect on some personal experience rather than to read up something before the lecture begins. Previous experience provides a broad context for learning (Kolb, 1984), and thereby ensures that a wide range of information can be processed, whereas prior reading could lead to an early 'closure' and limit the possible expansion of the learner's knowledge.

During the lecture the lecturer should ensure the learners are as active as possible (Gibbs *et al.*, 1989; Jenkins, 1992). Partly this should result from the initial engaging of the learners through objective setting, posing questions, and showing illustrations. During the lecture the lecturer could pause for the audience to stop and think through a particular point, and perhaps to make some notes. Questions and answers could also be taken when relevant. In addition, members of the audience could, at certain points, discuss something in pairs, or perhaps with two people turning round to another pair immediately behind them and discussing something in a small group of four. The lecturer might then ask for comments arising from this activity before proceeding to present further information. Towards the end of the lecture, the lecturer might summarise the points that have been made, and suggest ways in which the audience could actively follow-up the lecture. This might include people reviewing their notes of the lecture, making links between this lecture and previous ones, applying some of the information they have gained, or solving some problem as a result of the lecture. Perhaps the most telling judgment on a lecture is the work it stimulates learners to engage in once it is over.

In these ways, the lecture can become a learner-centred activity. Very importantly, the learner is likely to come to see his or her task in a new way. No longer is the learner a passive recipient of information but rather an active participant in the learning process, albeit in a lecture.

Curriculum design

In what ways, can the principles of learner-centred education be embodied in designing a curriculum? This seems almost as much a challenge as attempting learner-centred lecturing. In many ways, the problems are the same, and so are the possibilities.

Frequently curricula for educating health professionals fall into the trap of teaching what are often called the 'basics' early on. Curriculum planners seem to hold the same belief as many lecturers that theory must be taught before practice. This is the basis for the so-called preclinical/clinical division of the undergraduate medical curriculum (Coles, 1985).

This view entirely misses the point that 'knowing' is achieved through 'doing'. While much of what is taught in health professional education is 'basic' in the sense that it underpins professional practice, we are wrong to assume that this should be 'basic' in the sense of being taught first. Paradoxically perhaps, the theory we learn makes much more sense once we have experienced situations in which that theory can be applied. At the Medical Faculty of the University of Southampton, since the inception of its curriculum in the early 1970s, students have been examined in their basic science knowledge at the end of their first clinical year rather than at the end of the preclinical phase, which is where it occurs in traditional medical curricula. The timing of this examination, one year later than in other medical schools, is not just unique but educationally inspired (Coles, 1990*b*). Students find, when revising for this examination, that they can relate the theory of the basic sciences which they acquired during the early years to the clinical experiences they have now received, and this 'reprocessing' helps them make much more sense of it than they had originally.

This suggests there is almost a case for inverting the curriculum, with the clinical part coming before the basic sciences. This has led, only half-jokingly, to the suggestion that all introductory courses should come at the end of the curriculum because it is only then that they really make sense!

More seriously, problem-based learning mentioned above provides a good example of learner-centred education as applied to the whole curriculum. Students are actively engaged in the learning process through the problems they are set which provide a basis for them to agree with their teachers on what they should learn. Then, information is made available through various resources, and students have the opportunity to handle the information in an educationally desirable way when, individually or in their groups, they begin to solve the problems set by the cases presented at the outset. The teacher's role in all of this is less to 'teach' but more to facilitate learning (Boud & Feletti, 1991).

Problem based learning, however, requires a major upheaval for its implementation, and health professional educators devising new curricula could introduce a learner-centred approach into their existing programmes by following some simple procedures which are suggested by the principles proposed earlier. Teachers should somehow negotiate the learning objectives with the learners. Relevant examples and illustrations, and even first hand experiences, should form the basis for learning theoretical information. Learners should be active and not passive. The examination system should reflect the curricular aims (Coles, 1987).

To achieve this teachers need to adopt the new role of becoming learning facilitators, and some kind of staff training is likely to be needed. Indeed, these kinds of changes are unlikely to come about unless teaching and curriculum development are recognised as important functions of the academic staff, and are suitably rewarded. Unfortunately, the current position is that other academic activities, notably research, are more highly regarded. Probably this is because research output is more highly visible and can be more readily recorded than teaching excellence or contributions to curriculum development. The profile of teachers (Gibbs, 1991) must be raised, and the educational contributions by academic staff must be as highly regarded as criteria for appointments and promotion as are research achievements.

Learner-centred patient education

So far learner-centred principles have been applied to health professional education. How can they be related to the education of patients, their relatives and non-professional carers?

Once a chronic condition has been diagnosed patient care is essentially educational (Coles, 1989). Whatever the health professionals do and say, the routine management of the condition is largely in the hands of the patient. Whether that management is successful depends on how well the patient learns what it means to have the condition, and whatever expertise the health professionals have, the true expert in dealing with the condition on a day-to-day basis is the patient. For all of this to happen, the health professional has to become an effective educator. Health professionals have to educate their patients to care for themselves.

This often does not happen at the moment (Ley, 1988). The reason is that when the diagnosis is obtained, the health professional is in reality solving patients' problems for them. Learner-centred education, on the other hand, requires that learners identify and solve their problems for themselves. In health care, the mental skill of diagnosing may help the health professional understand the problem but it may do very little to further the patient's understanding of it. The professional 'owns' the problem, but the person who needs to manage it, the patient, doesn't.

Indeed, studies have shown (Beckman & Frankel, 1984) that when patients are asked to say what's wrong, most health professionals quickly interrupt and start pursuing their own line of questioning. It has been estimated, too, that 80% of consultations carried out by general practitioners were 'doctor-centred' (Byrne & Long, 1984). In fact, direct questioning by the health professional may overlook what the patient has to say, and may even miss additional diagnoses (McWhinney, 1989).

This has led some writers to distinguish between the terms 'disease' and 'illness' (Levenstein *et al.*, 1989). A disease is something that has some identifiable clinical pathology. An illness, on the other hand, is something experienced by a patient. Clearly it is possible to have a disease without an illness, as in the case of hypertension. Equally, it is perfectly possible to have an illness without any identifiable clinical pathology. Someone may be suffering from, for example, panic attacks or chronic pain, and yet the clinicians may find no physical pathology. The clinician might announce 'there's nothing wrong with you' rather than more honestly saying 'we can find nothing wrong with you'. Even so, the patient can be left with a very distressing condition that might remain untreated or at least unresolved.

A 'transformed clinical method' has been proposed in which 'physicians delay the pursuit of their own objectives' (McWhinney, 1989). Perhaps more realistically there is a case for suggesting that a consultation should comprise two elements. The first would be for the health professional to arrive at an understanding of the patient's problem and its solution, and the second for the patient to do the same. Certainly, these would need quite different strategies. The first would require something akin to the orthodox diagnostic approach, although there might also be a much wider exploration by the health professional of the patient's experience of the illness. The second part of the consultation should take a more educational approach, and could usefully follow the learner-centred model described in Table 5.1. What is the patient's view of the condition? How is this different from the health professionals? What does the patient want to happen? What does the health professional think needs to happen? How are their perspectives different? Do any differences need to be negotiated? How can the patient share the objectives being set? What is the patient's role in meeting these objectives, and how can the patient evaluate his or her own progress?

The skill of the educator (or of the health professional) is to create a situation in which the learner (or patient and/or relative) is asking the questions (Roter, 1977; Coles, 1990). Health professionals will know that they are achieving some understanding once the patient's questions become 'deeper'. Rather than asking questions that are merely requests for information, patients will be progressing educationally when they begin to 'predict ahead', when they ask questions like 'what will happen when I start playing sport again?' or 'what about going on holiday?'

At the outset of this chapter learner-centred education was said to occur when teachers help learners achieve some educational objectives that have been agreed between them and which address the teacher's and the learner's agendas. Much the same could be said about patient education. Patient centred-health care occurs when health professions help learners achieve some health care objectives they have agreed between them and which address the health professional's and the patient's agendas.

Conclusions

In this chapter we have seen how learner-centred education differs from teacher-centred education. We explored its roots and saw its application in the training of medical teachers. We then saw how this model could be applied in a number of situations regarding rehabilitation education involving health professionals and patients.

Learner-centred education (and patient-centred health care) emphasises the importance of agreed objectives. Central to this is the help the health professional/teacher provides the patient/learner. People learn best when they are helped to define their own problems, reflect on their own situation, understand and accept their strengths and weaknesses, and as a result define some educational objectives that combine their perception of what they want to learn and their teacher's perception of what they need to learn. The teacher's task is to help the learner achieve these objectives, largely through his or her own effort, and to encourage learners to crystallise their achievements by articulating what is being learnt. All learning should lead to further education. As a result of each piece of learning and every interaction between a learner and a teacher, new learning goals should be set, new tasks identified and ways identified as to how these new learning outcomes could be evaluated. The teachers' role is to enable this to happen. They should so arrange the situation and create such a conducive environment that self-learning occurs. Successful learning rests on the learners evaluating their own performance. Successful teaching is concerned with facilitating this process of self appraisal.

References

Allen, I. (1988). *Doctors and their Careers*. London: Policy Studies Institute.

Ausubel, D. P., Novak, J. S. & Hanesian, H. (1978). *Educational Psychology: a Cognitive View*, 2nd ed. New York: Holt, Rinehart and Winston.

Becker, H. S., Geer, B., Hughes, E. C. & Strauss, A. (1961). *Boys in White*, Chicago: University of *Chicago Press*.

Beckman, H. B. & Frankel, R. M. (1984). The effect of physician behaviour on the collection of data. *Annals of Internal Medicine*, **101**, 692–6.

Biggs, J. (1989). The preregistration years 1983–1988. *Medical Education*, **23**, 526–33.

Boud, D. & Feletti, G. (eds). (1991). *The Challenge of Problem-based Learning*. London: Kogan Page.

Broadbent, D. E. (1975). Cognitive psychology and education. *British Journal of Educational Psychology*, **45**, 162–76.

Byrne, P. S. & Long, B. E. L. (1984). *Doctors Talking to Patients*. London: Royal College of General Practitioners.

Coles, C. R. (1985*a*). Differences between conventional and problem-based curricula in their students' approaches to studying. *Medical Education*, **19**, 408–9.

Coles, C. R. (1985*b*). *A study of the relationships between curriculum and learning in undergraduate medical education*. PhD thesis, University of Southampton.

Coles, C. R. (1987). The actual effects of examinations on medical student

learning. *Assessment and Evaluation in Higher Education*, **12**, 209–19.
Coles, C. R. (1989). Diabetes education: theories of practice. *Practical Diabetes*, **6**, 199–202.
Coles, C. R. (1990*a*). Elaborated learning in undergraduate medical education. *Medical Education*, **24**, 14–22.
Coles, C. R. (1990*b*). Diabetes education: letting the patient into the picture. *Practical Diabetes*, **7**, 110–12.
De Volder, M. L. & De Grave, W. S. (1989). Approaches to studying in a problem-based medical programme: a developmental study. *Medical Education*, **23**, 262–4.
Dowling, S. & Barrett, S. (1991). *Doctors in the Making. The Experience of the Preregistration Year*. Bristol: SAUS publications, University of Bristol.
Dudley, H. A. F. (1990). *Creating a Teaching Portfolio*. Oxford: Technical and Educational Services.
Gibbs, G. (1991). *Creating a Teaching Portfolio*. Oxford: Technical and Educational Services.
Gibbs, G., Habeshaw, S. & Habeshaw, T. (1989). *53 Interesting things to do in your lectures*. Bristol: Technical and Educational Services.
Grant, J., Marsden, P. & King, R. C. (1989). Senior House Officers and their training. *British Medical Journal*, **299**, 1263–8.
Hunter, S. (1991). Doctors in the making: how to resolve problems in the preregistration year. *British Medical Journal*, 303.
Jenkins, A. (1992). Encouraging active learning in structured lectures. In *Improving the Quality of Student Learning*. ed. G. Gibbs. Bristol: Technical and Educational Services.
Knowles, M. S. (1986). *Using Learning Contracts*. London: Jossey-Bass.
Knowles, M. S. (1970). *The Modern Practice of Adult Education. Andragogy vs Pedagogy*. New York: Association Press.
Kolb, D. A. (1984). *Experiential Learning: Experience as a Source of Learning and Development*. Englewood Cliffs, New Jersey: Prentice Hall.
Levenstein, J. H., Brown, J. B. & Weston, W. W. (1989). The patient-centred clinical method: a model for the doctor–patient interaction in family medicine. In *Communicating with Medical Patients*. ed. M. Stewart & D. Roter. London: Sage.
Ley, P. (1988). *Communicating with Patients: Improving Communications, Satisfaction and Compliance*. London: Croom Helm.
McWhinney, I. (1989). A need for a transformed clinical method. In *Communicating with Medical Patients* ed. M. Stewart and D. Roter. London: Sage Publications.
Maddison, D. C. (1978). What's wrong with medical education? *Medical Education*, **12**, 97–106.
Munn, N. L. (1956). *Psychology: The Fundamental of Human Adjustment*. London: Harrap.
Murgatroyd, D. S. (1985). *Counselling and Helping*. London: The British Psychological Society and Methuen.
Pitts, J. (1991). *Change in Attitudes to Consulting and Teaching after a General Practitioner Trainer's Course*. MSc dissertation. University of Wales, Cardiff.
Polyani, M. (1958). *Personal Knowledge*. London: Routledge & Kegan Paul.
Rogers, C. (1961). *On Becoming a Person*. London: Constable.
Rogers, C. R. (1969). *Freedom to Learn*. Columbus, Ohio: Merrill.

Roter, D. L. (1977). Patient participation in patient-provider interaction: the effects of patient question-asking on the quality of interaction, satisfaction and compliance. *Health Education Monographs*, **5**, 281–315.

Royal College of Physicians Education Committee. (1991). *Education and Training for Senior House Officers*. London: RCP.

Schon, D. A. (1983). *The Reflective Practitioner: How Practitioners Think in Action*. San Francisco: Jossey-Bass.

Schon, D. A. (1987). *Educating the Reflective Practitioners: Towards a New Design for Teaching and Learning in the Professions*. San Francisco: Jossey-Bass.

Simpson, M. A. (1972). *Medical Education: a Critical Approach*. London: Butterworth.

Walton, H. J. (1973). *Small Group Methods in Medical Teaching*. Medical Education Booklet 1, Association for the Study of Medical Education, Dundee.

Woolf, B. (1987). Experiential learning in workshops. In *Coping with Crisis Research Group* ed. The Open University *Running Workshops*. Beckenham: Croom Helm.

6

Work occupation and disability

TED CANTRELL

Hypothesis

Rehabilitation is incomplete if the programme ignores the disabled person's own occupation plan.

Introduction

Clarke (1982) in his book *Work in Crisis* tries to analyse the significance of work, as a prelude to a study of the problems of the many unemployed people in the United Kingdom (UK). He says:

> Work is important because it provides us with a social arena in which a number of basic human needs are met.

He then emphasises eight particular functions of employment that may appeal to people, and explains why people continue to work. Some of his ideas overlap with a list of six functions of work presented by Hayes & Nutman (1981) who were also concerned with unemployment. These two lists have been put together, with some more that I have added (Table 6.1). It is very significant that ten of the 11 functions can equally apply to people busy with occupations (hobbies, interests and voluntary work) where they still gain a great deal of benefit from what they do, without regular payment. Money is not the only result of work. If we therefore study the importance of occupation to people, and include paid or unpaid work, then the subject becomes much wider than the political and economically-determined one of employment. My hypothesis relates to occupation in this *wider* sense, rather than simply paid work.

Income

A job is the 'key to the kingdom of consumption, it is the admission ticket by which the individual gains entrance to the goods and services the society

Table 6.1 *The functions of work/occupation*

Clarke	Hayes/Nutman	Cantrell	Apply also to unpaid work
Income	Income	Income	–
Social honour	Status	Respect	+
Adulthood	Identity	Identity	+
Life script	Time structure	Time structure	+
Something for others		Usefulness	+
Sociability	Identity	Company	+
Decision-making		Group voice	+
	Activity	Being busy	+
	Mastery	Achievement	+
	Purpose	Ambition	+
Power		Choice	+

produces' (Cox, 1966). Money must be a major reason why people continue to do difficult or demanding jobs. Although some paid employment may result in wages less than people would get on welfare benefits, the large majority of people who are unemployed are poorer than those in work.

The 'poverty trap' is a phrase used often to describe those who are not working (often because of disability) because it is claimed they will get more from welfare than from the jobs for which they might apply.

Respect

Social standards and public opinions seem to favour those who are regularly working more than those who are on the dole, or not working. Clarke (1982) reviewed the history of the 'Work Ethic' (a Calvinist approach) and also the considerable stigma attached to the unemployed in Roman, Elizabethan and Hebrew societies in the past.

In some housing estates where 25–50% of adults are unemployed the social norm may be towards accepting the lack of paid work as inevitable; but there are still likely to be many voices heard complaining about various national groups or figures who have deprived people of the right to work. It is likely that people out of work will feel they have no personal worth because they rely on charity (welfare) rather than earning their living. Respectability is therefore partly a concern about what others may feel about us, partly what value we put on our own lives.

Identity

Finding a job means a chance for a young person to have reason to stop being 'one of the kids' and to go out of the house daily, find a place in society and wear a badge of adulthood. Many forms of dress and behaviour are uniforms for such identity. In the middle years people are usually introduced to each other by what they do, more than for personal qualities. A professional or identifiable work label may mean more than whether a person is doing a useful piece of work (e.g. voluntary) or 'just a mother or housewife'. Unfortunately status is more available to those who have a widely recognised label than to those who simply care for others. There is very little status in being unemployed, disabled or a housewife.

Time structure

Although it can become overwhelming, the job or occupation can provide (or impose) a definite plan of demands on the time and the progress of each day. It is a reason to struggle out of bed, it reduces the need to try and decide each day what to do. There are timetables, deadlines, expectations, work schedules and many forms of public or financial accountability that drive the day, and can easily leave no free time. For many whose children have left home, or who have retired, or are severely disabled, this structure doesn't exist and can easily lead to apathy and boredom. It requires greater discipline to keep to a timetable that is entirely your own.

Usefulness

For many people, a great deal of job satisfaction comes from the fact that they have been useful to other people, particularly if there is praise or gratitude. One feature of the nursing and remedial professions that tends to make jobs easier is when patients (or colleagues) are grateful. It is extremely discouraging to be disabled and therefore unable to help anyone else, to have to rely on charity and to need physical help from other people. Welfare benefits may pay some of the bills, but they deny any feeling of being valuable.

Company

When people retire they can suddenly find themselves without the usual crowd of people at work that has been their source of regular company. They can even miss people they disliked or opposed. They cease to be one of the crowd. Some will have adapted long before by belonging to sports clubs, churches or interest groups, but occupation provides a very real sense of belonging for many. Premature retirement because of disability can be much worse if combined with the blocks of poor mobility, pain, speech defects or deafness. These can suddenly take people from their work group and isolate them at home; they may lose all reason for going out. Sociability is much harder because of disabling problems.

Group voice

The employed often belong to work-related groups that may have some influence on local or national decisions. Even if there are obvious power-brokers in finance, politics or military systems, a place in a professional body, or an industry or union does allow participation in public debate.

The unemployed have no such voice, except perhaps in the negative sense of violence that comes from boredom, or the alcoholism of despair. The Centres for Independent Living (CIL) movement, which disabled people started in California, are now a means for some British disabled people to voice their opinions and claim a say in the way society runs. They would prefer absolute power and control of resources (Oliver, 1991) but then so would most of the other ethnic and gender groups in society who want to be in charge. The most disadvantaged are those who have dysphasia, dysarthria or are intellectually unable to speak for themselves, particularly if they are also unemployed.

Being busy

Work provides physical and/or mental activity and although most people will complain about being too busy and exhausted, they would probably be much worse if they were forced into inactivity. Very busy people sometimes take time to adjust to the destructuring of a holiday, but would soon change if this process was to last for years or a lifetime. Smith (1987) has analysed many papers on the apathy, depression and ill health that follow loss of a job. This includes the effects of anticipated loss of work (two years ahead) in a Calne factory, where closure plans affected sickness rates in the employees (Beale & Nethercott, 1985) or in Marienthal (Jahoda, 1982) where the only factory closed down. Being reasonably busy can be stimulating and prevent atrophy of the body or mind; being inactive all the time rarely produces health.

Achievement

Many jobs do provide challenges and results, and if the work objectives are met, then success. Certainly the structure of work in some professions can lead to much greater energy if there are large or small achievements. Actors play better to a cheering audience and everyone likes praise. It is possible that politicians even thrive on confrontation! For those who have no work, achievement is more difficult and every day can be like the last with nothing to be good at, no results.

Ambition

Hours spent in study, practice, research or skill-training can be worth it if they lead to a qualification or an end result that gives public recognition. These are examples where current behaviour is fired by a specific goal, public acclaim or recognition, and is a driving force. For those who are unable to see such goals, or cannot meet their own objectives, each day can be a grey murk of uniformity and loss of self-respect.

Choice

Those who are wealthy or regular wage-earners have more choice over what they can do or buy than those in poverty. Purchasing power cannot be ignored in a society where there are great variations in finance but it is a noticeable absence for those who have to live on pensions, welfare benefits or charity. Choice can also be reduced if financial reduction is associated with the expensive needs of being disabled, and being short of transport, independence and lifestyle options. Isolation may be the only choice for some who are short of money.

The features of a working life can be contrasted with the status of those people who are unemployed or unoccupied as shown in Table 6.2.

Smith (1987) has reviewed the wide range of health problems associated with unemployment, and particularly depression, a higher suicide rate, obesity and several medical problems (e.g. heart disease and smoking-associated disorders). There is a problem that is difficult to study scientifically, namely how to prove whether less healthy people are those who are more likely to lose their jobs, or whether ill health is a common result of unemployment in otherwise fit people. The study in Calne is significant because the factory closure was an economic problem of business failure, and affected a whole village population. What is even more important is the fact that ill health figures started to rise as soon as closure was announced, even though the actual event was not going to occur for another two years (Beale *et al.*, 1985).

The list of the damaging effects of unemployment (Table 6.2) indicates the wide range of problems faced by a person who moves from a regular steady

Table 6.2. *The effects of being unoccupied*

Occupied	Unoccupied
Income	Poverty, shortages
Respect	Ignored by others
Identity	Nobody, no status, no self-esteem
Time structure	No reason to do anything
Usefulness	Beggar, role, pity
Company	Loneliness, isolation
Group voice	No place in debate, anger, alienation, fantasy
Being busy	Boredom, unstimulated, stagnation
Achievement	Failure, guilt, jealousy, loss of hope
Ambition	Frustration, apathy, no challenges
Choice	Passive receiver, parasite

job, to a life of wondering what to do at home, with no prospect of working. It is also a serious problem for four specific groups of people whose ability to find employment is denied or impossible because of problems in the society or a recession. This can be represented on a graph (Figure 6.1); the vertical scale of inspiration is used to summarise the range of positive effects mentioned as the benefits of work or occupation.

Retirement

Whatever the retirement age, and however well recognised as a specific time in a person's calendar, the process of officially ceasing to be useful in the work-force is very often a time of upheaval, distress and ill health. Some companies try to prepare staff well in advance, by running retirement courses for their employees, but the change in status is still one to which many people do not adjust easily, however much they protest that they are glad to give it all up and 'have some free time at last'.

For some the process is less painful because they have started planning years ahead, and can ease themselves into hobbies or voluntary work that has been well established, and so the change is one of positive anticipation. For many more, particularly those who leave highly paid, exciting or influential posts (or are voted out of office) the change can be one of bitterness, recrimination and decline. For most it is a period of sadness, not opportunity.

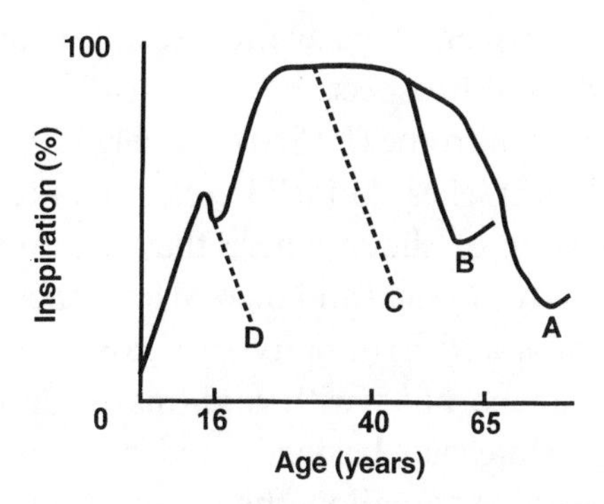

Figure 6.1. Inspiration, i.e. effects of unemployment in relation to age. A: retirement; B: redundant mothers; C: disability/sudden premature retirement; d: congenital disability/work unknown.

Redundant mothers

Another group whose change of occupation is predictable, but who may have less awareness at the time of status change are mothers with children whose children grow out of parental care. This can be a painful rejection, and may be a traumatic separation, but some may try to blur the edges of change by variations of 'looking after' young adults at home. Whatever the process, a woman may well have started child-rearing at an early age before obtaining qualifications for employment, and as a mother finds that her status rapidly or slowly disappears over 15–30 years. This is a kind of premature retirement that can be very difficult to accept, and it may merge into a life of acceptance of house management, gardening and flower arranging, or it may result in great restlessness and the need for a second career.

It is possible that many women adjust better to their first retirement than men, because they started to look for alternative training, a career or occupation at a younger age. They certainly have a higher life expectancy.

Disability : sudden premature retirement

For the person who is suddenly struck down with a stroke, or had the early signs of severe arthritis or multiple sclerosis, the loss of work can be a sudden disaster, that could not have been anticipated. Not only may they have the pain of the illness, and the struggles to get up and dress themselves, but they also face the bleak prospect of being unable to work. If the illness is a myocardial infarct, the problem may be fear more than genuine inability to work, but that will only be answered by a positive rehabilitation programme.

For many other disabilities (e.g. traumatic tetraplegia) the awareness of loss of work potential may be a very sudden and total prospect.

Work carried out on post-traumatic stress syndrome (PTSS) (Turner, 1991) has shown that after major disasters (train crashes, landslide, earthquake) most victims (and relatives) may enter a state of shock where they are too dazed to sort out their lives. There can be many physical and mental complications from a lack of concentration, tiredness and irritability to a complete inability to organise themselves. Nights can be filled with nightmares and broken sleep. Coming out of this mental state can be facilitated by good listeners who will accept the anger and questions and allow the victim's mind to explore out loud the distress and loss that follows. The private disaster of an individual who becomes disabled is no less than the public problems of a Clapham rail crash victim, but it can be far more difficult to deal with the results alone where no surge of public sympathy is available. It is very hard to have to fight with the trauma (or ignore it) alone in an intensive care unit, or after leaving a shattering clinic session where a diagnosis has been given.

The readjustment to a sudden loss of work potential may be made more difficult by the agendas of the personnel who surround the newly disabled person. An obsession with clinical signs and pathologies (doctors), bowels and hygiene (nurses), painful physical jerks (physiotherapists), and the learning of self-care tasks (occupational therapists) may take precedence over the agenda and concerns of their patient. Self-care activities are important goals but do not constitute quality living, just as they do not for adults who do not have a physical disability. The functions of work listed in Table 6.1 are more likely to be achieved by productive occupation and purposeful activity than by success in transfers or dressing.

Meaningful occupation, however, may be of low priority to the surrounding professionals, who thereby transmit the message 'There will be nothing interesting that you can do for the rest of your life'. Some therapists claim that conversations focusing on what the newly disabled person is going to do are too overwhelming when added to the stress of the traumatic injury and its other implications. There is often no one who is prepared to listen to the anger and uncertainty and respond with humour or sympathy or practical alternatives to a life of unwelcome discomfort and frustrating helplessness. It might be beneficial and helpful to some patients if future options for meaningful occupation were routine topics during rehabilitation, especially if there is an opportunity to explore the alternatives. Planning for the future may prove to be less overwhelming than ignoring it altogether.

Congenital disability : work unknown

The real tragedy for many children born with handicaps (spina bifida, cerebral palsy, epilepsy) is that community support and expectations may be raised while they are at school, but dashed when they leave and cannot find work. They may have the full support of teachers, therapists and educational psychologists while at school, which they lose when they return home. The danger is that they can return to a solitary life of being a dependent 'child' with their parents, lose touch with their own age group and sink into apathy or anger as they fail to join the independent adult world. The situation is much worse if the school emphasises academic work and ignores vocational needs altogether, as if to say 'employment is unlikely when you leave here'. If, however, their school curriculum has identified skills that could develop into occupation or jobs, then they have a chance to move to a training unit, day centre or sheltered workshop and become part of a working group with some independence. If the whole emphasis has been on school examinations, the effort is wasted unless they have a real potential for college and higher or vocational education.

Types of work and occupation

In the context of this study there are three basic types of activity that can be called work or occupation.

Paid work

Most people would be reluctant to describe their regular activity as work unless it is paid, in salary or wage. The amount of payment may bear little relation to the amount of physical or mental effort required, but it is part of some contract system. Most employment statistics relate to people who are paid for their work, but ignore those who use their own existing resources in gambling or playing the money-market (very similar activities).

Unpaid and voluntary work

Many people gain no wage or salary for what they do, particularly mothers of children, carers of relatives and those who do voluntary work. There are several thousand listed voluntary associations in the UK, and most of them are staffed by people who are paid nothing. Sometimes the gain is to work on behalf of relatives or children who suffer from some specific condition (e.g. cerebral palsy) rather than live with the anger of watching them suffer the indignities of their particular illness or disability. For others the gain is to do useful work, what Clarke calls the 'contribution' ethic, and so be involved in something that is socially useful and valued by the community; a feature of the community activities of traditional Hebrew society.

Creative work

In both paid and unpaid work there can be a very important dimension of creativity, where people can put something unique of themselves into the job and gain recognition or fascination for what they do. This is a major feature of the types of people (and jobs) that are least likely to result in burn-out (Roberts, 1986) in that there are ways of getting regular achievement, positive feedback, appreciation and fascination from what they do.

For some the job is routine, boring and exhausting, but does provide finances for creative enthusiasms in off-duty periods (sport, fishing, art, literature, theatre, music). For others the pay is non-existent or inadequate but the work involves activities that are totally absorbing and give great inspiration.

The key feature of creative work is that it stimulates energy and interest, and the effects of this can colour the rest of existence. For some disabled people such personal interest can be a powerful antidote to all the other painful, distressing and exhausting efforts that they have to make to cope with their disabilities in a community that may ignore them. A rehabilitation programme can be very tiring, but it can be much more bearable if it is associated with a plan to develop the real personal creative enthusiasms of the disabled person. Without a creative goal or interest what else will provide the incentive to get moving each morning, struggle with a dysphasia, wrestle with uncontrollable clothes and put energy into difficult training routines?

'Apathy is our main option' said one severely disabled person at a conference on employment. Most studies show that disabled people are much more likely to be unemployed, hence the need to search carefully for creative occupation from the outset of any training programme and for every person who is disabled.

Types of disability

Before trying to help a disabled person to match up their needs with possible occupations it is important to examine the different types of disability that exist, particularly their natural histories and prognosis. Disease or injury can affect people's working potential in four ways (Figures 6.2 and 6.3). Each pattern may have a very different implication for the individual, but the

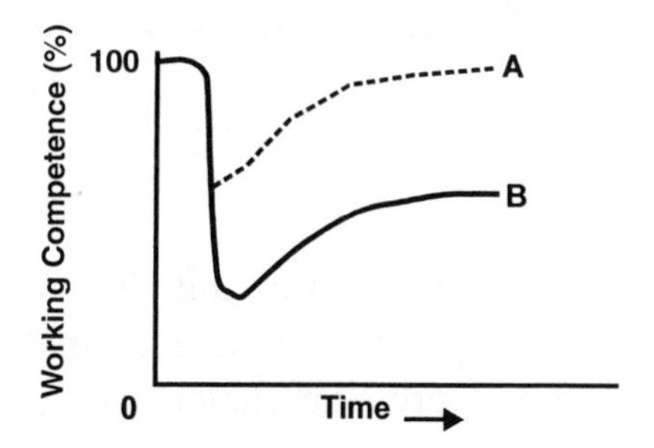

Figure 6.2. Recovering disabilities in relation to working competence A: temporary disability; B: severe recovering disability.

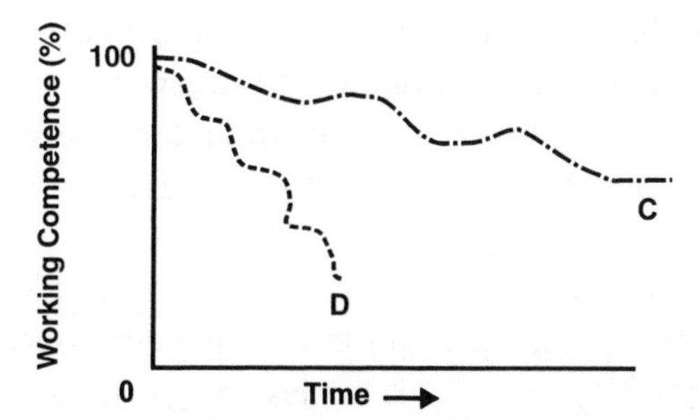

Figure 6.3. Worsening disabilities in relation to working competence. C: slow, worsening disability; D: severe worsening disability.

condition may make it difficult for him or her to return to the original work, or to find a job. Clearly the business of matching an individual to possible work is a very complex process, but it is important that potential future changes are considered.

Temporary disability

For many people who have a myocardial infarct, the medical condition may heal totally in a week, and they can soon recover to a state of symptom-free health. They can even train to a level of fitness far greater than their unfit precoronary state. This recovery may be seriously affected by a lack of counselling and in fact far too many people may leave hospital crippled with fear, totally lacking confidence, waiting for the next attack and unable to return to work. This cardiac anxiety can usually be overcome by adequate informed discussion and formal retraining and progressive self-awareness of recovery and confidence.

Such people are examples of a condition that need not result in permanent disability, and if the employers are advised in the first week, the job may be kept open for later return, provided the victims of the illness are given a good retraining programme, and time to recover.

Severe recovering disability

Many conditions result in a level of disability that is very severe initially, but has potential for partial or full recovery over a long period of time. Examples are head injury, stroke, cerebral palsy, back pain, depression, major hand or limb trauma, severe burns, spinal cord injury and many cancers. In all these examples, the difficulty in matching person to work lies in the problem of knowing the extent of recovery and how long it will take.

Brain damage may go on improving for years, but employers will probably want an appraisal after a few months. The public demand is for answers in a condition that may need much more time to allow relearning and adaptation. There is always a chance in these conditions that permanent disabilities may be lifelong.

In these instances of possible slow recovery the (potential) employer still needs to be encouraged to try and keep a place open in the working environment, either the original post (if optimistic) or to look for less physically or mentally stressful work. Trying to keep options open for one to two years is very difficult for them, but the presence of a chance of return to work can influence the recovery process, and make many clients more hopeful, although others may have no strong attachment to the last job.

Slow worsening disability

Sometimes the natural history of a condition such as multiple sclerosis, arthritis, glaucoma, deafness or Parkinson's disease is known to be one of steady or periodic deterioration, but the levels of severe incapacity may not be obvious until well into retirement age. This means that in the early stages the threat of disability can be an anxiety affecting the individual much more than the actual physical problems that present. Work potential certainly is often affected, but this can result far more from worry about things that could be adapted than to the actual inability to continue work. People with these problems may welcome regular long-term support and a review of adaptive measures or equipment.

Severe worsening disability

In a condition such as advanced cancer or motor neurone disease, the expected outlook may be for quite rapid progression towards incapacity or even death.

Work and social life are bound to be affected, but absolutely nobody can predict precisely how quickly or in what way. The need for a positive short-term achievable occupation is most essential for this group, to provide them with daily achievements and support. Far too often the result of diagnosis is to produce only pity or avoidance from professionals and public acquaintances who have no resources to cope with impending severe disability or mortality. This group above all needs to have the option of the company of others, if they wish it, and of activities they can do which allow them to see results, feel useful, contribute to family, or even to explode some of their anger and despair into creative energy.

Assets needed for employment

Most employers are likely to prefer to employ people who are basically able to work efficiently and fast, remain flexible to be used in different parts of the organisation, never cause trouble, and are socially compatible with the rest of the workforce. This may include many features of life that may be assumed to be present without featuring in any formal job description.
For example:

Socially mobile (housing and family)
Capable of independent transport to and from work
Well dressed and well behaved (perhaps even deferential)
Easy to talk to, conforming to anonymous 'norms' and socially acceptable
Capable of hearing and remembering any instructions or practical advice (e.g. safety rules)
Enthusiastic and full of energy
Cooperative in all changes imposed by management or the economy
Fully mobile upstairs, through heavy fire doors, and past all the hazards of the workplace
Good vision and hearing
Cheerful, reliable and without anxieties, moods or strange behaviour
Fully skilled and experienced (but not too old).

The trouble is that most of these imply that businesses want to make no allowances to integrate each person into the achievement of productivity and financial success, especially if a cost will be entailed. Something like dystonia can immediately cause social problems. The peculiar movements may in fact cause no difficulties in the job, but other staff may be intolerant of the grimaces or movements and interpret them wrongly as signs of mental illness. The problems may result from public ignorance and from a management structure that is unwilling to educate other workers to be more tolerant. For many disabilities the apparent problems (needing some adjustment in others) may be more important than the real ones of whether they can really do the job. Deafness can intrude in many aspects of work, particularly in picking up the conversations of others or the inadequately prepared instructions of management. Anxiety after a coronary may reduce concentration and increase fatigue. Those who have had severe childhood disabilities may be capable of skilled work but lack some training through having an education that was regularly interrupted by periods of treatment or therapy.

John (1981) carried out a study of epilepsy and employment and uncovered many serious examples of prejudice about the condition, false assumptions about higher insurance premiums (not needed) and in some companies a complete refusal to consider any person with epilepsy, however mild, for employment in the company (John & McLellan, 1988). Any admission of back pain in a job application is likely to have the same effect of blanket refusal to consider people for jobs.

A major problem is that employers are increasingly inclined to seek people for whom they need make no allowances whatever, in the pretext of being cost effective and making maximum profits. This means that many people with disability problems have little chance of being considered when competing with more active and apparently uncomplicated people. This is a bigger problem in a recession and with high unemployment, even when some companies make massive profits.

Statistics at work (UK)

It is difficult to find accurate figures for the number of people who are in paid work in the UK (probably about 22 million) compared with the number of people in the population as a whole (approximately 55 million), or for different age groups. Currently the highest rate of unemployment is in the 18 to 24-year-old age group. Regular figures are given for the claimant-registered unemployment rate (2.4 million in the UK in August 1991). This gets frequent publicity, but in fact the rate is a fairly carefully massaged piece of information relating to certain categories of people who are officially accepted for unemployment benefit and excluding a whole variety of people such as housewives who are for some reason not regarded as part of the politically-defined working population. The actual proportion of the population defined as capable of working (registered workforce) therefore is only about 50% of people in the UK, and although theoretically anyone in the 16 to 65-year-old age group is capable of employment, many of this group are not actually doing paid work and a large number are not regarded as employed or even unemployed in the official statistics. The labour force survey tends to give a larger figure for the total numbers of unemployed workers in the UK.

Even more elusive are the figures for job vacancies. This is difficult to pin down because many vacancies are only advertised in local or trade publications, by personal contacts, or by casual enquiries, and never reach Job Centre statistics. In spite of this, the official figures are of great concern, showing a downward trend:

Registered vacancies: 248 000 (1988) > 108 000 (1991)
Registered unemployed: 1.8 million (1988) < 2.4 million (1991).

It is unacceptable to condone the cynical way in which some regard unemployment as a justifiable means to try and keep the economy going, to reduce pay rises and ignore employment conditions for the average members of the workforce. When the information about unemployment is further broken down it is clear that people in ethnic minorities have twice the national unemployment rate for any district in which they live, and that disabled people according to various definitions of disability probably have three or four times the national unemployment rate.

Figure from the Bridge Agency (specialising in placing disabled people in work) and extracted from the Office of Population Censuses and Surveys (OPCS) (1988) show that there are:

Over six million disabled adults in the UK (14% of the adult population)
41.2% of disabled people are in the working age group (16–65 years)
5.8% of disabled people are in the 16 to 30-year-old age group
In the working age group of disabled people: 64% of men are not working; 69% of women are not working; 52% of men under 30 years of age are not working.

The quota

In 1944 the Disabled Persons Act (employment) placed a duty on employers of any workforce of more than 20 people to accept a quota of 3% of disabled people. The theory of this positive discrimination was good in that it made a claim for this group of people in the population (10%) to have a chance of being considered for employment. There are four aspects of the idea that have limited its value:

1. It is almost unenforceable, as there is no official body that has the resources to establish how many employers take any notice of the quota, or the power to

extract any penalties from those that don't. The German system offers a choice of taking disabled people or paying towards a central fund for sheltered work (Floyd & North, 1984).

2. Many employers if challenged say that they have no work suitable for disabled people, but seldom does this mean that they have investigated the range of disabilities they might consider, and rarely have they taken the trouble to establish sheltered work, even for their own employees when they are ill or disabled.
3. High unemployment rates mean that there is a huge body of healthy, sometimes skilled, people to take up the precious vacancies.
4. Many disabled people do not like to risk the stigma of being registered disabled so the Job Centres may only have a small proportion of the most severely impaired to offer the few interested employers.

Figures from the Registered Disabled in Employment Gazette (1991) show some very poor results for quota, especially from the National Health Service (NHS) and County Councils which are very large organisations with big varied workforces. Overall figures for percentage quota fulfilled are shown in Table 6.3.

These figures are disappointing because nearly all these organisation have a high proportion of jobs involving office work that could easily suit people with poor mobility (10% of the population: OPCS survey, 1986). It does, however, beg the question as to whether enough disabled people are able to gain the desired skills and qualifications to compete with able-bodied competitors, particularly in office, management and computer skills.

Institutional alternatives to paid work

In most parts of the UK there are day centres and some sheltered workshops providing part-time or full-time opportunities to get out of the house and find a community of people and some activities. The best of such centres offer a busy working environment, creative outlets and some opportunity to achieve results from a day of activity. They will also seek to have a choice of activities that allow for the very different needs of the variety of disabled people who may want to join in. For those who cannot drive, or have no family car, some centres also have their own transport to collect people from their homes. Sheltered workshops usually rely on batches of secondary work from other local factories, and can make some profit to supplement the official subsidies and therefore allow each worker to receive a weekly wage packet. Most day centres offer interesting activities, and company, but not money.

It has been shown (Nhekairo-Musa, 1988) that the opportunity to encour-

Table 6.3 *Overall figures for percentage quota fulfilled*

Employers	*Total numbers*	*Workforce (%)*
Regional Health Authorities (all)	165	0.5
Wessex	1	0.1
SW Thames	15	1.2
BBC	71	0.2
Post Office Corporation	1884	1.0
County Councils (all)	5637.5[a]	0.7
Hampshire	110	0.4
Wiltshire	138	0.9
Dorset	271	1.9
District Health Authorities (all)	2621	0.3
Southampton	4	0.0
Merton/Sutton	65	1.0

[a] 0.5 included part-timers.

age disabled people to spend two to three days at a day centre every week has real benefits for the carers, who can have some relief from a 7-day week of being in a state of constant on-call. It has also been shown (Moyo, 1989) that the clients of a day centre may also gain real advantages from being at the centre regularly rather than just staying at home all week. This is most likely to be time when each person can develop his or her own special interests. McLeod (1991) showed how disabled people's skill can be matched to the workshop or factory equipment in an industry.

The worse types of day centres are simply large understaffed parks for too many people who are failing to manage at home. If inadequately funded, then the few staff members are rushing around coping with some urgent needs and failing to show the energy and enthusiasm to develop a wide range of interesting activities. They do not offer much choice of company, other than a difficult mixture of serious mental and physical disabilities; they certainly are not stimulating, and they can be centres of boredom for people who have little choice but to stay there. They encourage segregation from able-bodied people, rather than the challenge to return and function in normal society.

The place of work in psychiatry

Rowland & Perkins (1988) have reviewed the theory and practice of work in psychiatric patients, both from the theoretical descriptions of what work means to the practical effects it can offer to hospital patients. They also lay claim to the enormous need to explore work centres/day centres for the same type of disabilities during this current national trend to close down long-stay hospitals, and to promote community care. In 1968 there were 122 psychiatric hospitals in the UK, and 100 of them had industrial therapy units. What is the equivalent priority to offer people useful occupation now that many of these institutions are closing?

Their review of the benefits of work-related activities showed particular concerns for the special needs of mental illness, and some examples are important in this field:

Providing structure to the day
Concentration
Social interaction
Exercise in relating perception and reality
Providing limits to achieve goals
Balancing social expectation and reward
Decreasing dependency
Offering a sense of achievement.

Although there are only a few detailed studies of the place of work activities in the total programme of treating people with temporary or long-term mental illness, they did present evidence that the workshop provided as much, if not more, benefit to the patients as the medication or social structure of the hospital. To quote William Cowper (Rowland & Perkins, 1988):

> the absence of occupation is not rest, a mind quite vacant is a mind distressed.

Rehabilitation services

It is very easy for the major activities of hospital rehabilitation services to be directed at getting people home, without always having the perspectives of family or community staff to be sure that this home going suits the carers, family or housing situation, or the client's own needs. The emphasis of treatment can be related to professional interests, e.g:

Mobility	activities of daily living	speech
transport	independence	medical needs

The end-point can therefore be an empty hospital bed for the next emergency, and a disabled person 'placed' at home with nothing to do except survive. Alternative outcomes for the more severely disabled may be a nursing home, rest home or Cheshire home, though use of the word 'home' is challenged as inappropriate by the more verbal clients. This must be a grim existence for the restricted person without occupation, and provides little incentive to keep trying to gain more function or independence. This situation has been called 'social death' (Oliver, 1991).

Matching problems with assets: personal plan

There has traditionally been a tendency for rehabilitation professionals to establish goals for their patients, to expect compliance, cooperation and gratitude. After perhaps many months of adopting this behaviour, the newly disabled person is discharged to the community and expected to demonstrate independence, creative problem solving and realistic goal setting (Tucker, 1980). Involvement in decision-making from the earliest possible time, establishing goals that are mutually agreed on and consideration of future occupation through the rehabilitation process will ensure both the relevance of the programme to the individual and will also help to foster the very behaviours that are survival skills following discharge to the community.

One way round the indifference to client interests is to use a personal plan (Figure 6.4) that is a one-page summary of all that can be found about the negative and positive sides of the person and the disability. From this can be drawn some specific objectives, preferable personal wishes balanced by what can be achieved in therapy, equipment or financial restraints.

The exercise only makes sense if the client's personal priorities are clearly labelled (*) and acted on. If he or she is expected to consider only the plans of the professionals the result may be totally negative. Clients have the right to attempt goals even if they fail, but they are unlikely to try so hard if the objectives ignore their own wishes.

Problem lists are widely used in hospitals, nursing procedures and therapy departments, but they can very easily be worded to be specific to the type of work carried out by the professionals. Stroke victims with dysphasia can be extremely miserable because they cannot speak their minds, but the external labels may be depression (leading to the use of mind clouding drugs), or a lack of cooperation in therapy. What may be essential (but very difficult) is to find ways in which they can start to express their biggest needs, even if they can only use the non-verbal signals of anger and tears. The speech therapist may be the most important person to help define client priorities for a dysphasic, and observation by nursess and family can identify these, e.g:

Need to get into the garden	Dislike of hospital
Friends don't visit	Desire for quiet
Fear of the future	Desire for music
Financial worries	Anxiety about home.

Hospital No: **Date:**

Disability Assessment

Name........Red Joint.............................. **GP**................Dr Turnover................

Age...........50.. **Consultants**..Dr Hectic....................

Address.....17 Acacia Avenue................ **Occupation**...Builder.......................

.................Woodstoke.........................

Diagnosis **Prognosis** **Improve / ?Worsen** (Worsen circled)

Rheumatoid Arthritis

*=Client choices

Clients Problems	Assets	Objectives
1. Insomnia (pain) 2. Weakness of grip : Can't lift 3. Unable to bricklay or build 4. Finance short (mortgage doubt) 5. Depressed, bad tempered	*Sea Fishing *Fuschias Music Pools	A. OT review of tools Could adapt B. Industrial workshop assessment → DEA C. Night analgesic + antidepressant D. Welfare advice E.* ? Day centre gardening (time away from home) F.* Fishing boat trips + adapted gear
Family Carers		
Wife back pain 3 young children High anxiety levels	Helpful neighbours Church links	Home visit to look at adaptations *Regular local contact for counselling

Destination

Adapted house/equipment
Retraining for alternative work

Long Term Plans

Figure 6.4. Disability assessment.

The problem list presented (Figure 6.4) defines specific family and home needs as well as those of the individual, but some of the statements may reflect the perspectives of those who can see serious difficulties that may be obvious only to those who have clinical experience with the disease or disability presented, e.g:

pressure sore risk	lack of insight	memory loss
contracture risk	tendency to fall	comprehension loss
inattention dangers	insulin balance	
perceptive chaos	toxic drugs	

The medical perspective may also include an element of prophesy, an attempt to judge the prognosis. This really can be no more than broad ideas of (a) likely to improve, (b) variable outlook, or (c) likely to deteriorate. In some instances (e.g. MND) the time scale may be much more definite (e.g. three years) and have serious implications for the family.

Assessing assets (interests and abilities)

It makes a great difference to a rehabilitation programme if part of the time is spent in looking for all examples of interests, skills, abilities and knowledge that can form the basis of future occupation or work. Examples of significant assets are:

music	computing	sports	sculpture
gardening	academic studies	business	craftwork
fishing	cars and driving	nature	writing
painting	electronics	ecology	pottery
sailing	photography	stamps	poetry

There are four practical approaches to this process:

1. *Willingness to listen* is a crucial part of the work of all rehabilitation staff because although an individual may have many thoughts and ideas about the future, if the disability has been a sudden and severe change, all ideas may be submerged in despair, anger and shock. For those who can see potential in any previous interest, however scatty or impractical in the present, there is a great need to make time available and to encourage the disabled person to talk freely about past enthusiasms and future ideas. This is sometimes left to the obvious counsellors (social worker, Disablement Employment Advisor, psychologist) but may actually be more successful if the keen listener is involved in everyday nursing tasks, in physiotherapy training, during medical procedures, as part of an occupational therapy programme or when the ward orderly is cleaning the floor. Listening needs to start on day 1 of any disability. If all staff are prepared to listen, and any ideas come back to a personal plan for the case conference, then casual comment can be followed up and tested out more formally. The only exception is when the client talks in confidence and does not wish the information spread around.

2. *Client's choice*. It is one thing to know about interests, but quite another to push them forward regardless. There has to be a willingness in the disabled person to develop a work option, and it can only succeed if he or she agrees to be enthusiastic. Sometimes an idea (e.g. sea-fishing) might be discarded because the individual cannot see how to overcome practical problems of doing it again (transport, getting into a boat, controlling ataxia, handling equipment, keeping warm). If these are the only reasons for a fading interest in a past activity, they can often be solved by inventive therapy, social and engineering answers, or by voluntary societies with special interests.

   If, however, a past activity is discarded because of genuine dislike (a tedious job, personality clashes or association with painful memories, e.g. colleagues lost or injured in an accident), then the ideas for return should be dropped. There is no point in forcing an individual towards activities that are distasteful, depressing or produce antagonism and apathy.
3. *Brainstorming*. There is some value in asking an individual formally to think aloud about all the possible jobs, hobbies and interests they could possibly enjoy learning to take part in and creating an options list. This is also easier to do in an industrial rehabilitation unit and/or day centre of activities including many they have never tried before, to see if any of them are of special interest. The Hexagon Day Centre (Hampshire Social Services) can offer about 40 different activities from domestic to crafts, from horticultural to industrial, and for some people this allows room to expand and experiment with things they could try later. Any one of the many options could develop into a viable future occupation.
4. *Actual skills*. Sometimes a person will defy all 'expert' predictions and prove totally capable of doing a job they want to do in spite of all predictions. It is, however, important that some of the trial practice at chosen activities is guided by a team of people who can establish the real level of ability that a person has (or could have) and to ensure that skills really are what will be practical, but this assumes:

   Enthusiasm is not the same as insight
   Single-minded application is not the same as safety
   Conviction can be flawed by cognitive failures
   Application can sometimes mimic obsession
   Experts are often wrong.

If a person expresses keenness to try and learn a new skill or follow an old trade, it is essential that experienced people or colleagues are available to carry out work studies and see if the skills are safe, capable of application without supervision or are likely to be associated with whatever equipment or help is needed in the intended workplace. Whether this is paid work or unpaid occupation, the abilities need to be assessed with future employers or family in mind.

Table 6.4 *Job Description*

EMPLOYER		PRODUCTS
ADDRESS		NO: OF EMPLOYEES
		LOCAL TRANSPORT
PHONE NO:		LIAISON PERSON
	Access problems through plant/WCs/public access	
PLANT		
	Factory design	
PAY	Pay system (piece/wage/salary)	
	Qualifications	
TRAINING		
	Expected	
WORK	*Work type*	Special Needs
	Day/night/alternating shifts	Hearing
	Unskilled/semi-skilled/	
	skilled/professional	Vision
	Work cycle	Bending
	Sitting/standing/movements	Lifting
	Description	Ladders
		Dust
	Tools used	Driving
		Inside/outside
	Special skills needed	Heat/cold
STAFF	*Management structure*	
	Method of instruction	
	Expectations of senior staff	
	colleagues	
POLICY	What do company feel about employee?	
	-previous work record	
	-what is known about condition?	
	Any alternative (lighter) jobs available?	
ACTION	*Rehabilitation plans*	

Assessing a job (job description)

If return to work is a remote possibility, and a welcome one, then a full job description should be completed. This sometimes appears from personnel departments as a dreary list of activities and management-speak that is more conceptual than practical. Table 6.4 illustrates a check list of specific questions that may be far more relevant than the usual job description because it does not assume any of the features of mobility, transport, social acceptance or basic skills that a personnel handout might include.

Doctors are often put in the absurd position of having to sign a person's 'fitness to work' while having absolutely no idea what they really do. Job titles may be so technical as to be meaningless to all outsiders (e.g. CAD (computer-aided design) operative) or so familiar that they give no idea of what the work actually entails (e.g. kerb-layer). Too often a decision may be made that a person can go back to 'light work', in a factory with all heavy work, or to sign someone as fit when they have fallen far below the physical levels of exercise tolerance needed for a job. This type of uninformed decision can be helped by:

1. Better liaison with employers directly on what they expect.
2. Using a job centre DAS (Disability Advisory Service).
3. Using a checklist of specific questions that assume nothing about what a person is expected to do at work, or even how to get to work.

Assessing loss of work

If a disability precludes return to specific work, or the particular occupation has gone (e.g. factory closure) then the enquiries need to start at the more basic level of matching assets/interests with the available occupations, employment openings or training facilities that exist locally or nationally.

Assessing assets (p. 135) shows a wide range of options which are worth exploring with the disabled person to see if some may lead to an acceptable and practical form of work. Clearly with the UK in a major recession, the chances of open employment for disabled people are much worse than for the other two to three million who are registered unemployed.

The DEA at the job centre can be a vital link between health, social or education services and the possible openings in local employment. Successive government restrictions on the way the DEA service can operate, and on the availability of adequate assessment or the retraining that can be achieved, does mean that the adequacy of Department of Employment facilities is becoming seriously compromised.

Summary chart = Team review = Personal plan

Figure 6.4 represents an example of a one-page Rehabilitation Plan using a matrix of problems and assets for the disabled individual and their carers or family from which short- or long-term objectives can be decided. This information needs to be brief and represent the conclusions for assessment of all professionals involved, and particularly the ideas and plans of the individual for whom this programme is designed. It also needs to identify the disabled person's own plans and those which are being imposed (even if with good reason). The items mentioned may be headings only in that they do not include all the details that each professional therapist is concerned with, but enough to allow all the rest of the team to know what is going on. It is also essential that the disabled person is afforded the choice of what is useful public (team) knowledge and what he or she regards as private (Cantrell, 1978), so that personal details that would be embarrassing or distressing are left out. It does make a great difference for all staff to be widely informed about the insights of other team members, but personal problems must be left to the most relevant person (e.g. social worker) if that is the client's choice. The best team plan is one the individual accepts, where remotely possible.

Case conferences based on such summary charts can then focus on what can be achieved (objectives) and how to reach short-term targets. They can avoid endless hours of detailed reviews if the rehabilitation matrix is the result of detailed assessment before the group meets. They can also benefit greatly from peer support groups helping to encourage the most defeated disabled people back to decision-making.

Any plans can only become genuine personal plans if they are based on the conclusions of questions about what people want to do. Not only do their future self-images matter in theory but plans made for them are unlikely to succeed if they have not decided to accept them. Anything less, which is only a team decision, is a disposal plan.

Destination?

What is projected by staff as likely beyond hospital or rehabilitation unit can be classified in four grades. Unfortunately ward rounds and staff discussions often concentrate on the first (sometimes the second):

1. *Zero*: the label is a purely medical one (e.g. multiple sclerosis). No discussion refers to home or what the disabled person might do in the future.
2. *Vegetable*: future plans are confined to site of 'replanting' (after discharge) only, an address perhaps.
3. *Animal*: some discussion includes the human support and care that will be needed in future.
4. *Soul*: the client is introduced as a person with specific work/enthusiasm/occupation as a main goal and all other objectives are to that end.

It is sad that people are usually known only by the work they do, unless they are TV stars, sports personalities, professionals or writers. It is even more tragic that once people are ill or disabled they are labelled by their diagnosis (e.g. C5/6 tetraplegia or stroke). It seems far more logical to start with even a provisional label of how they might like to spend their next few months or years (work/occupation) and then work backwards to the practical objectives they need to achieve this result.

Difficulties for employers willing to enrol disabled people

There is a very real need for agencies who promote the need to employ disabled people, and for rehabilitation or training centres, to look carefully at the preparation of employers as well as clients for job applications and employment. There will not only be a need to tackle discrimination and misunderstanding, but there is a strong need to take part in the education of all their fellow workers. Employers are by no means well-informed about disability.

John (1981) in a study of industry's attitude to epilepsy found that most employers were unaware of the practical ways of allowing for the needs of epileptics, that many sufferers had very few fits, or of how to cope with fits. Even the fact that most insurance companies would accept epilepsy as having no extra cost to insuring a workplace or employee was something that no one was aware of. Such details can only reach employers if some group (such as the British Epileptic Association) make a clear objective to educate all levels of industry to the practicalities of accepting most people with epilepsy as totally employable.

The sort of questions that employers may need help with are:

- how to reduce the indifference of other workers
- practical assistance with access (ramps, doors)
- adaptation of heavy fire door controls
- redesign of equipment for lifting, movement reaching circles (McLeod, 1991) and safe lifting statistics
- equipment to help those with poor hearing, sight or speech disorders
- special transport, parking and mobility facilities
- safety features of the workplace
- grants to allow adaptations (especially when the business is short of money)
- the differentiations of involuntary movements (e.g. dystonia, Parkinson's disease) from antisocial behaviour
- the practical management of weakness, pain and ataxia in employees
- methods for reducing spine pain (neck and back) in employees, pain prevention programmes, chair design, ergonomics
- retraining of people returning to work after illness, e.g. coronary patient's loss of confidence (positive feedback)
- the handling of cognitive/memory problems (memory aids)
- alternative ideas for redeployment, if a company is likely to lose a market (e.g. Lucas Aerospace, as described by Clarke, 1982)
- informed medical advice to "fitness to work".

In the national job centres, the purpose of the DAS is really to liaise with all local employers, and essentially help them to retain workers whose skills are compromised by recently-acquired illness or disability. The more difficult job of getting them to accept new employees who are disabled is still the work of a non-carer grade of civil servant, the DRO (Disabled Resettlement Officer) who has a very uphill struggle. They have neither the time nor the resources for all the education and marketing needed to change the minds of employers in modern Britain. Perhaps this is why the Bridge Agency is so necessary.

Personal choice occupation

People whose lives have been changed by disability, whether suddenly or gradually, are in danger of losing many of the benefits of work/occupation outlined in Table 6.1. The three factors that can reinforce this loss and keep them in premature retirement are:

1. The major shortages of finance, with loss of earnings and an increasing demand for money to pay for the complications of being disabled (transport, special equipment, isolation).
2. The difficulties of breaking through the post-traumatic stress syndrome and taking over decisions from the professionals who are liable to make the substantive conclusions unless overridden.
3. The attitudes of society that give so little value to 'Useful work' (Clarke, 1982) and so much to paid work and its associations with prestige, power and market force related status.

The (COPM) Canadian Occupational Performance Measure system does allow a set of questions and priorities to be set by the disabled individual, but this does not guarantee to facilitate involvement of all professionals in the total personal plan that represents the person's own preferences and interests (Law *et al.*, 1990).

Personal choice may only be achieved if any rehabilitation, nursing, clinical or therapy programme makes a priority of prefacing every document or action plan with a provisional or definite occupation label for the future, which the person accepts, e.g.:

Jones the carpenter	not the C5.6 tetraplegic
Collins the artist	not the CVA/stroke
Smith the caterer/cook	not the rheumatoid

If the client changes the label, we accept the change, but because we (the professionals and family) can so easily let the diagnosis dominate our thinking, this priority of occupation can easily get lost in ward rounds and case conferences.

Pete Seeger sang about people in 'little boxes', perhaps disabled people are not better off if they remain labelled as 'little diagnoses'. The new life of recovery starts with a new inspired image of occupational plans.

References

Beale, N. R. & Nethercott, S. (1985). Job loss and family morbidity : a factory closure study. *General Practice Journal, Royal College of General Practitioners*, **35**, 510–14.

Cantrell, E. G. (1978). Privacy : the medical problems. In *Privacy* ed. J. B. Young, pp. 195–219. Chichester: John Wiley.

Clarke, R. (1982). *Work in Crisis, Dilemma of a Nation*. Edinburgh: St Andrews Press.

Cox H. (1966). *The Secular City*. SCM Press.

Floyd, M. & North, K. (1984). *Disability and Employment*. Conference papers: Anglo-German Foundation for the Study of Industrial Society. Printed by George Over, Harrow, Middlx.

Hayes, J. & Nutman, P (1981). *Understanding the Unemployed*. London: Tavistock.

Jahoda, M. (1982). *Employment and Unemployment*. Cambridge: Cambridge University Press.

John, C. A. (1981). *Opportunities for Employment for People with Epilepsy*. Fourth year project, Southampton Medical Library.

John, C. A. & McLellan, D. L. (1988). Employers' attitudes to epilepsy. *British Journal of Industrial Medicine*, **45**, 713–15.

Law, M., Baptiste, S., McColl, M., Opzoomer, A., Polatajko, H. & Pollock, M. (1990). The Canadian occupational performance measure. *Canadian Journal of Occupational Therapy*, **57**, 82–7.

McLeod, F. A. (1991). *A Study to Evaluate the Match of Employees to Task at Enham Alamein Village*. MSc Project, Southampton Medical School.

Moyo, A. M. (1989). *The View of the Clients and Staff of the Function of the Hexagon Day Centre*. MSc Project, Southampton Medical School.

Nhekairo-Musa, P. A. (1988). *Do Day Centres Benefit Carers?* MSc Project, Southampton Medical School.

Office of Population Census Studies. (1988). *Surveys of Disabilities Among Adults*. London: HMSO.

Oliver, M. (ed.) (1991). *Social Work: Disabled People and Disabling Environments*. London: Jessica Kimpsley.

Registered Disabled People in the Public Sector. (1991). *Employment Gazette* (Feb), 81–6.

Roberts, G. (1986). Burnout: psycholobabble or valuable concept? *British Journal of Hospital Medicine*, **36**, 194–7.

Rowland, L. A. & Perkins, R. E. (1988). You can't eat, drink or make love eight hours a day: the value of work in psychiatry. *Health Trends*, **20**, 75–9.

Smith, R. (1987). *Unemployment and Health*. Oxford: Oxford University Press.

Tucker, S. J. (1980). The psychology of spinal cord injury: patient–staff interaction. *Rehabilitation Literature*, **41**, 114–22.

Turner, S. W. (1991). Post-traumatic stress disorder. *Hospital Update*, **17**, 644–9.

7

Management in rehabilitation

KEITH ANDREWS

Introduction

To cope with our daily lives we find strategies and tactics that in the broadest sense can be termed 'management'. It is the buzz word in the organisation of any health system and is something that clinicians moving up the career tree becomes anxious about as they move from clinical care to taking responsibility for organisation of resources and other people.

Management

There are a number of definitions of 'management' but most include certain elements that have been described by Levey & Loomba (1987) as being 'simultaneously the judicious use of resources, the motivation of people, the provision of leadership, planning, controlling and the guidance of an organisation or system toward a set of goals and objectives'. Fayoul (1949), 40 years ago when management as such was in its infancy, described the four basic functions of a manager as planning, organising, coordinating and controlling. By planning he meant looking to the future and drawing up a plan of action; by organising, the building up of a structure of the available resources; by coordinating, the bringing together, unifying and harmonising of all activity and effort; and by controlling he meant seeing that everything occurs in conformity with the established rule and expressed demand.

Over the last few years there has been an explosion of books on how to manage. There are, however, only a few basic principles concerning the role of the manager and these have been summarised by Mintzberg (1975) as falling into three major functions: the leadership role (the figurehead, the leader and the liaison role), information role (monitoring, receiving and sending information and being the spokesman) and the decisional role (the entrepreneur, handling problems, allocating resources and negotiating). To these can be added counsellor and the management of change.

Griffiths, when interviewed (May, 1993) about his recommendations for the management restructuring of the National Health Service stated that there are a standard set of templates which are applicable to any large organisation: how well you look after your customer (patient and community), how well you look after your staff, and how well you look after your shareholder (taxpayer). He then went on to suggest that there are three basic things for an organisation to consider: the quality of the goods or services provided, how economically that quality can be provided, and how to motivate staff. It is these elements that will involve managers in health services as well as in industry.

New managers in clinical subjects often find difficulty in adapting to the different philosophies between clinical practice and management practice. Kurtz (1987*a*) has pointed out that clinicians are basically 'doers', prefer one-to-one interactions, making decisions, valuing autonomy and independence, and requiring immediate gratification. Managers on the other hand are planners, interact with many people, delegate, value collaboration, are participitive and interdependent and accept delayed gratification. In view of this difficulty of changing from clinical to management mode it is important to decide whether management really is important in our clinical work. Douglass (1988) has suggested the following reasons why management and planning are important:

it leads to success in achieving goals and objectives
it gives meaning to work
it provides for effective utilisation of available personnel and facilities
it helps in coping with crisis situations
it is cost effective
it is based on past and future, thus helping reduce the elements of change
it can be used to discover the need for change
it is needed for effective control.

The need for effective management is epitomised in the study (Wilson, 1993) of the running of an outpatient clinic. When asked what time the clinic started 'the doctors felt it began when they arrived, the nurses felt it began when the patient arrived, and the clerks felt it began at the time of the first appointment'. In recognising that there is a problem is half way to solving it.

The management styles

There is no single successful management style. Look at the range of mega-successful businesses and you will find a wide range of personality types at the top of the tree. What they all have in common is that they have used their own strengths to the maximum.

Sims (1990) has suggested that those aspiring to high levels of health-care management competence need to know how to function effectively in several learning modes in various environments. He has suggested that Kolb's (1984) experiential learning model provides a suitable framework for this. This model basically considers combinations of management concepts that are opposites: active and reflective; and concrete and abstract. The combination of concrete and reflective produces a learning process known as divergence : people who are strong in this style excel in situations that call for imagination and 'brainstorming'. The combination of abstract and reflective produces an activity termed assimilation, which is associated with abilities to observe, analyse and conceptualise, excelling in reasoning but being less interested in people. The combination of abstract and active results in convergence which is strong in the ability to theorise and experiment as a result of being able to select between alternatives, focus efforts, evaluate plans and programmes, to test hypotheses and make decisions. Finally, the combination of concrete and active results in effective implementation. This requires the ability to advocate positions or ideas, set objectives and implement decisions.

One other way of understanding these management functions is the approach used by Jung (1971) who tried to simplify the complex process of our response to situations by describing four methods of processing information : thinking, intuition, doing or empathising. He suggested that each of us has one of these approaches as our predominant method of coping, while one or two of these traits act as secondary influences on our approach to situations. These can be seen in management styles:

1. *The Thinker* enjoys the intellectual approach of sorting out problems with logic, resisting any project which is not backed up with rational arguments. This personality type is particularly effective with facts, figures, research, system analysis and the financial control of the organisation though may be weak on producing solutions.
2. *The Doer* is usually energetic, 'practical' and thrives on preferring action to words. Although often impatient during the planning stage they enjoy routine work and are usually very well organised, are excellent for getting the project off the ground once the decision has been made about the goals. They are good at negotiating and transforming the 'concept' into the 'deed'.
3. *The Intuitor* is creative, enjoying the concept of 'ideas'. This manager is excellent at the overview of the situation, is creative and responds to 'gut feelings' that have the irritating tendency to work out. This type of personality

is good at long-term planning, brainstorming, lateral thinking and is the person who makes an organisation 'special'.

4. *The Empathiser* is the great conciliator of the team. Warm and sympathetic he or she is very sensitive to the moods of others and is good at keeping the team together. This is the person who is entrusted with negotiating where there are conflicting views with the team, who others turn to for support and when they are in difficulties at home or at work, who is able to communicate as easily with the porter as with the senior physician, and who is the excellent 'front' person in public relations.

You will recognise your own trends and those of your colleagues in these descriptions with the qualifying 'but . . .' because there is a mixture of each of these traits in all of us. It is, however, essential to recognise that a successful organisation is only 'successful' when it has a combination of these managerial styles as part of its senior team.

Strategic planning

Strategic planning has been defined (Drucker, 1973) as 'a continuous systematic process of making risk-taking decisions today with the greatest possible knowledge of their effects on the future; organising efforts necessary to carry out these decisions and evaluating the results of these decisions against expected outcome through reliable feedback mechanisms'. The main components of the planning process are design, delegation, education, development, implementation and follow-up (Ratcliffe & Logson, (1980). These components are involved in the following stages of strategic planning.

The Mission : 'why are we here?'

This is a basic statement of the purpose of the unit or organisation. This could be a simple statement such as 'To provide a comprehensive physiotherapy service in the community within the area covered by X Health Authority'.

The Strategic Plan : 'where do we want to be?'

This is the identification of what is to be achieved within a defined period, say ten years. This can be broken up into short-term (next three years), medium-term (next six years) or long-term (next ten years) objectives. These are generally statements of goals to be achieved.

The Business Plan : 'how do we get there?'

This examines how the goals can be achieved. The process of the business planning for a new development, for instance, has been described by Nylen (1985) as:

define the problems and opportunities the new project will present
define the competitive position of the 'product' and set objectives to meet the anticipated problems and opportunities
detail work steps, schedules, assignments or responsibilities, budgets and the other elements of implementation
describe the monitoring plan.

This type of approach is often shortened in management circles to SWOT : Strengths, Weaknesses, Opportunities and Threats. Using these four titles for analysis of the planning will go a long way to ensuring that most areas are covered. This approach identifies where we are now, where we want to be, what we need to do to get there and the resources required. Resources can be examined under the four main headings of money, manpower, equipment and buildings.

Action Plan : 'who does what and by when?'

The Action Plan takes each of the objectives set out in the Business Plan and makes a statement of specific actions that have to be taken to achieve the objectives, how the success of the action can be judged, who is to take responsibility for ensuring the action is carried out, the time scale for achievement of the action and the time for review of progress being made. This is the day-to-day working programme plan.

Management of change

Health services throughout the world are undergoing major changes. Any change to the status quo results in anxiety, stress, resistance and uncertainty, and can be a demotivating factor for staff. Management of change is therefore an important part of the manager's role. There are a number of approaches (Redin, 1969; Welch, 1979; Spradley, 1980; Hunt & Rigby, 1984) put forward for the management of change. Putting these together a number of logical steps evolve.

there has to be a recognition that there is a rational need for change, i.e. that the change will result in advantage over the present system
staff need to be informed that a change will be made, why it is being made and how it will take place

setting objectives with relevant members of staff (involvement and 'owning')
analyse possible approaches and solutions to the problem
identify the strengths, weaknesses, opportunities and threats (see above)
select the method to be used and plan the changes
keep staff informed of the progress being made
review progress and identify obstacles.

It is not unusual to have some resistance to change. A recognition of the reasons for resistance will go a long way to overcoming the resistance. Some staff see change as a threat because it upsets the comfortable and secure way of their present working, including the opportunities for promotion, whether it will increase the workload or even whether there will be a place in the new system for them.

Management of resources : staff

Appointment of staff

The greatest investment a manager makes is in the appointment of good staff. The manager may be fortunate enough to have a Personnel Department that will assist in drawing up the job description and specification of the type of employee required, prepare the advertisement, make a short-list of the applicants, interview and following-up the references.

If the manager does not have the assistance of a Personnel Department then there are a few basic principles that may be of some help:

Identifying what is required

A new vacancy is an ideal opportunity to review whether the original post is still required or whether there should be a change in emphasis in the job description or in the type of grade of person required to do the job.

Job description and job specification

Some managers find these confusing. The job description lays down the duties involved. In general these should be relatively broad to allow some flexibility within the job, although it is important to recognise that the job description will be the basis of the Individual Performance Review (see below).

The Job Specification is the list of characteristics of the type of experience or training, the time since qualification or other characteristics that you would find beneficial for the applicant to have. In other words, the Job Description describes what the job is about; the Job Specification describes the type of person you want for the job.

The advert

The advertisement is the first impression the applicant will have of your organisation and should give sufficient information to interest a potential candidate by describing what is on offer, what you are looking for and the strengths of your organisation, i.e. what makes this job special. It is usually worthwhile indicating a closing date for applications in the advertisement.

Applications

It is always polite to confirm that you have received the application, telling the applicant when you expect to have the short-list decided and the date when the interviews will be held.

It is worth offering the candidate the opportunity to look around the department and to discuss the position with you informally. Some doubt must be raised about the candidate who applies without knowing anything about the position or the people they will be working with, especially at the more senior staff appointment levels.

Seeking references

Managers need to know why they are seeking references as this will influence the information requested from the referee. In health care it is important from a legal point of view that you have checked that the applicant is qualified for, and capable of carrying out, the job and that there is nothing in his or her history which would alert the manager to any qualities that may create a danger to patient care.

When asking for a reference give the referee as much detail as possible about what information you require, along with a copy of the job description. The referee may not know your hospital or department, so some background information may be worthwhile adding.

The interview

The manager has a major responsibility to ensure that applicants have the opportunity to show themselves in the best light, to the organisation in appointing the best candidate for the job and to oneself in the knowledge that the interview was run efficiently giving the best opportunity for a successful appointment.

Do everything possible to make the candidate comfortable and relaxed. I usually tell the candidates in advance who will be interviewing them and the official position of the interviewer.

If several people are involved in the interview, plan in advance the areas of questioning for which each will be responsible. Also decide in advance how long the interview will take. It is not necessary for all members of the interview panel to ask questions just for the sake of asking a question.

Some interviewers find it helpful to draw up a profile by identifying in advance certain characteristics such as personality, presentation, general experience, specific experience, knowledge of the patient group to be treated, and other features on which they will make a decision. They can then score these out of five or ten. This gives some comparison between candidates, especially as it is too easy to forget what impression the first candidate made by the time we get to the sixth.

Allow the candidate to ask questions. This means that you should be prepared with answers on condition of service, preferred date of start of the appointment, salary range, availability of accommodation and other local factors.

Specific conditions before acceptance

Make it very clear to the candidate that any offer is subject to evidence of good health, professional qualifications, any registration procedures which may be required, and any professional insurance indemnity that may be required for some posts.

Letter of Offer/Contract

The exact format of the letter of offer or contract will vary from one employing authority to another. There are usually common elements including:

- a statement of the conditions to which the offer is subject (see above)
- starting date
- hours of work
- duties (usually the Job description)
- probationary period
- pay grade, salary, starting incremental point, the incremental date and the number of incremental points, and any special allowances or deductions
- statement of annual leave
- details of sickness arrangements*
- grievance and disciplinary procedures*
- health and safety regulations*
- terms and conditions of service*.

those marked with an asterisk will probably be presented in a separate staff handbook.

Motivation

Once an appointment has been made there is then the need to get the best out of staff. In reality you can't motivate people, you can only help them to motivate themselves.

There is a considerable amount written about motivation. Probably one of the most widely quoted theories is that of Maslow (1970) and its variations (Hertzberg *et al.*, 1959) which recognise an hierarchy of needs. The first level is that of 'hygiene factors' such as safety, belonging, basic creature comforts and financial reward. The second level is that of the 'motivating factors' such as ego or status and self-fulfilment. It is generally recognised that the hygiene factors are not motivators in their own right but their absence can act as a demotivating factor. The ego factors have been further classified (Kurtz, 1987*b*) as those needs relating to self-esteem such as need for self-confidence, independence, accomplishment, capability, success and knowledge base; and those relating to reputation such as recognition, status and respect by others.

The above are regarded as 'contents theories of motivation'. Another approach has been termed 'process' theories of motivation based on the concept that motivation is a learned behaviour and can therefore be influenced by behaviour modification or operant condition theory (Gibson *et al.*, 1988); or that behaviour is controlled by the individual and can therefore be used in conscious motivation.

So what motivates people? Although many will immediately respond in terms of financial reward, this is usually very low on the list of the motivating factors. The factors which play an important, and suggested actions that can be taken by the manager are as shown in Table 7.1.

Communication

One of the more difficult areas of management is communication within the organisation. Tourish (1993) has pointed out that 'organisations significantly improve their effectiveness, efficiency and quality of service delivery if their internal communications are working well'. About 80% of a managers time is spent in communication, so this is a skill that needs to be nurtured.

One component is keeping staff informed, which even in industrial settings has been shown to reduce the rate of absenteeism and other indicators of stress (Aeillo, 1983; Scweiger & Denisis, 1991).

There are several approaches to communication methods including holding staff meetings, oral communication (verbal communication has been said to be 7% word choice, 38% articulation and 55% facial expression (St John, 1985),

Table 7.1 *Motivating factors and potential action by managers*

Motivating factor	Action by manager
A sense of belonging	Getting to know the staff as individuals and being aware of what is happening to them
	Keep them informed of what is going on and involve them in decision making
A sense of achieving	Understand what motivates the individual in their work and in their out of work activities
	Being aware of their strengths and weaknesses, playing to the strengths; training and supporting in areas of weakness
	Help them achieve their personal aims: you need to know what they are
A challenge	Specifically identify challenges for the individual but monitor carefully to ensure that they are not getting out of their depth
Being recognised	Provide immediate recognition of good work done; praise has a greater reinforcing effect than criticism
	Ensure that other, especially your superiors, are informed how well your staff are doing
A sense of responsibility	Being prepared to delegate tasks (see below)
To feel supported	Help them resolve difficulties and being prepared to listen
To have a happy work environment	A small amount of spending on the environment can go a long way
	Look at whether the position of furniture or equipment in the office or department can be moved to make it more 'user friendly'

written communication, reports, having an 'open door' policy or management by walk about. Communication is, however, more than simply keeping staff informed but is a two-way process recognising Meerloo's (1968) quip that 'between two beings there is always the barrier of words'. Communication is therefore as much about listening and receiving feedback as it is about informing. In a review of 27 studies on communication Levenstein (1984) found that feedback was associated with increased productivity in nearly all the studies.

Delegation

Delegation has a bad reputation. It is often regarded as getting someone else to do the jobs you don't want to do. This concept fails to recognise the positive aspects and responsibilities of delegation. Although responsibility is passed on to another person this does not absolve the manager from overall responsibility. In delegating a duty it is important to recognise that you must also delegate the authority to carry out the task. There is no point continually stepping in and undermining the authority of the member of staff.

There are certain aspects of a manager's work that can be delegated (Jenks & Kelly, 1990):

1. *Routine tasks.* These are the tasks that occur frequently and by which a statement of 'rules' can allow others to carry out your wishes.
2. *Essential tasks.* These are the tasks that have to be carried out as part of the organisation of the department. Examples of this category include keeping a record of the number of patients attending the department, the recording of income and expenditure, or the checking of the amount of materials held by the department.
3. *Minor activities.* It is only too easy for time to be taken up on trivial activities that require few skills or little decision-making. Before delegating these tasks it is important to question whether they need be done by anyone.
4. *Those requiring special skills.* It is rare for a manager to have all the skills required. There are some tasks that will be much better carried out by someone else in the department. Which activities fall into this category depends on the strengths and weakness of the manager but may include financial management, setting up the information technology or creating the departmental newsletter.
5. *The jobs you like to do.* This is not so silly as it seems. Many managers spend a considerable amount of time doing things that they like to do but which are not an essential part of their real role. This is particularly true of new managers who cling onto the activities they were doing before promotion. We tend to spend more time on the things we like to do; these activities are ripe for consideration for delegation.

It is important to also recognise that there are certain tasks which should not be delegated. These include:

1. *Authoritative tasks.* By this I mean those that require your position of authority either as the spokesperson or the presenter. Even simple activities such as farewell speeches to departing members of the department should not be delegated. Purchasers are more impressed by meeting the 'boss' rather than as assistant or deputy.
2. *Personnel matters.* Matters related to discipline, staff evaluation and disputes should not, in general, be delegated to others unless it is part of their job description.
3. *Policy decisions.* No matter how much you involve your staff in decision-making the final responsibility for the policy is yours. You can delegate to others how tasks are to be carried out; what those tasks are remain your responsibility.
4. *Confidential information.* Rehabilitation is full of potential areas of confidential information, much of which is available on a 'need to know' basis. There are several forms of information, however, either related to the organisation or about people, that you should not delegate. These include confidential reports, attending certain meetings and staff matters which should remain firmly within the manager's responsibility and not be delegated to others.

The manager has the responsibility for the supervision of the delegated task. The manager must first of all make clear what is being delegated, the purpose of the delegated task, what results are expected, the deadline for the completion of the task, the resources that will be available and at what stage the member of staff should report back to the manager. The manager is responsible for the outcome of the delegated task. The delegatee should receive the credit when the delegated task is successful : the manager the blame if it is not. In other words, as the manager carries the responsibilities of delegation, it has to be planned carefully, supervised thoroughly and the member of staff supported throughout without the manager being overbearing and inhibiting initiative.

Staff appraisal : Individual Performance Review (IPR)

The performance review is one of the more difficult management tasks. Managers do not like doing them and staff see them as a threat. The main purpose should be to assist the members of staff to maximise their performance, create job satisfaction, identify their training needs, identify potential for further development and to identify those areas where the member of staff has concerns or worries.

The IPR gives the opportunity to discuss all areas of the job, the strengths of the individual and how these can be fully used, weaknesses and how these can be overcome, and to set plans for the future. At the end of the session it should be possible to identify not only what the member of staff should do but also what the manager and the organisation should be doing to help the member of staff.

There are several Don'ts about IPRs:

- the IPR is not about promotion or salary increases
- they should not be rushed and squeezed into a spare moment
- they are not a one-one conversation of the manager telling the member of staff what has gone wrong and what has to be done to correct the problems
- they are not paperwork for the sake of paperwork; this means that the manager has a responsibility to follow through on the actions to be taken and not to file the results away until the next IPR
- they are not about working harder, they are about effectiveness, i.e. working smarter not harder.

Disciplinary action

Disciplinary action is one of the most distressing functions of a manager. By far the most effective form of management is to set up procedures that prevent disciplinary action being required. For instance, employees must be aware of what is expected of them in carrying out their duties and their conduct of work.

Be aware of the danger signals that something is wrong, such as an increased sickness rate and staff beginning to perform badly, producing substandard work, not communicating with others, being late, not producing reports on time, lack of interest in team activity and becoming irritable or withdrawn.

At this stage it is important for the manager to step in and provide a counselling service. It is important to make it clear that you are aware that something is wrong and encourage the members of staff to talk about their problems.

Absence of staff is a particular problem and is higher in the National Health Service than in most other industries (CBI, 1993). There are several steps that can be taken in dealing with staff absence (Seccombe & Buchan, 1993). The first is to measure the amount of absence, including the use of computerised personnel information systems. The second step is to monitor the absence with the line manager and the third step is to identify the reasons for the absence, some of which may require support (e.g. domestic problems or stress at work), others require training or a change in the working practice whereas some may require disciplinary action.

If the situation cannot be resolved by counselling or the misdemeanour is more serious, then disciplinary action may be required.

In rehabilitation services we are dealing with a very vulnerable population. An employee is expected to conduct him/herself in a way that maintains the confidence of the public, and at all times the care and welfare of the patient takes priority.

Examples of misconduct requiring disciplinary action are shown in Table 7.2. These are only some of the potential areas for informal or formal disciplinary action. Managers should make sure that they are aware of the Disciplinary and Appeals procedure for their own hospital.

There is a particular need to be aware of those activities which can be regarded as Gross Misconduct that may result in summary dismissal because of the special nature of health care when working with vulnerable people. In a rehabilitation environment these could include: theft, malicious damage to property, dishonest or fraudulent offences (including failure to disclose convictions, giving false information when applying for an appointment or falsifying record sheets or clock cards), wilful action seriously threatening the health and safety of others, physical violence, sexual offences at work, excessive consumption of alcohol or misuse of drugs, unauthorised disclosure of a confidential nature, criminal offences outside the employment and taking on paid employment elsewhere during periods of paid sickness.

Disciplinary procedures

The management of disciplinary procedures is complex and in most health-care facilities will be carried out in collaboration with the Personnel Department. Some basic principles apply to most situations:

- the procedure should be seen to be fair
- disciplinary action should not take place until the case has been fully investigated.
- the employees must be informed of the nature of the offence and given the opportunity to state their case before any decision is made
- the employee should have the right at all stages to have in attendance a work colleague or a union representative
- the employee has a right to appeal against any disciplinary penalty imposed at a formal hearing
- the employees should be given due warning of the time and date of the disciplinary hearing, and informed that they may have a representative present.

Table 7.2 *Examples of misconduct requiring disciplinary action*

Misconduct	Example
General conduct	Being abusive towards a patient, member of the public or another member of staff; discriminates against others on grounds of sex, marital status, religion, colour, race, nationality, ethnic or national origin; accepts fees, gifts, hospitality or other reward beyond that which is authorised; commit any act which is likely to offend decency
Working arrangements	Absence from work, reporting late, ceasing work before authorised finishing time without permission
Working procedures	An employee who disobeys, or omits to carry out, proper instructions
Documentation and communication	Making misleading or inaccurate statements deliberately or through neglect; altering entries with the intent to misrepresent the true position; destroying documents without sufficient cause, or communicating confidential information or documents to a third party without proper authority
Care of equipment and materials	Removal of property from the hospital; make use of items for unauthorised purposes and cause wilful loss, waste or damage: these include drugs, dressings and other medical items
Alcohol and drugs	Unfit for duty due to drugs or alcohol

There are four stages to disciplinary procedures:

1. *Informal warning*. This is used for minor breaches of discipline. At the interview the offence is explained and the action required to improve standards or conduct discussed. The employee should be informed that any repetition of the offence or failure to improve will result in formal disciplinary action. The informal warning should be confirmed in writing, normally within a week of the interview.
2. *Formal warning*. This should be carried out by the manager in the presence of a management witness, the employee and his or her representative. The employee is informed of the nature of the offence and presented with the

supported evidence. The employee is given the opportunity to explain his/her conduct and to question any witnesses.

If it is decided to progress to a formal warning the employee should be informed of the decision and of any action that is required to improve standards or conduct. This verbal warning is confirmed in writing within the next seven days.

The employee should have the right to appeal against the decision by a request in writing stating the reasons for the appeal. The appeal will normally be held by the manager's senior.

3. *Final warning*. This is used for those situations where there has been a failure to improve or if the misconduct is sufficient to warrant a final warning but not sufficient for an instant dismissal.

   The same procedure as for the Formal Warning is carried out but the employee will be told that if there is any repetition of the offence or similar offences then this will lead to dismissal. Again the employee has the right to appeal.

4. *Dismissal.* This procedure will be implemented if the employee has failed to improve or the offence is repeated. The hearing will normally be carried out by a very senior manager in the presence of a managerial witness along with the employee and his/her representative (if they so choose).

   As for the other Warnings, the employee is given the chance to explain his/her actions and to appeal against the decision. The dismissal will be confirmed in writing.

The main points to note are first to make sure you have all the facts, that the interviews are carried out in the presence of witnesses, that the employee has a right to be represented by a colleague or union representative, that the employee has the right to explain, that the decision should be confirmed in writing and that the employee has the right to appeal. Failure to meet these criteria can complicate the procedure and may make the decision invalid.

Conclusion

The day-to-day management of a department is basically about allowing others to succeed. The manager acts as the conductor of the team, making policy decisions and providing the right managerial atmosphere whereby others can carry out their jobs effectively and efficiently. While staff are encouraged to be part of the decision-making process the final decision is in the hands of the manager. The successful team therefore needs to know the parameters within which they work and the expectations of the manager if motivation is to be maintained and disciplinary action avoided.

References

Aeillo, R. (1983). Employee attitude surveys: impact on corporate decisions. *Public Relations Journal*, **7**, 21.

Confederation of British Industries. (1993). *Too Much Time Out*, London: CBI.

Douglass, L. M. (1988). *The Effective Nurse: Leader and Manager*, 3rd edn. Saint Louis: C. V. Mosby, pp. 95–6.

Drucker, P. F. (1973). *Management: Tasks, Responsibilities, Practices.* New York: Harper and Row, p. 125.

Fayoul H. (1949). *General and Industrial Management.* London: Pitman & Son.

Gibson, J., Ivanovich, J. & Donnelly, A. (1988). *Organisations: Behaviour Structure Processes.* Homewood, IL: Richard D. Irwin.

Hertzberg, F., Mausner, B. & Snyderman, B. (1959). *The Motivation to Work.* New York: John Wiley.

Hunt, R. E. & Rigby, M. K. (1984). Easing the pain of change. *Management Review*, September 1984, 41–5.

Jenks, J. M. & Kelly, J. M. (1990). *Don't Do, Delegate.* London: Kogan Page.

Jung, C. G. (1971). *Psychological Types.* London: Routledge.

Kolb, D. A. (1984). *Experimental Learning: Experience as a Source of Learning and Development.* Englewood Cliffs NJ: Prentice-Hall.

Kurtz, M. E. (1987*a*). Role of the physician as manager. *Physical Medicine and Rehabilitation State of the Art Review*, **1**, 185–96.

Kurtz, M. E. (1987*b*). Leadership styles. *Physical Medicine and Rehabilitation State of the Art Review*, **1**, 197–212.

Levenstein, A. (1984). Feedback improves performance. *Nursing Management.* October, 60–1.

Levey, S. & Loomba, N. P. (1987). Management and overview. *Physical Medicine and Rehabilitation State of the Art Review*, **1**, 177–84.

Maslow, A. H. (1970). *Motivation and Personality.* New York: Harper and Row.

May, A. (1993). Full circle. *Health Service Journal*, **103**, 24–7.

Meerloo J. (1968). In Anderson: What's blocking upward communication. *Personnel Administration*, Jan–Feb: 5.

Mintzberg, H. (1975). The manager's job: Folklore and fact. *Harvard Business Review*, **13**, 49–61.

Nylen, D. W. (1985). Making your business plan and action plan. *Business*, Oct–Dec, 12–16.

Ratcliffe, T. A. & Logson, D. J. (1980). The business planning process : a behavioural perspective. *Management Planning*, March–April, 32–8.

Reddin, W. J. (1969). How to change things. *Executive*, June, 22–26.

Scweiger, D. & Denisis, A. (1991). Communication with employees: a longitudinal field experiment. *Academy of Management Journal*, pp. 101–35.

Seccombe, I. & Buchan, J. (1993). High Anxiety. *Health Service Journal*, **103**, 22–4.

Sims, R. R. (1990). Ensuring competence in health care managers. *Journal of Health Care Quality Assurance*, **3**, 11–13.

Spradley, B. W. (1980). Managing change creatively. *Journal of Nursing Administration*, May, 32–7.

St John, W. D. (1985). You are what you communicate. *Personnel Journal*, October, 40–3.

Tourish, D. (1993). Don't you sometimes wish you were better informed? *Health*

Service Journal, **103**, 28–9.
Welch, L. B. (1979). Planned change in nursing: the theory. *Nursing Clinics of North America*, June, 307–21.
Wilson, M. (1993). No time like the present. *Health Service Journal*, **103**, 15.

8

Research and evaluation in rehabilitation

BARBARA A. WILSON

Introduction

For the worker in the field of rehabilitation the similarities between research and evaluation are likely to be of more interest than the differences. While this chapter aims to describe a wide range of research and methodologies, including the kind of grant-supported research that is conducted by academics and professional researchers, it is also written in the belief that the rehabilitation worker can make a difference to the quality of rehabilitation through self-or unit-directed research that is closely aligned to evaluation. The results of such direct research on the part of workers in the field of rehabilitation can lead to measurable improvements in the rehabilitation of patients in their immediate care. I deliberately avoid stating all patients because, owing to limitations imposed by lack of time, finance and sometimes expertise, much self-or unit-directed research will not be generalisable to other patients. Nevertheless, the kind of direct or 'action' research to be described in parts of this chapter can make an extremely important contribution to our knowledge, given the current situation in which there is as yet no adequate theory of rehabilitation and not much in the way of well funded, large research studies that are generalisable. Until we have a theory that can inform practice we should welcome any form of research that chips away at ignorance in rehabilitation. It is possible, after all, that any umbrella theory will include a place for action research on the part of professional workers.

Self-or unit-directed research that is closely aligned to evaluation is essential for people working in rehabilitation because it provides feedback on the productivity of their work. Without the knowledge provided by such research it would be difficult to assess the effectiveness of practice. Furthermore, such action research, rooted in practice, demands that the researcher looks at other work conducted by professional researchers and academics, thus encouraging the development of a broader theoretical framework on which to base one's work.

This chapter aims to provide an overview of the different kinds of research and methodologies available to academics and professional researchers with the objective of increasing understanding among the professional engaged in the field of rehabilitation. It also discusses a number of ways in which the professional workers can use some of the methodologies to engage in research studies of their own design based on the work of their own particular unit.

Some research will require large numbers of subjects and a research budget while other research can be carried out by the individual practitioner or a small group working within the same unit. The latter form of research does not necessarily require large numbers of subjects, huge amounts of time or expensive financial assistance. It is the kind of research that can be conducted by each and every therapist, teacher or psychologist engaged in the process of maximising the physical, social and psychological functioning of individual people who happen to be disabled by injury or disease.

Questions requiring answers that will inform both immediate and daily practice can be answered by focusing research on a single patient. For example, occupational, physiotherapists or speech therapists working with an individual patient will want to know whether their methods are effective. Is the patient's behaviour changing and, if so, has the change come about by the intervention or treatment on offer or is it simply the result of natural recovery or some other non-specific factor, such as increased attention or general stimulation? In much of the research I describe in this chapter it is possible, by the use of baselines, single case experimental designs and other observational procedures, to tease out the effects of natural recovery and general stimulation so that the effects of any particular intervention can be isolated and thus evaluated (Wilson, 1987*b*).

Although time is a factor for busy therapists to consider, it is worth reminding ourselves that the hours spent on unevaluated work that may in fact be of little or no benefit to a patient is a *waste* of time, and that research may inform us how to use our time more efficiently. Research should not be regarded as something extra to be added on to work but should rather be accepted as an essential part of clinical practice. Therapists who have a few minutes to write notes about patients and prepare for an individual patient's session (or group session) will be able to find time to evaluate the effects of their treatment. When therapy sessions are designed to treat patients *and* answer questions about the effectiveness of that treatment then research is already underway. Simply put, research is a procedure that enables us to answer questions. Different methods must be employed to answer different questions and there is no single or absolute way to conduct research into rehabilitation. Research will be governed by the patients we treat, the questions we ask, the facilities available, the time we *make* available, any reading round a subject we can manage (particularly from current professional and academic journals), and of course considerations of an ethical nature.

Asking questions

Asking the right question in an investigation is of paramount importance. If the question is appropriate, timely, relevant and, most importantly, specific to the particular patient or patients and situation being examined then we might obtain some useful answers. It is of little use posing questions that cannot be answered. 'Does rehabilitation work?' or 'Is occupational therapy worthwhile?' for example, are not good questions because they are too broad to answer as they stand. At whatever level such questions are asked, whether it be at a tea party or in politics, they remain unanswerable, so there is no point in starting with such questions in research. Indeed, questions of this nature may be used politically because there are no ready answers! A much better question would be something like: 'Do brain-injured people with problem solving deficits improve their scores on neuropsychological tests following specific problem solving training?' (Von Cramon *et al.*, 1991).

Suitable questions for individual patients might include: 'Is visual imagery better than rote rehearsal for teaching names to Mrs. Smith?' or 'Does this child with cerebral palsy exercise better when given feedback from a computer than when given feedback from a physiotherapist?' (Mackey, 1989).

Types of research

Broadly defined, research can be described as '. . . trained observation and inquiry directed on any department of knowledge with a view to the discovery of new information' (Webster's Dictionary, 1975 : 1233). The three main ways in which such enquiry can be conducted are through surveys, observations and experiments. Each is described below.

Surveys

See Bryant & Machin Chapter 9 for further discussion of surveys. Drummond (1990) suggests there are five reasons for choosing to conduct surveys.

To identify a problem in a preliminary study

Wilkinson *et al.*, (1989), for example, surveyed the numbers of severely head injured (SHI) people in the Southampton Heath District to identify their needs. They found that over 50% of those identified had multiple impairments including those that could be described as physical, cognitive and behavioural. The authors recommended prospective outcome studies at a district level, as less than 10% of those predicted to have disability following SHI were identified.

To establish the size and extent of a problem

Levin *et al.*, (1991), for example, surveyed 650 closed head injury patients to determine the numbers discharged in a persistent vegetative state (PVS). They found there were 84 (14%) such patients.

To provide a baseline so that the effects of a subsequent intervention programme can be monitored

For example, Rusk *et al.*, (1966) surveyed 127 head-injured patients and found 40 pressure sores, 200 joint contractures and 30 frozen shoulders. This situation would now be very uncommon in Western Europe and North America because of the services that are now provided for head-injured people (Greenwood & McMillan, 1996).

To evaluate treatment when a randomised control trial (see Bryant & Machin Chapter 9) is not possible

It is sometimes unethical or impractical to withhold treatment, in which case the survey method may be the best alternative. Wood *et al.*, (1993), for example, describe a sensory regulation method for managing patients in coma. The unit in which the patients were treated was designed to maximise sensory regulation, making use of a control group virtually impossible. To evaluate the success of their programme Wood *et al.* compared their patients with those in the Traumatic Coma Data Bank Study (Levin *et al.*, 1991). The survey conducted by Levin and his colleagues showed that 52% of the PVS subjects had recovered consciousness after one year. In contrast, 93% of those on a sensory regulation programme had recovered consciousness at a much earlier stage. There are of course problems in using this kind of comparison as the two sample groups may differ in other ways.

To provide data for audit purposes

Wilson (1981), for example, carried out a survey of patients referred to the clinical psychology department during a nine month interval at a rehabilitation centre to determine the reasons for referral, the nature of the treatment given and the success or otherwise of each treatment.

The practical problems of subject selection, outcome measures, design and so forth faced by those conducting surveys are essentially no different from those carrying out observations or experiments, and these matters will be discussed later in this chapter.

Observations

Observations are defined as 'the acute watching and noting of phenomena as they occur in nature with regard to cause and effect or mutual relations' (*Concise Oxford Dictionary*, 1990: 818). They can be carried out to describe phenomena with a view to generating an hypothesis, or to support or disprove an hypothesis. In addition, they can be helpful in evaluating the effects of treatment procedures. Observational procedures may also be conducted in simulated settings by participant or independent observers.

Naturalistic settings

Rehabilitation is partly concerned with returning people to their own social and vocational environments, so it is often important to observe how a subject behaves or manages in those environments. Observations would need to be conducted when a subject is at home, at work, on the ward or in other places where he or she may spend time. Haynes (1978) gives three reasons why natural observations are important. Firstly, they often reveal behaviour that cannot be reported in interviews, questionnaires, checklists or tests. Secondly, they avoid interference, often inherent in many assessment procedures. Thirdly, they may be less subject to bias than other measures. Hammond (1987), for example, videotaped rheumatoid arthritic subjects engaged in two domestic tasks (making a cup of tea and preparing a snack). She did this before and after the subjects joined a group to learn about joint protection principles. A colleague scored the videotapes 'blind', i.e. she did not know which of the tapes were from before or after the group treatment. There was no significant difference in the behaviour of the subjects regarding joint protection after attending the group sessions that had lasted for two hours each week over a period of six weeks. Nevertheless, on a questionnaire the subjects *thought* they had changed their behaviour and were thereby protecting their joints.

Hammond's study is a good example of the use of observations to assess the effect of a particular treatment regimen. As a consequence of her evaluation it will now be possible to make testable predictions as to how to improve the learning of joint protection principles for people with rheumatoid arthritis.

For example, it will be worthwhile hypothesising that improvement will follow if real life tasks are incorporated into treatment sessions, or if generalisation of the tasks from hospital to home are taught, or if people are in fact *not* taught in groups but taught individually. Whatever the results of such further investigations, their long-term effect on therapeutic practice is likely to be beneficial, possibly leading to a concentration of workable treatments, thus saving time and effort by avoiding less successful programmes. Such changes may also bring about a significant improvement in the subjects' attitude towards joint protection.

Another example of observation in natural settings, aimed at assessing the behaviour of patients with subtle planning and organisational problems, was that by Shallice & Burgess (1991). They asked patients to go to a shopping centre to buy a number of items and find out certain things (such as checking a newspaper to find the coldest place in the UK the day before) while following certain rules. The patients, who all scored at the normal level on standardised tests aimed at testing their particular problems, had great difficulty in completing real life tasks whereas control subjects did not.

Some behaviours are impractical to observe in the natural environment. For example, although return to work on the part of certain subjects may be prevented by their inability to cope with complex situations, it remains very difficult to observe these subjects *in situ*. In such cases it is likely to be more appropriate to simulate the situations.

Simulated settings

Observations in simulated settings are often less time consuming, particularly when the behaviour being observed is infrequent in everyday life, or when the subject can be seen only in a limited range of situations. Simulated settings can be subdivided into analogue and role play. Occupational therapists use analogue situations regularly. For example, many occupational therapy departments have a mock flat or apartment to observe whether patients have the skills required for activities of daily living (ADL). They may also have a workshop or mock office to test vocational skills. The Shallice & Burgess task in the shopping precinct could perhaps be adapted to a rehabilitation centre or occupational therapy department. This would certainly be possible in the USA where some hospitals have an analogue miniature town with a shop, an office, a theatre, a bus and so forth.

Role playing can be employed to evaluate change over time or before and after treatment. This method is widely used in social skills training (Spence, 1980) when some form of social interaction is taking place, and has also played a part in the treatment of head-injured people (Godfrey & Knight, 1989).

Evans & Wilson (1992) found role playing helpful in their memory group for brain-injured people. Sometimes patients are asked to role play how they would explain to others the nature of their problems. On other occasions they might be asked to role play a receptionist at their place of work, taking telephone messages. One of the ways to evaluate the effectiveness of a patient group would be to see if there is any improvement in the members' ability to perform certain tasks over time. To perform such observational assessment successfully, certain measures would have to be taken to ensure that any changes were not simply the result of recovery. A control group might be included, or several baselines could be taken to demonstrate the stability of the behaviour being observed. It must be recognised, however, that it is hazardous assuming that behaviour observed in an analogue or role play situation will necessarily be the same when observed in a real life setting.

A participant in a naturally-occurring situation, such as a relative at home, an employer at work, or a nurse on a ward could take on the role of observer. Sometimes independent observers can be brought in to the situation and might be drawn from students or visitors to the unit. The main advantage of having a participant observer is that the familiarity that has been built up between the observer and the patient(s) will encourage more natural behaviour. The main disadvantage of participant observation is that the observer may be too busy in the participant role to be able to observe sufficiently carefully.

Independent observers have more time to observe in detail but their very presence might affect the behaviours being observed. Sometimes video cameras have been employed to reduce this problem, as happened in a direct observational study to assess patients in and emerging from coma (Horn *et al.*, 1993). It is unlikely that filming affected the behaviour of the patient, even if staff involved found it difficult to act naturally.

The kind of rehabilitation questions that might be appropriate for research involving observational procedures are illustrated by the following two examples: 'What is the nature and frequency of accidents sustained by right hemisphere stroke patients in a rehabilitation ward over the course of a month?' 'Is the nature and frequency of accidents on a rehabilitation ward different for right and left hemisphere stroke patients?' For those interested in pursuing similar kinds of questions Carr (1991) provides some useful guidelines.

Experiments

An experiment is a test or trial set up to test a hypothesis or demonstrate a fact. If the task is, for example, to find out whether people learn a new motor skill better with continuous (massed) practice or with distributed (spaced) practice, it would be possible to design an experiment to answer the question. Such an experiment was in fact conducted as long ago as 1930 by Lorge. He was interested in the learning of a mirror tracing task, a difficult operation in which the subject is required to trace a pattern (for example, a star) while only being able to see the pattern and his or her hand through a mirror. Lorge studied three groups, one of which was given 20 consecutive trials with no break between them, the second was also given 20 trials but had a one minute interval between each trial, and the third was given one trial each day for a period of 20 days. The outcome measure was the length of time required to trace the pattern, the shorter the time the better the performance. Subjects who had the 20 trials without any rest performed worst, while subjects who had one minute intervals scored second. The best performers were those in the group who had a 24 hour rest between trials.

Another study involving alternative ways of teaching postmen to type (Baddeley & Longman, 1978) also showed that spaced or distributed practice leads to faster learning. Both these experiments are of considerable relevance to rehabilitation yet their findings are virtually unknown by most therapists.

Although Lorge's investigation involved three groups of subjects, experiments can be conducted with any number of groups and also with individuals. We can classify experiments into group studies or single case experimental designs.

Group studies

Designs

The majority of group studies probably use a two group design although they can be conducted with any number of groups including just one. Some care is needed with one group designs because it is very difficult to assess whether any changes that have taken place have been caused by interventions which have been built into the research or whether they have been caused by some other influence. For example, any subjects in a single group who may have improved in some way or other over a period of time may have done so because of a particular treatment or because of some other factor outside the research design, such as natural recovery or practice effect. A solution to this problem might be to reassess several times before introducing the treatment thus ensuring that performance was stable prior to treatment. The main difficulty here is that although it is a device used frequently and successfully in single subject designs, it is somewhat impractical to make multiple baselines on a group of subjects.

A single group (or within subjects) design is appropriate when the purpose is to compare one group of subjects under two or more conditions, such as different treatments or programmes. Wilson (1989), for example, wanted to know which of four presentation methods was best for enabling health service professionals to remember information about patients. Each subject in the group was required to listen to tape recorded summaries of four health-related problems. Each summary was presented in one of four ways. The order of presentation was counterbalanced across subjects. Following a distracter task, the subjects were asked to write down as much as they could remember. The written responses were scored 'blind', i.e. by other subjects who did not know whose paper they were marking. Simplifying and categorising the information resulted in superior recall to other methods. Similar designs could be employed in a number of rehabilitation situations.

An alternative is to use a two group design to evaluate treatment efficacy. A typical design involves an experimental and a control group, one of which is exposed to treatment and the other is not. Assessments are taken before and after treatment. Care must be taken to ensure that the only difference in the circumstances of the two groups is indeed the application of the treatment being evaluated, otherwise you might get results that do not truly apply to the treatment itself. For example, if the control group receives no attention whatsoever, the treatment group might respond to the extra attention rather than to the treatment itself. The answer is to ensure that the control group receives a similar amount of attention, although not the treatment being evaluated. It is also possible to have two control groups if circumstances permit, one of which would be a 'no treatment' control and the other would be a 'placebo' control. This would enable a researcher to look at the effects of treatment compared with attention and with no treatment.

The number of groups can be expanded if necessary and if appropriate. Suppose, for example, the aim is to compare the effects of a symmetrical approach to the treatment of hemiplegia with a non-symmetrical approach. It is possible to have four groups distinguished in the following manner:

Group 1 symmetrical treatment
Group 2 non-symmetrical treatment
Group 3 placebo control (e.g. relaxation training)
Group 4 no treatment control (on waiting list).

A variation on the above is to employ a 2x2 (or 3x3 or some other variant of this) design. The purpose might be to consider two different kinds of treatment with two different levels, styles or variations. For example, as a treatment for unilateral visual neglect, it would be useful to know whether training in scanning is better than training in the use of an anchor point (Weinberg *et al.*, 1979). Additionally, it could be asked whether training with feedback made any difference. Thus the design could be as shown in Figure 8.1.

In some cases it may seem unethical or indeed impossible to withhold treatment even though such an omission may be the only effective way to evaluate the treatment's usefulness. In such circumstances it might be worth considering a cross-over design whereby treatment is given to all subjects but at different time intervals. Wilson & Moffat (1992) describe the use of a cross-over design in the evaluation of a memory group. All patients at a rehabilitation centre were expected to attend a group session each afternoon, the memory-impaired patients duly attending the memory group session organised by the clinical psychology department. In these circumstances it would have been very difficult to withhold treatment for certain patients. Instead, the first cohort of patients attended the daily memory group for three weeks and then attended a daily problem-solving group for the next three weeks. The second cohort attended the problem-solving group for the first three weeks and then switched to the memory group. This was repeated for cohorts three and four so that everybody in the four cohorts received memory group training for some of the time. The problem solving group thus acted as a control. While this method has the advantage of ensuring that all patients receive treatment, it cannot allow comparisons on long-term outcome of treatment with no treatment.

Randomised controlled trials

(See Bryant & Machin, chapter 9 for further discussion of randomised control trials (RCTs). An RCT requires that subjects are randomly allocated to the treatment (experimental) or control condition along the lines discussed by Bryant & Machin (Chapter 9). The rationale of RCTs is that individual differences are expected between subjects, the intention being to spread the differences out fairly across the groups.

RCTs are an obvious and important choice for seeking answers to certain questions. In many drug studies one group of subjects is randomly allocated to the drug in question and the other group to a placebo. This design is applicable to investigations where some factor is introduced, or is already present, and is likely to bring about changes in subjects. For example, an RCT could be employed to investigate the effects of a new surgical procedure, or to determine which of a number of background noise levels causes most disruption to learning.

Although many scientists and researchers regard RCTs as the 'gold standard' for testing treatments in clinical medicine, it should be noted that they are not always necessary or indeed appropriate in the field of rehabilitation. As

	With feedback	Without feedback
Scanning training	Group 1	Group 2
Training in the use of an anchor point	Group 3	Group 4

Figure 8.1. A 2 × 2 Design.

Andrews (1991:5) reminds us, the RCT 'is a tool to be used, not a god to be worshipped'. He argues that the RCT is an excellent tool in research where 'design is simple, where marked changes are expected, where the factors involved are relatively specific and where the number of additional variables likely to affect the outcome is few and can be expected to be balanced out by the randomisation procedure'.

Unfortunately most rehabilitation research is more complex and randomisation may not always be possible. We saw earlier how in one centre designed to provide sensory regulation to comatose patients (Wood *et al*., 1993) it would have been impossible to randomly allocate to a no treatment or different treatment regimen as the staff and the environment would not have been able to accommodate this.

Furthermore it is not particularly sensible to allocate subjects to rehabilitation versus no rehabilitation, or to treatment versus no treatment without specifying more precisely the nature of the rehabilitation or treatment. Some studies (e.g. Cope *et al*., 1991) have asked if patients attending rehabilitation centres do better than those who do not. As we have discussed above, this does not help us understand which aspect of rehabilitation results in any change. Is it general stimulation or greater encouragement or something specific to the therapy itself that is responsible?

We can make the questions more clear cut by specifying (a) the patients, (b) their problems, (c) the strategies employed, and (d) the circumstances in which rehabilitation is offered. When questions have been delineated in this way it is safe to assume that RCTs can be carried out.

Von Cramon *et al*. (1991), for example, showed how this could be carried out in treating brain-injured patients. Subjects had difficulties with planning, organisation and problem solving as measured by tests, observations and rating scales. They were alternately allocated to specific problem solving training (PST) or to memory training (MT). The procedures used were specified and those in the PST group benefited to a significantly greater degrees than those in the MT group, as measured by post-test assessment. Berg *et al*. (1991) also used a RCT design to evaluate the effects of memory rehabilitation. RCTs are possible in rehabilitation but they need to be carefully thought out and are not the only way of evaluating effectiveness.

Many health economists, managers, scientists and others believe there is only one way to truly evaluate the effectiveness of intervention and that is through the use of a double-blind RCT, i.e. when neither the person receiving nor the person giving treatment knows what the treatment is. This would be possible in a drug study where both the experimental and placebo drugs can be made to look alike with an independent person keeping a record of who is receiving what, but would be impossible to achieve for many rehabilitation procedures. Therapists must know what therapy they are giving, and patients are of course able to observe differences in the treatment they and others receive.

Nevertheless a single-blind trial (as described above by Hammond, 1987) is usually desirable in rehabilitation studies. In other words, an independent assessor who does not know which subjects have been seen under what conditions is preferable to an assessor involved with the patient who may (albeit unconsciously) desire a particular outcome.

Practical considerations for group designs

Subjects

It must be clear from the outset as to which subjects will be included in any particular study. This may sound obvious but the inclusion and exclusion criteria must be specified nevertheless. If, for example, stroke patients are to be included then it should be specified (a) whether right or left hemisphere strokes or both are to be included, (b) whether all kinds of stroke or only those with subarachnoid haemorrhage or intracerebral haemorrhage or infarction are to be included, (c) whether anyone who has had a previous stroke will be excluded, and (d) whether upper and lower age limits will be imposed, and so forth.

Furthermore, the number of subjects required for the study and the number expected to be enlisted during the course of the study must be assessed with a reasonable degree of accuracy. As a general rule, I would suggest that initial numbers, based on early predictions, can be halved. It is fairly safe to assume that many of the subjects thought to be available to the researcher will disappear once research begins. The numbers required for any particular trial will depend on several things that are covered by Bryant & Machin (Chapter 9). It is worth remembering, however, that a statistician will probably advise a fairly large number of subjects whereas a research psychologist will probably suggest that adequate results can be obtained from a much smaller sample. A useful and encouraging book to have available is *Experimental Psychology: a Small-*N *Approach* (Robinson & Foster, 1979).

The source of the subjects will also need to be considered. Dependence on just one source should be avoided as several things, such as illness or departure of a therapist with access to a particular group of patients, can lead to that single source 'drying up'.

Consideration must be given to possible 'drop-outs' or refusers that may be encountered as research progresses. If nearly all drop-outs are from one of the conditions, or if over half of the subjects drop out or refuse then a study will be very seriously weakened. There are statistical procedures to cope with some missing data but a statistician will need to be consulted about this, and it should be remembered that statistics are only as good as the data and research design allow. As far as possible it will need to be ascertained whether the drop-outs are similar to those subjects who do not drop out, and whether there are differences in the drop-outs from different groups.

Allocation to groups

Is allocation to be random, pseudo random by matching, or by some other procedure? If allocation is strictly random then it will be just as well to flip a coin or use a table of random numbers to determine subject allocation to groups. Such methods can lead to unequal numbers in each group, which in turn can cause problems when analysing results where statistical procedures require equal numbers in each group.

If there is a sufficiently large group of subjects, say 100 or more, then randomisation will probably balance out more or less evenly over time, but if the number of subjects is 20 or less, random allocation could unbalance an experiment to the extent that there could be 15 in one group and five in another.

Another potential problem is that subjects may know each other and could talk to each other about the study. In some circumstances this could confound the effects of treatment. For example, suppose we wanted to know if payment of £10 was better than payment of £1 for cooperation with an exercise regimen; then subjects who knew they were receiving a lower rate than their friends could get angry and refuse to cooperate. We would not then know the uncontaminated effects of the lower rate.

The problem of unequal numbers may be solved by alternate allocation provided this does not in itself cause bias (e.g. if alternate patients come from Dr X and Dr Y, the two doctors could have different referral criteria). Cohort or block matching can also be considered, i.e. the experiment can be run in a series of cohorts or blocks. The memory group experiment described above (Wilson & Moffat, 1992) is an example of this. Each group required five or six people and only one group could run at any one time, so the first cohort began with the memory group and the second with the problem-solving group.

Another procedure is to use matched groups whereby all subjects are assessed on measures assumed to be relevant, such as age, sex, IQ, socio economic class, etc., and then allocated to ensure all groups are approximately equal on these measures. The problem with this method is that the groups may differ in other ways (such as motivation or previous exposure to rehabilitation) that have not been measured but which might affect the results. As with all experiments we should use common sense to eliminate as much bias as possible.

Having allocated subjects it may be necessary to check that there are approximately equal numbers and that groups are similar in ways considered by the researcher to be important, and that there are no obvious biases. For example, if group 1 one has 90% men and group 2 has 90% women, or most people in one group are on anticonvulsants and those in the other group are not, it will be necessary to consider whether it is legitimate to balance out these biases through a pseudo random procedure.

Definition of treatment/therapy/rehabilitation/intervention

When investigating or evaluating some aspect of therapy it will be necessary to specify what is meant by this. Questions to be answered include: what procedures are being used, how frequently and for how long? what instructions will be given to the subjects? will it be possible to correct for missing data?

Outcome measures

How is success or improvement to be measured? Will this be achieved through a questionnaire, rating scale, testing or direct observation? Whichever method is used, we may need to consider incorporating an operational definition of success, e.g. 'success means an increase in the test score of 3 or more points', or 'means the subject can walk across the gym at least 10 seconds faster'.

Finally, who is going to evaluate or assess the outcome? Will the subjects themselves decide whether improvement has occurred? This is how some pain relief treatments are assessed and this method might be appropriate for some rehabilitation questions. For example, 'Does counselling result in less depression?' Will care staff or relatives do the assessment, or is an 'expert' assessor such as a neuropsychologist required to see if there has been any change in neuropsychological test scores? Will the assessor need to be trained to evaluate properly? For example, for evaluating change in behaviour following coma stimulation it might be necessary to teach somebody how to observe and record subtle changes that could be missed by the untrained eye.

There are no right and wrong answers to these questions. Experimenters need common sense to reduce or overcome bias and to take into account alternative explanations for their results such as spontaneous recovery or changes over time through maturation or repeated practice.

Summary of the main characteristics of group studies (adapted from Robinson & Foster, 1979)

1. Group studies use many subjects. It is recognised that each subject is unique and the experimental design makes allowances for the differences between subjects.
2. Randomisation is used to share out or spread these differences as equally as possible between groups.
3. Control groups are often used as part of the randomisation process.
4. Statistics are an important part of the analysis of the results. They help the experimenter to decide whether the differences result from individual variations or the variable being tested.
5. As a rule only one or two measures are taken from each subject.
6. Data are usually analysed at the end of the experiment to avoid or reduce experimenter bias.

Limitations of group studies

Wanting to know how many subjects have benefited from a particular treatment is a question applicable to groups, the results apply to groups and we would use a group design to answer the question. We cannot, however, assume that an individual patient will benefit from the same treatment given to those in the group study. The individual might be different from the subjects included in the group study, perhaps having milder or more severe problems, or additional problems. If 99% of subjects in the group study benefited and our individual patient is very similar to those subjects in the group study, then there is a good chance our patient will also respond. In practice, however, the situation is typically less clear cut. Group studies are usually concerned with average performances so individual differences are masked. Ten subjects each scoring 10 points would give an average score of 10, but so would ten subjects with scores of 4, 4, 6, 6, 10, 10, 12, 12, 18 and 18. Suppose the average score for a control group was 4, there would be a statistically significant difference between the two groups, yet two people in the experimental group scored the same as the average control subject. How do we know our individual patient is not like one of these two?

Thus group studies may confuse clinical and statistical significance. A statistical difference does not mean every individual does better, nor does it mean that the difference is clinically important or relevant. Suppose we give biofeedback to teach control of a shoulder muscle in a patient with hemiplegia, and suppose biofeedback proves to be statistically superior to a traditional physiotherapy exercise. If the patient is still unable to use her arm, the result will not be clinically significant.

To take another example, suppose we know that a particular cognitive test is failed by 95% of people with Alzheimer's disease and 60% of people with multi-infarct dementia. This is likely to be a statistically significant difference, i.e. not due to chance, but in clinical practice we cannot use the test to diagnose Alzheimer's disease or multi-infarct dementia because an individual subject who fails the test could have either one of these conditions or even another.

A further problem with some group studies is that it is easy to confuse the *numbers* of people changing with the *amount* of change. For example, we may find that there is a 75% change in the treatment group compared with a 35% change in the control group. Does this mean 75% of the treatment subjects improved or that each improved by 75%? We are rarely told how many individuals improved, how many stayed the same and how many became worse.

Group studies also cause problems if we are working with someone with a rare syndrome, such as visual object agnosia, where it would be difficult to get together a group of subjects to evaluate treatment for object recognition disorders.

Certain theoretical questions are also difficult to answer with group studies. In theoretical studies of memory, for example, one of the sources of evidence to support the distinction between short-term and long-term memory comes from brain-damaged patients. Most memory-impaired people have damage to the long-term or delayed memory system with relatively normal short-term or immediate memory. To demonstrate that there really are two distinct systems it was necessary to find patients with impaired immediate memory functioning together with normal delayed memory. Although rare, such patients do exist (Vallar & Shallice, 1990). In large group studies of memory-impaired people such double dissociations would have been missed.

Luria (1981) describes a soldier who received a gunshot wound many years earlier. The text is an account of the soldier's life and struggle in overcoming his many problems. Such detailed individual studies are valuable in helping us to understand aspects of recovery and compensation but would be almost impossible to carry out in large groups.

Finally, group studies are of limited value in evaluating an individual's response to treatment. They do not allow us to see the *pattern* of change over time, they do not make allowances for adjustment during the therapy process and they do not allow us to tailor our treatment to the individual patient. Yet every good therapist will be looking for a pattern of change, e.g. is the patient slow to learn initially but then learns how to learn and so speeds up? A good therapist will also make adjustments as necessary: does the patient do better if instructions for exercises are written down or if guided through a sequence of exercises first, or if allowed to rest for a few minutes between exercises? So even if the treatment of choice is a particular exercise regimen, this would be tailored to the individual patient's needs.

Single case experimental designs avoid many of the problems inherent in group studies. They are often the method of choice when trying to evaluate an individual's progress in rehabilitation. They are perfectly respectable scientific research methods (Hersen & Barlow, 1982; Kazdin, 1982; Gianutsos & Gianutsos, 1987) and provide complementary information to group studies. Neither is better or worse; rather it is a question of 'horses for courses'. Large group studies need many people because of individual variations that need to be shared out. Single case and small group studies do not have to be so concerned with these individual differences. Instead, each subject is monitored for a period of time and acts as his or her own control. Secondary or non-specific variables can be controlled for during the baseline period. Baselines then are used instead of control groups.

Types of single case experimental design

ABAB (and variations on this) or reversal designs

Among the simplest designs are the ABAB designs, where A = Baseline and B = Treatment. Mackey (1989) used an ABA design where following a baseline period (A) children with cerebral palsy were given computer feedback on their spasticity inhibiting exercises (B). Exercising improved. They then returned to the baseline condition (A) to see if it really was the computer feedback that helped. Each of six children in the study improved during computer feedback and deteriorated when this was withdrawn. This suggests that the treatment rather than maturation or attention was responsible for the improvement. These designs are also called reversal designs because of the reversal to baseline conditions.

There are a number of variations to the basic design. Alderman & Ward (1991), for example, implemented an ABACACD design with a brain-damaged women exhibiting severe behaviour problems. As always A is the baseline, B refers to the first treatment, C the second treatment and CD a combination of the second treatment and a further treatment.

Wilson (1994) also describes an ABAC design to evaluate a remedial reading programme in a man who became alexic, i.e. completely unable to read, following a gunshot wound to his brain. Although these designs are simple, they are limited in rehabilitation for three main reasons. Firstly, it is often impossible to revert to baseline conditions. If the patient has learned to do something such as walk or read or shave during the B phase then he or she cannot 'unlearn' this. Secondly, it may not be ethical to revert to baseline conditions, as would be the case if the patient is a self-injurer. Thirdly, it is not always practical to revert to baseline conditions. If you have managed to reduce a severe behaviour problem, the other staff may be very unwilling to revert to the earlier state of affairs. Nevertheless, it is worth having this design in your repertoire for those occasions when it is appropriate.

Multiple baseline designs

These are probably more useful evaluative procedures in rehabilitation as they are more adaptable to a range of problems and situations. The major characteristic of these designs is that the introduction of treatment is staggered.

Multiple baseline across behaviours (or problems) design

In this design several problems or parts of a problem are selected for treatment. Baselines are taken on all, but only one behaviour or problem is treated at any one time. Treatment for the remaining problems is staggered. For example, if we wanted to improve three different exercises (long sitting, bridging and trunk rotation) in a patient who was very unwilling to exercise, we could take baselines (e.g. the number of seconds the patient will engage in these exercises). In stage 2 we could 'treat' one exercise, for example by telling the patient how well she did the day before, asking her to manage a few seconds more today, and if she succeeds allowing her to rest or to do an activity she enjoys. We would then keep records (baselines) on the remaining exercises but not 'treat' these. Having performed this daily for a few days, we might move on to stage 3 where we begin 'treating' a second exercise, so that now we are treating two in the same way and keeping baselines on the third exercise. Eventually we can also treat this one. Wilson & Powell (1987) report an example of a treatment very similar to this.

If improvement results from natural recovery of non-specific factors then it will not occur consistently with the introduction of treatment. If the treatment is responsible, then change should occur only after the introduction of the treatment phase.

Multiple baseline across behaviours designs have also been used in the rehabilitation of memory and reading problems (Wilson, 1987*a*) and attention difficulties (Gray & Robertson, 1989).

Multiple baseline across settings designs

Here only one problem is tackled but the effects of treatment are investigated in one setting at a time so once again treatment is staggered to tease out the effects of natural recovery or non-specific factors. Suppose we wanted to teach a patient to use an electronic memory aid. We might take baselines on the extent of its use in occupational therapy, woodwork, lunch and tea breaks and at home. If the aid were used very little, we could teach its use in occupational therapy first, continue taking baselines in the other settings but not encourage or teach its use there. As with multiple baseline across behaviours design, we could then teach its use in one other setting at a time. This design was used by Carr & Wilson (1983) to teach a man with a spinal injury to lift from his wheelchair in four different settings.

Multiple baseline across subjects design

This design can be used when you use a small group of subjects and wish to evaluate a particular technique. Wilson (1987*a*) looked at a visual imagery technique for learning people's names. Four memory-impaired men (three with stroke and one with a cerebral tumour) were included in the study. The first subject started treatment following two baseline sessions, the second following four baselines, the third following six and the fourth following eight baselines. Thus, once again, treatment was staggered and again each man only improved once the visual imagery technique has been introduced.

Other single case designs

The three multiple baseline designs can be applied to a wide range of patients and problems, and are valuable tools for monitoring intervention strategies. Other single case designs include alternating treatment designs where two or more treatment strategies are employed in the same treatment session. Wilson (1994) for example compared four different remedial reading strategies in each session for a letter-by-letter reader. Three of the four worked equally well and one made him slower. Embedded designs are another variation. Here reversal and multiple baseline designs are used together (Wong & Liberman, 1981).

Finally, one can compare two or more treatments directly within a single subject design just as one would in a group study. Instead of two groups of subjects one could compare two procedures on a number of occasions. Wilson (1987*b*) for example compared two methods for improving verbal recall in a brain-injured subject with a severe amnesia. These methods were PQRST (Preview, Question, Read, State and Test) and Rehearsal. Sixteen passages were selected and randomly allocated to one of two conditions (eight in each). The subject was seen on six occasions and each time was asked to work through two passages. For one he followed the PQRST strategy and for the other he used Rehearsal, i.e. he went over the passage four times. The order of presentation was counterbalanced and the same amount of time was spent on each passage. Comparisons were made between the amount recalled on each occasion under each condition. PQRST proved to be superior to rehearsal for delayed recall but there was no difference between the two for immediate recall.

Statistics in single case designs

Statistics are less often used in single case designs than in group studies. Indeed, some people question whether they should be used at all. They argue that if statistics are needed to determine whether intervention is effective then there is little chance of the results having clinical significance. Effective intervention will be immediately obvious without the need for statistics. An example would be from Wilson (1987*a*, Chapter 6, experiment 1). A memory-impaired patient was unable to learn names prior to using visual imagery but once a drawing was provided for each name, he learned them. The results were very clear cut without the need for statistics.

There are occasions, however, when statistics are useful in single case designs. If, for example, comparing two or more treatments both of which appear to have some effect but the results are not 'all or none', then statistics can determine whether one is significantly superior to the other. The PQRST experiment described above was just such an example. Although the patient scored better on the PQRST, there was a considerable variation among the results and it was not as clear cut as we had hoped, so a statistical analysis was used.

The test used in this case was a Wilcoxon matched pairs, signed ranks test. This is a non parametric test often used in small group designs or in studies where one would not expect a normal distribution. This and other non parametric tests such as the sign test and the chi-square test are useful tools for the researcher using single case experimental designs. Alderman & Ward (1991) used a non parametric analysis of variance, a Kruskal–Wallis test, to analyse their ABACACD design. Siegal (1956) and Edgington (1982) discuss non parametric tests in more detail.

Other tests that are appropriate for single case studies include time-series analyses (Tryon, 1982). The essence of time series analyses is a periodic measure of an individual prior to and following the introduction of an experimental change. Analysis is concerned with whether the rate of change is different before and after the experimental intervention.

Hersen & Barlow (1982) and Kazdin (1982) both provide more detailed discussion of the use of statistics in single case experimental research.

Despite the kudos attached to statistics, they are, even when applied to large group studies, only one of several pieces of evidence to evaluate the effectiveness of treatment. Robinson & Foster (1979: 129), in their excellent book on small groups, concluded that 'Statistical tests are given a much greater role than they deserve in determining the effects of an independent variable'.

Generalisability of results

One criticism that is often made about single case and small group studies is that one cannot generalise from the findings, i.e. the findings only apply to the single subject. This is not entirely true. Firstly, it is incorrect to assume that generalisation can only occur if large numbers of subjects have been used in a study. This may happen but it does not always happen and it is certainly not the only way to achieve generalisation (Sidman, 1960; Robinson & Foster, 1979; Gianutsos & Gianutsos, 1987; and many others).

In most large *N* experiments attempts are made to select subjects who fulfil certain criteria, e.g. they have had a unilateral left hemisphere stroke, are aged between 50 and 65 years, score above or below certain points on particular tests of IQ and language, and so on. The results of the study with these patients might then be assumed to generalise to other left hemisphere stroke patients. This might be true, but these patients would have to be people with the same characteristics as those included in the study. We cannot assume that the results will apply to people who had more than one stroke, who were older or younger, or had other conditions along with the stroke, such as a previous head injury or a history of alcohol abuse. The list is virtually endless. Even for those people who do have all the characteristics present in the experimental subjects, the results have been averaged out over a large group so that the findings are not typical of any single individual, yet it is to individuals we wish to generalise.

Secondly, it is incorrect to assume we cannot generalise from individual subjects to others. One of the earliest studies in neuropsychology (Broca, 1861) was of a single subject known as 'Tan', so called because this was the only 'word' he could utter. On postmortem, he was found to have a lesion in the anterior section of the left hemisphere. This type of language deficit became known as Broca's aphasia. Numerous people with lesions in this area have developed a language disturbance similar to that originally described by Broca. There are many other examples that could be described. In 1920 Watson & Rayner used a single subject, a young boy called Albert, to condition fear to a harmless stimulus. The results have proved to stand up to generalisation and have been used to explain conditioning to other stimuli. Indeed, experimental psychology began with in-depth investigations of individual subjects. Wundt *et al.* and others used themselves and a few other individuals as subjects (Hergenhan,1992) and their findings are still applicable today.

Hersen and Barlow (1982: 57) point out that 'To increase the base for generalisation from a single case experiment, one simply repeats the same experiment several times on similar patients, thereby providing the clinician with results from a number of patients'.

Gianutsos & Gianutsos (1987) go even further and argue that generalisability can be directly addressed only in single case designs. Limits of generalisation can be established through systematic replication with controlled changes in variables across which generalisation might be expected.

As well as generalisation from one subject (or one group of subjects) to another, one can consider generalisation from one setting to another, from one behaviour to another, or even from one therapist to another. These applications, however, are usually ignored in large *N* and single case designs. It is probably true to say that evaluation of the extent to which they occur or ways in which generalisation can be improved will probably be easier to measure in single case than in large group studies.

Advice on planning your own research project

Before you start your project ask yourself *why* you are interested in the topic or question. Be clear in your mind as to what question it is you want an answer. Once the question is correct it will be easier to select an appropriate design. You may want to state a hypothesis (a testable proposition) such as 'Right hemisphere stroke patients have more accidents than left hemisphere stroke patients'. For statistical purposes it is easier to use a 'null hypothesis', i.e. in this case assume there is no difference between the two, so the proposition would be 'There is no difference in the accident rate between right and left hemisphere stroke patients'. The statistical test will help to determine if you can accept or reject the null hypothesis.

Hypotheses and null hypotheses are not essential, however, to research designs. It is quite legitimate to set out the main purpose of the study or the most important questions you wish to answer.

You might find it helps to define operationally the concepts that you are using. For example, if you are concerned with improvements in patients undergoing rehabilitation you could operationally define 'improvement' by saying that in this study it meant 'increases the number of points obtained on a motor assessment scale' or 'walks across the physiotherapy gym at a faster rate'. Operational definitions specify clearly and precisely what you are measuring, they enable others to repeat the study and they decrease the likelihood of misunderstanding.

Reading books and journal articles on research design is helpful. You should familiarise yourself with the terminology, and take note of any theoretical discussion that illuminates the area on which you aim to focus. Follow the advice presented earlier in this chapter and above all do not be intimidated. If you are *treating* a patient then you should be able to carry out a research project. Research should be part of one's own clinical practice.

Communicating the outcome

There is little point in conducting research if you do not tell others about it. The logical questions you should ask in any paper you wish to present to others are: (a) Why did you start? (b) What did you do? (c) What results did you get? and (d) What does it mean? (Bradford-Hill, 1965).

Choose your means of communication with care. Ask yourself 'Who do I want to read this?' If you want to tell your own profession choose a journal read by members of that profession. If you want to persuade other professions then choose one of their journals.

Have you used a single case design? If so, this will restrict you to journals that accept such designs. Among these are the *Journal of Applied Behavioural Analysis*, the *Journal of Clinical and Experimental Neuropsychology*, *Clinical Rehabilitation*, *Neuropsychological Rehabilitation*, *Physiotherapy Practice*, *Aphasiology* and the *British and American Journals of Occupational Therapy*.

Use simple language and do not make claims which cannot be substantiated by your data. Ask your colleagues to read and comment on your earlier drafts, and be prepared to redraft.

Andrews (1993) provides a helpful guide to writing for medical journals and his advice will also hold good for rehabilitation and non-medical journals. He points out that you should check the Guidelines for Authors provided by the journal of your choice, and ask yourself whether your paper fits into the stated objectives of the journal. Is your paper presented in a way that is compatible with the style of presentation offered by the journal? You must ask yourself how long should your paper be, and what should be its format? A very important issue is the way in which references should be presented. There are two main ways, known as the Harvard and Vancouver styles (see Andrews, (1993) for an explanation).

Andrews gives some general points, including the need for a meaningful and clear title. The abstract should give the main point of the research and include a description of the area studied, how it was studied, the main findings and what conclusions can be drawn. Your paper should include an introduction and literature review. A method section should describe the subjects, the environment of the study and the procedure adopted. The results section will be your pride and joy and you must spend time getting it right. Figures and tables must be clear and unambiguous and should not contain too much information. If your paper raised questions on an earlier stated hypothesis then your results should answer these questions. You must of course state any method of statistical analysis chosen. In the discussion section the findings should (as Andrews states) 'be put into perspective and related to the findings of others, the hypothesis and the limitations of the study' (Andrews, 1993: 95).

Finally, for those of you who might be anxious about your own written style may I suggest that you can always call on friendly colleagues to help you in the redrafting process. I believe far too many people leave school thinking they cannot write and this is often a reflection of the way writing has been taught in the school rather than on individual ability. The best way to learn to write is to write. And the best way to write well is to write for a real purpose. With the aid of computers and word processors it is now possible to get your initial ideas written up quite quickly and so spend plenty of time redrafting your text for the audience you have in mind. It is at the later redrafting stages that you can aim for clarity, correctness and coherence. I see computers and word processing packages as a boon to would-be writers; they are machines that can actually help you improve your writing skills. They are also useful for presenting text to colleagues who can then also assist in changing the odd word, spelling or expression. Indeed, computers are being used in the best schools these days to make writing a more communal activity in which the more able help the less able. We should follow suit. The thing is to get started, take the plunge and surprise yourself by your own cleverness.

References

Alderman, N. & Ward, A. (1991). Behavioural treatment of the dysexecutive syndrome: reduction of repetitive speech using response cost and cognitive overlearning. *Neuropsychological Rehabilitation*, **1**, 65–80.

Andrews, K. (1991). The limitations of randomized controlled trials in rehabilitation research. *Clinical Rehabilitation*, **5**, 5–8.

Andrews, K. (1993). Writing for medical journals. *Clinical Rehabilitation*, **7**, 91–8.

Baddeley, A. D. & Longman, D. J. A. (1978). The influence of length and frequency on training sessions on the rate of learning to type. *Ergonomics*, **21**, 627–35.

Berg, I. J., Koning-Haanstra, M. & Deelman, B. G. (1991). Long-term effects of memory rehabilitation: a controlled study. *Neuropsychological Rehabilitation*, **1**, 97–111.

Bradford-Hill, A. (1965). The reasons for writing. *British Medical Journal*, **2**, 870–2.

Broca, P. (1861). Nouvelle observation d'aphémie produite par une lésion de la moitié postérieure des deuxième et troisième circonvolutions frontales. *Bulletin de la Société Anatomique de Paris*, **6**, 398–407.

Carr, E. K. (1991). Observational methods in rehabilitation research. *Clinical Rehabilitation*, **5**, 89–94.

Carr, S. & Wilson, B. (1983). Promotion of pressure relief exercising in a spinal injury patient: a multiple baseline across settings design. *Behavioural Psychotherapy*, **11**, 329–36.

Cope, D. N., Cole, J. R., Hall, K. M. & Barkan, H. (1991). Brain injury: analysis of outcome in a post-acute rehabilitation system. *Brain Injury*, **5**, 111–39.

Drummond, A. (1990). Surveys. *Clinical Rehabilitation*, **4**, 255–9.

Edgington, E. S. (1982). Nonparametric tests for single-subject multiple schedule experiments. *Behavioral Assessment*, **4**, 83–91.

Evans, J. J. & Wilson, B. A. (1992). A memory group for individuals with brain injury. *Clinical Rehabilitation*, **6**, 75–81.

Gianutsos, R. & Gianutsos, J. (1987). Single case experimental approaches to the assessment of interventions in rehabilitation psychology. In *Rehabilitation Psychology* B. Caplan ed., pp. 453–70. Rockville, MD: Aspen Corporation.

Godfrey, H. P. D., Knight, R. G., Marsh, N. V. & Moroney, B. (1989). The relationship between social adjustment, social skill and cognitive deficit in poor outcome closed head injury patients. *Psychological Medicine*, **19**, 175–82.

Gray, J. & Robertson, I. H. (1989). Remediation of attentional difficulties following brain injury: three single case studies. *Brain Injury*, **3**, 163–70.

Greenwood, R. J. & McMillan, T. M. (1993). Models of rehabilitation programmes for the brain injured adult.*Clinical Rehabilitation*, **7**, 248–55.

Hammond, A. (1987). *Joint protection behaviour of patients with rheumatoid arthritis following an education programme*. Unpublished MSc thesis, University of Southampton.

Haynes, S. N. (1978). *Principles of Behavioral Assessment*. New York: Gardner Press.

Hergenhahn, B. R. (1992). *Introduction to the History of Psychology*, 2nd edition. Belmont: Wadsworth Publishing Company.

Hersen, M. & Barlow, D. J. (1982). *Single Case Experimental Designs*. Oxford: Pergamon Press.

Horn, S., Shiel, A., McLellan, L., Campbell, M., Watson, M. & Wilson, B. A. (1993). A review of behavioural assessment scales for monitoring recovery in and after coma with pilot data on a new scale of visual awareness. *Neuropsychological Rehabilitation*. **3**, 121–37.
Kazdin, A. E. (1982). *Single Case Research Designs*. New York: Oxford University Press.
Levin, H., Saydjari, C., Eisenberg, H. M., Foulkes M., Marshall, L. F., Ruff, R. M., Jane, J. A. & Marmarou, A. (1991). Vegetative state after closed-head injury: a traumatic coma data-bank report. *Archives of Neurology*, **48**, 580–5.
Lorge, I.(1930). Influence of regularly interpolated time intervals upon subsequent learning. Quoted in Johnson, H. H. & Solso, R. L. (1971). *An Introduction to Experimental Design in Psychology: A Case Approach*. New York: Harper & Row.
Luria, A. R. (1981). *The Man with a Shattered World*. Harmondsworth: Penguin.
Mackey, S. (1989). The use of computer-assisted feedback in a motor control task for cerebral palsied children. *Physiotherapy*, **75**, 143–8.
MRC News. (1993). Why do we need large trials? Summer, no. 59.
Robinson, P. W. & Foster, D. F. (1979). *Experimental Psychology: A Small-N Approach*. New York: Harper & Row.
Rusk, H. A., Loman, E. W. & Block, J. M. (1966). Rehabilitation of the patient with head injury. *Clinical Neurosurgery*, **12**, 312–23.
Shallice, T. & Burgess, P. (1991). Deficits in strategy application following frontal lobe damage in man. *Brain*, **114**, 727–41.
Sidman, M. (1960). *Tactics of Scientific Research*. New York: Basic Books.
Siegel, S. (1956). Nonparametric Statistics for the Behavioural Sciences. Kogakusha: McGraw-Hill.
Spence, S. H. (1980). *Social Skills Training with Children and Adolescents: A Counsellor's Manual*. Windsor: NFER Publishing Company.
Tryon, W. W. (1982). A simplified time-series analysis for evaluating treatment interventions. *Journal of Applied Behavior Analysis*, **15**, 423–9.
Vallar, G. & Shallice, T. (ed.) (1990). *Neuropsychological Impairments of Short-Term Memory*. Cambridge: Cambridge University Press.
Von Cramon, D. Y., Matthes-von Cramon, G. & Mai, N. (1991). Problem solving deficits in brain injured patients: a therapeutic approach. *Neuropsychological Rehabilitation*, **1**, 45–64.
Watson, J. B. & Rayner, R. (1920). Conditioned emotional reactions. *Journal of Experimental Psychology*, **3**, 1–14.
Webster's Universal Dictionay. (1975). New York: Harver Educational Services.
Weinberg, J., Dilles, L., Gordon, W. A., Gerstman, L. J. *et al.* (1979). Training sensory awareness and spatial organization in people with right brain damage. *Archives Physical Medicine and Rehabilitation*, **60**, 491–6.
Wilkinson, S. M., Fisher, L. R. & Bromfield, P. (1989). Survey of severely head injured people in the Southampton Health district. *Clinical Rehabilitation*, **3**, 317–28.
Wilson, B. A. (1981). A survey of behavioural treatments carried out at a rehabilitation centre. In *Brain Function Therapy*, ed. G. Powell Aldershot: Gower Press.
Wilson, B. A. (1987*a*). *Rehabilitation of Memory*. New York: Guilford Press.
Wilson, B. A. (1987*b*). Single case experimental designs in neuropsychological rehabilitation. *Journal of Clinical and Experimental Neuropsychology*, **9**,

527–44.
Wilson, B. A. (1989). Improving recall of health service information. *Clinical Rehabilitation*, **3**, 275–9.
Wilson, B. A. (1994). Syndromes of acquired dyslexia and patterns of recovery: a 6–10 year follow-up study of 7 brain-injured people. *Journal of Clinical and Experimental Neuropsychology*, **16**, 354–71.
Wilson, B. A. & Moffat, N. (ed.) (1992). *Clinical Management of Memory Problems*, 2nd ed. London: Chapman and Hall.
Wilson, B. A. & Powell, G. (1987). Treatment of neurological problems. In *Handbook of Clinical Adult Psychology*, ed. S. Lindsay & G. Powell, pp. 632–48. Aldershot: Gower Press.
Wong, S. E. & Liberman, R. P. (1981). Mixed single subject designs in clinical research: variations of the multiple baseline. *Behavioural Assessment*, **3**, 297–306.
Wood, R. L., Winkowski, T. & Miller, J. (1993). Sensory regulations as a method to promote recovery in patients with altered states of consciousness. *Neuropsychological Rehabilitation*, **3**, 177–90.

9

Statistical methods

TREVOR N. BRYANT AND DAVID MACHIN

Introduction

Clinical measurements on humans, whether healthy or ill, rarely give exactly the same results from one occasion to the next. It is often quite difficult to appreciate the magnitude of this variability and therefore assess its influence on the conclusions that one may wish to draw from any investigation. Thus, although penicillin was one of the few miracle cures in which little dispute of its benefit remained after use in only a few cases, variable levels of benefit achieved when patients with rheumatism are given gold therapy are much more common in clinical practice and therapeutic research. With such variability present, it follows that differences are almost bound to occur in any comparison between patient groups. These differences may be due either to real effects, for example, the two groups have received treatments that really do differ in efficacy, or to random variation, for example, the different responses in diagnostically similar patients to gold therapy as indicated earlier, or these differences could arise from a combination of both. Such variation is just as likely to be present in patients who require some form of rehabilitation therapy.

The presence of variation means that choosing the correct design for any study is crucial. A well-designed study which is then carefully carried out but poorly analysed, can be rescued by a more appropriate re-analysis. A flawed design, however, may not provide the answer to the question posed, no matter how detailed the analysis. Consequently, such a study is wasteful of resources. It is a sad fact that many clinical studies fail in their objectives, either through poor design or the lack of (patient) numbers. A good design is one that minimises the number of subjects required to answer the question(s) posed.

The appropriate statistical analysis depends on the study design and the nature of the data. Complex analysis should be avoided, if possible, especially in situations where a clear graph, figure or table can summarise the results of a study concisely. It is important, however, that the magnitude of the inherent variability referred to above is reported in some way.

Ideas relevant to good design and analysis are not always easy and we encourage investigators to seek the advice of a medical statistician at the early stages of a study, whatever its nature.

Study design

As indicated earlier, it is important to get the design right. It is worth first asking the following questions. What is the major objective of the study? Is it clinically or scientifically a worthwhile question to pose? Is the primary objective clearly defined? Are there any secondary, but nevertheless important, objectives?

Thus, before conducting a clinical study of any kind, one must first specify the questions to be answered very clearly. It is usually beneficial to talk these through with a colleague who is not so familiar with the subject area. Of course one should also seek appropriate specialist advice. In most situations several questions may be relevant. For example, if one were to investigate the value of a new approach to avoiding bedsores, a key question is: Is the new approach better than the current method(s) used to avoid this condition? It is then necessary to define how this can be assessed, and in such a way that it can be measured in all patients.

A clinical study requires careful planning as well as execution and it is usually worthwhile to put the design in a formal protocol. In the protocol it is necessary to define all the aspects of the study from the design to an indication of the form of the final analysis. The protocol then provides the reference document as the study progresses.

A useful check at the design, analysis and reporting stages of any clinical study is provided by guidelines for contributors to medical journals by Altman *et al.* and checklists in assessing the statistical content of medical studies by Gardner *et al.* both of which are reproduced as Chapters 9 and 10 in Gardner & Altman (1989). In particular these authors stress the important distinction between clinical and statistical significance; the latter indicating that either a difference between groups may have been detected following statistical analysis but the size of that difference perhaps having no clinical importance, or alternatively that a study may have failed to demonstrate a clinically important difference between two groups merely because the study was too small in size to make a reliable assessment. These authors also stress the importance of quoting confidence intervals, a topic we discuss in some detail later.

Surveys

Suppose an investigator wishes to determine the **prevalence** of Raynaud's disease, then an appropriate design may be a **survey** of the **population** by means of a self-completed **questionnaire**. If such a design were chosen then considerable attention should be given to the design of the questionnaire itself. The survey may be conducted, for example, at town, county or national level. The necessary prerequisites before such a survey is conducted are the precise definition of the target population, for example, all adults in a particular locality above the age of 18 years, and the **sampling frame**, which is a list of all the individuals in that population. Once the sampling frame has been obtained it may be possible to send a postal questionnaire to all individuals so identified. The questionnaire is then completed by the recipient and returned to the investigator. More usually, as the list may be very extensive, one may wish to draw a **sample** of individuals from the list and send the questionnaire only to this sample. Their replies are then taken as representative of the target population. If this is to be so then an essential requirement is that the selection from the list is made by an appropriate **randomisation** technique.

To assess the prevalence of disability among the elderly in the community, Lundgren-Lindquist & Jette (1990) took a **systematic sample** of men and women aged 70 years and above living in Gothenburg, Sweden. Their **sampling fraction** of 1148 individuals represented 30% of that age group resident in the city at that time.

A systematic sample is derived by first dividing the sampling frame into equal sized and successive **blocks** of individuals within the list, taking the number of blocks equal to the size of sample required. For example, to choose eight individuals from a numbered list of 200, choose eight blocks of 25 individuals. An individual is then chosen at random from the first 25 which are numbered beforehand 01, 02, to 25. This can be performed by using random number tables. Although these are usually computer generated, they are similar to what would arise from repeatedly throwing a ten-sided die, with faces marked 0 to 9. Such tables can be found in many statistical texts. The tables are used by first choosing a point of entry, perhaps with a pin, and deciding the direction of movement from that entry, perhaps along the row or down the column. Suppose the pin chooses the entry in the tenth row and 13th column and it had been decided to move along the rows. This then gave the first ten digits as 54 13 52 05 67, which are paired here for convenience. We search along these pairs to find the first with a value not exceeding 25 (the block size). This search gives subject 13 as the first member of the sample. To identify the remaining individuals we add 25 to 13 repeatedly to obtain the numbered individuals 38, 63, 88, 113, 138, 163 and 188 to complete our systematic sample of eight individuals.

This procedure can be adapted to other situations. Thus, if equal numbers of men and women are required in the sample, all that is necessary is to produce two (men and women) lists and to take a systematic sample from each list of the relevant size.

Of the 1148 individuals chosen from the elderly in Gothenburg and invited to participate in the survey, 85% (the **response rate**) completed the required battery of tests and examinations. A low response rate, albeit not the case here, can cause considerable difficulty in interpretation of the results as it can always be argued (whether true or not) that non-responders are atypical with respect to the problem being investigated. In which case, the estimate of the prevalence of the condition of interest in the survey, necessarily obtained from responders only, will be inherently **biased**.

In a good survey, every attempt should be made, both in the design and conduct phases, to keep the number of non-responders to a minimum. In some situations a personal interview rather than a self-completed questionnaire may be more sensible. This may be costly both in time and money, however, and may require the training of interview personnel. As a consequence, such a study will usually involve a smaller sample than that possible by means of a postal questionnaire. One sensible compromise is to attempt to follow up postal non-responders (or a random sample of them), both to try and improve the response rate, but more importantly, to see if they do indeed differ from the responders.

Mobility disability was identified in 69 men from among the sample of 449 tested in Gothenburg. This gives an estimated prevalence of this disability as $p_M = 69/449 = 0.1537$ (15.4%) in the male population. To assess the reliability of p_M we need to calculate a **confidence interval (CI)** for the population prevalence. Loosely speaking, a 95% CI establishes a plausible range of values for the (true) population value of the prevalence , although there remains a 1 in 20 (5%) chance that the real value falls outside this range. The true or population prevalence could only be determined if ALL the males in the age group in Gothenburg were assessed. A more careful and detailed definition of a CI is given by Gardener & Altman (1989).

The expression for a 95% CI is given by

$$p_M - 1.96 \times \mathrm{SE}(p_M) \text{ to } p_M + 1.96 \times \mathrm{SE}(p_M)$$

where

$$\mathrm{SE}(p_M) = \left[\frac{p_M(1 - p_M)}{n}\right]^{1/2}$$

is the estimated **standard error** (SE) of the prevalence and n is the sample size.

With the data from the Gothenburg males the SE $(p_M) = 0.1537(1-0.1537)/449]^{1/2} = 0.0170$ and the 95% CI is 0.1204 to 0.1870 or 12 to 19%. Thus the investigators could conclude, in broad terms, from this that the prevalence of mobility disability in the males is unlikely to be less than 10% or more than 20%. The investigators have clearly established that mobility is a problem for, at the very least, approximately 10% and may be a problem for as many as 1 in 5 (20%) of elderly males.

It is worth noting that as the size of the sample, n, increases the SE decreases and consequentially the width of the CI decreases. One method of determining the appropriate survey size is to specify the width of the CI in advance using a reasoned guess for the prevalence p. Using this given width one can then back calculate to obtain a value for n. This then provides a guide to the appropriate survey size when discussing all aspects of the projected survey.

It has become something of a convention to calculate 95% CIs rather than, say, 99% CIs, but it is only a convention. If a 99% CI is required, all that is necessary is to change the 1.96 in the expression above to 2.58. For the males the 99% CI is 0.1098 to 0.1976 or 11 to 20%, which is always wider than the corresponding 95% CI because this increases the chance of this range including the true (population) value.

Randomised controlled trials

A **clinical trial** is a prospective study comparing the efficacy of one or more **test** therapies (or interventions) against a **control** (often standard) therapy in human subjects. The assignment of a subject to test(s) or control is made at random. The simplest design is a **two group parallel** trial in which equal numbers of subjects are allocated to each group. Such a design is illustrated in Figure 9.1 which summarises an intervention trial conducted by Stowe *et al.* (1982) in patients requiring bath aids in their rehabilitation.

Figure 9.1 defines the type of patient eligible for the trial, the allocation procedure, the intervention options and the assessment to be made. In this trial the control patients received bath aids through the usual channels following discharge from hospital. The intervention group were provided with bath aids immediately on discharge and were instructed in their use at home by a peripatetic occupational therapist. All patients were assessed some 3–6 months later to see if they were safe bathing in a seated position. The design could have been improved if this time 'window' for assessment had been narrower.

The (mandatory) need for **randomised allocation** of patients to treatment is

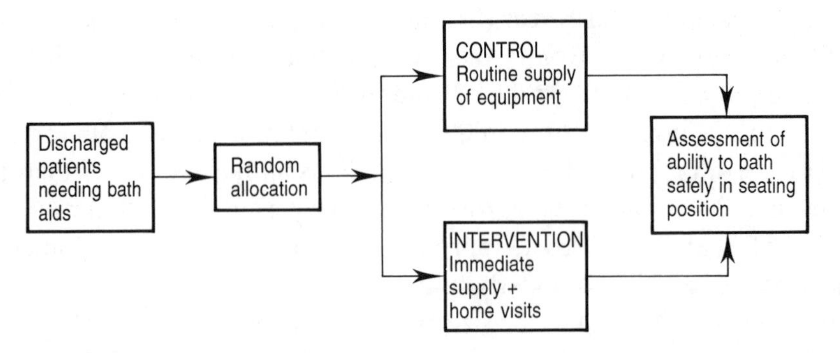

Figure 9.1. Design of a randomised controlled trial to test the value of intervention to assist in the provision of bath aids for patients requiring rehabilitation. After Stowe *et al.* (1982).

often not appreciated; neither is it always understood that allocation must take place after the patient's eligibility for the trial is determined.

It is important to recognise that **haphazard** allocation is not acceptable. A typical haphazard allocation procedure is to assign test or control therapy to alternate patients as they enter the clinic. The argument is that, as patients arrive at random (Is this really true?), then treatment allocation is also random. The problem here is that one knows the treatment the patient will receive even before they are screened for **eligibility** to the trial. This knowledge may then influence the investigator when determining which patients are eligible for the trial and which are not. The resulting (selective) exclusion of patients for treatment-related reasons will **bias** the final treatment comparisons. The clinician's job (in the context of a therapeutic clinical trial) is to determine whether both (all) treatment options are appropriate for the patient being examined and (provided he or she does not know which is best for the patient) to randomise, with the patient's consent, the allocation. This is known as the **uncertainty principle** in this context. If on the other hand he or she knows, or thinks he or she knows, which option is best for the patient, then the patient should receive that option. The problems associated with patient consent are usually different (and not always appropriate) for intervention trials.

The number of patients recruited to the study of Stowe *et al.* (1982) by diagnostic group is summarised in Table 9.1, and there were 50 patients randomised to each intervention group. The simplest randomisation device is a coin which if tossed will land with a particular face upwards with **probability** one-half. Thus one way to assign treatments at random in a clinical trial would be to assign control whenever a head (H) occurred and test whenever a tail (T) occurred. Such a procedure is termed **simple randomisation**. As indicated

Table 9.1 *Number of patients recruited by diagnostic group by allocated intervention and the percentage safe bathing in each group*

	Randomised Group		
Diagnosis	No intervention (Control)	Intervention (Test)	Total
Rheumatoid arthritis	18	12	30
Osteoarthritis	12	13	25
Strokes	12	17	29
Other	8	8	16
All patients	50	50	100
Number (%) safe bathing in a seated position	20 (40%)	45 (90%)	65 (65%)

Source: Stowe *et al.* (1982).

earlier randomisation can be generated using random number tables rather than a coin.

Suppose we use the random number sequence introduced earlier, i.e. 54 13 52 05 67. Then if even numbers, 0 is regarded as even, are assigned to control (C) and odd numbers to intervention (I) this would generate the allocation list IC II IC CI CI. Thus the first patient would receive the intervention (I) as would the tenth. This process continues until the allocation for the required number of patients for the trial is complete, for example, for the 100 of the Stowe *et al.* (1982) trial.

Although simple randomisation gives equal probability for each patient to receive C or I it does not ensure that equal numbers of patients will in fact receive each of the options. Indeed, in our example, of the first ten patients four would receive C and six I and there is no guarantee that this will even out by the 100th patient. One way round this is to use a **restricted** randomisation scheme that ensures equal numbers per treatment group in successive blocks of patients. In our example, we might require equal numbers of C and I in each successive ten patients. To do this we count up from the start of the block and once half (here five) of the patients have received C (or I) then the remainder are given I (or C). Thus in our example, patients 9 and 10 would both receive C as once patient 8 is recruited to I then five patients have now received I and we must give the remainder C to achieve balance.

In some situations it may be desirable to allocate equal numbers within subgroups of patients. Thus in the trial of Stowe *et al.* (1982) it may have been appropriate to have equal treatment allocation (as far as possible) within each of their four diagnostic groups. To do this they would have had to choose a relatively small block size, say four or six, and as there will always be some uncertainty about the patient mix in the 100 anticipated, such a **stratified** randomisation would not guarantee equal numbers to each treatment within each diagnostic group. It would, however, reduce the imbalance, between 'No Intervention' and 'Intervention', in the rheumatoid arthritis and stroke groups of Table 9.1.

It is advisable to generate a randomisation list in advance of recruiting the first patient that is then kept by someone other than the assessing clinician. Once eligibility is determined, the responsible clinician then asks this colleague for the treatment to be given. This apparently cumbersome procedure has several advantages. It removes the possibility of the clinician not randomising properly, it will usually be more efficient in that the list may be computer generated very quickly, and it allows modifications from simple randomisation to be more easily implemented.

It should be recognised that a randomised controlled trial will provide information about the average effect of a treatment in a selected population. This information cannot necessarily be applied to a single patient, because in clinical trials some patients may do better on one treatment and others on the alternative. Faced with a patient with a chronic condition, in which symptoms are stable, a physician may try out different treatments to see which one is best for an individual patient. Rather than do so in an uncontrolled fashion Johannesen (1991) has advocated the use of a rigorous clinical trial approach, that includes randomisation, double blinding and use of controls, but where the units are treatment periods within an individual, rather than separate individuals. These, so called - **n of 1 trials**, have also been discussed by Lewis (1991) who commented on the difficulties that arise when such designs are extended beyond the individual patient. A clearly positive result in an n of 1 trial shows that the intervention or treatment is effective, but tells us nothing about the average effect, or about the variation in effect from patient to patient. A series of n of 1 trials will usually be less efficient than a conventional (parallel or cross-over) design for the whole series. In fact n of 1 trials are an extreme form of **cross-over** design (see Senn (1993) for a full description of these) and problems with cross-over designs, such as carry-over effects, apply with equal force to n of 1 trials. Thus they may be of use in deciding whether a patient would benefit from alternative treatments that are well established, but are unlikely to be useful in generalising the results from the individual to the population.

The results of the intervention trial (Table 9.1) show that the proportion safe bathing in the intervention group, $p_{\mathrm{I}} = 45/50 = 0.9$ (90%), is higher than that amongst the controls, $p_{\mathrm{c}} = 20/50 = 0.4$ (40%). The difference $d = (p_I - p_C)$ $= 0.9 - 0.4 = 0.5$.

The 95% CI for a difference in two proportions is

$$d - 1.96 \times \mathrm{SE}(d) \text{ to } d + 1.96\mathrm{SE}(d)$$

or

$$(p_\mathrm{I} - p_\mathrm{C}) - 1.96 \times \mathrm{SE}(p_\mathrm{I} - p_\mathrm{C}) \text{ to } (p_\mathrm{I} - p_\mathrm{C}) + 1.96 \times \mathrm{SE}(p_\mathrm{I} - p_\mathrm{C})$$

where

$$\mathrm{SE}(d) = \mathrm{SE}(p_\mathrm{I} - p_\mathrm{c}) = \left[\frac{p_\mathrm{I}(1 - p_\mathrm{I})}{n_\mathrm{I}} + \frac{p_\mathrm{C}(1 - p_\mathrm{C})}{n_\mathrm{C}}\right]^{1/2}$$

This is an extension of the expression used earlier for the 95% CI for a prevalence survey. Substituting the values of p_I and p_c in these expressions and noting $n_\mathrm{I} = n_\mathrm{c} = 50$, gives the estimated standard error of the difference.

$$\mathrm{SE}(d) = \left(\frac{0.9 \times 0.1}{50} + \frac{0.4 \times 0.6}{50}\right)^{1/2} = 0.0812$$

and the 95% CI as 0.34 to 0.56 or approximately 35 to 55%.

The investigators could reasonably conclude that the intervention has indeed improved the proportion safe bathing although there remains considerable uncertainty about the magnitude of the improvement as the 95% CI for this difference is wide.

This plausible range of values of the difference between the interventions does not include a zero difference. A zero difference would represent the situation in which the two interventions (here essentially passive and active interventions) do not differ in their influence on the proportion safe bathing. In such a case, any difference observed would be ascribed to **chance** and the CI would also include the zero difference within it.

An alternative way of expressing the benefit to the intervention group is to report the ratio of the **odds** of safe bathing in the intervention group (45 to 5), to the odds of safe bathing in the control group (20 to 30). These two odds indicate that for a patient a *better bet* to safe bathing is to receive the intervention. In summary, we calculate the **Odds Ratio (OR)** as (45/5)/(20/30) = 13.5 to describe this advantage. If there was no difference in the proportion safe bathing then OR = 1 in such circumstances. Further discussion of the OR is given by Campbell & Machin (1993).

Comparison of two means

In some situations in a clinical trial one may be interested in measuring a continuous variable such as weight, blood pressure or pain measured on a linear analogue scale. In these cases the summary of that variable over a group of patients is the **mean**, $\bar{x}$, and a measure of the variability between subjects the **standard deviation (SD)**. The **standard error** (of the mean), **SE**, measures the precision of the mean and is calculated as

$$SE(\bar{x}) = SD/\sqrt{n}$$

when n is the number of patients in the particular group. This should be compared with the SE of a prevalence given earlier.

Wigram *et al.* (1986) describe a small controlled trial in 34 patients undergoing upper abdominal surgery who were randomised to receive either papaveretum on demand (control) or electroacupuncture and papaveretum on demand (test) for pain relief. Patients estimated pain using a visual analogue scale every eight hours for the two postoperative days, and mean levels were calculated for each patient group as time progressed.

The electroacupuncture patients reported more pain at each assessment over the 48 hours yet received almost the same amount of analgesia as the control group. Two patients asked for the acupuncture needles to be removed. In this example, the intervention group appeared to fare worse than the controls. This is clearly illustrated in Figure 9.2, albeit the authors should have presented some measure of the inherent variation at each plotted point. The fact that the test therapy fared worse than the control is not as rare as it may seem and illustrates the need for randomised trials when new therapies are proposed.

In some situations comparisons between groups may be required where random allocation is either inappropriate or not possible. Thus Sackley (1990) compared the balance coefficients, BC, in left and right affected hemiplegics to see if this differed in the two groups of patients. Their results are summarised in Table 9.2 and indicate a higher mean BC in those patients with a right hemiplegia. In contrast, the SDs are approximately equal for the two groups indicating that patient variability about the mean is similar in both groups.

The 95% CI for a difference in two means is given by the usual expressions

$$d - 1.96 \times SE(d) \text{ to } d + 1.96 \times SE(d)$$

but here $d = \bar{x}_R - \bar{x}_L$ and

$$\begin{aligned} SE(d) &= SE(\bar{x}_R - \bar{x}_l) \\ &= \left(\frac{SD_R^2}{n_R} + \frac{SD_L^2}{n_L}\right)^{1/2} \\ &= \left(\frac{0.13^2}{52} + \frac{0.16^2}{38}\right)^{1/2} = 0.0316 \end{aligned}$$

where the suffices R and L refer to right and left hemiplegic groups.

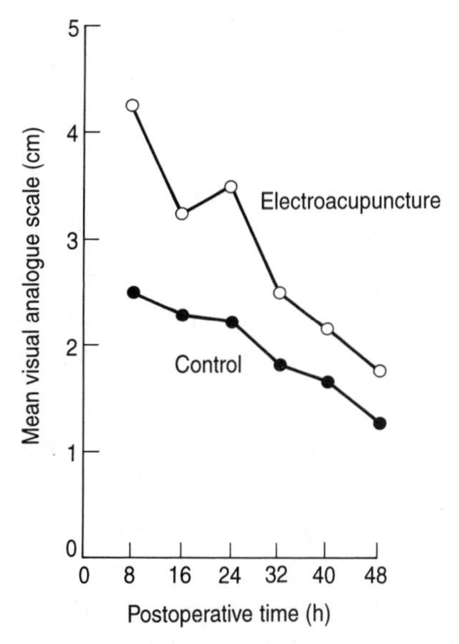

Figure 9.2. Mean postoperative pain profiles by treatment group. Reproduced from Wigram *et al.* (1986).

Table 9.2 *Difference in mean Balance Coefficient (BC) following right and left-sided hemiplegia*

		Side of hemiplegia		Difference, *d* (Right - Left)	
		Right	Left		
Number of subjects		52	38	–	
n	Mean	0.62		0.36	0.26
Standard deviation	SD	0.13			0.16
Standard error of difference	SE(*d*)	–		–	0.03

Source: Sackley (1990).

The 95% CI is 0.20 to 0.32 and does not include a mean BC difference of zero between the right and left-sided hemiplegic patients. The results therefore confirm a higher BC in those with a right-sided hemiplegia.

There are alternative approaches for calculating the SE of a difference in means to the method given here. It is usually advisable to seek help with this.

Survival methods

The major outcome variable in some studies is the time between successive **critical events**. Thus Mayo *et al.* (1991) determined the recovery time from stroke to full and independent sitting function in 45 poststroke victims who were not self-sitting following the stroke and investigated its relation to perceptual impairment caused by the stroke. The time to recovery of this ability (the second critical event) was measured from the date of the stroke (the first critical event). The time between the two events is often referred to as a **survival no-to-mild time** as the techniques used to analyse such data have often been applied to patient survival times following, say, diagnosis of cancer.

Suppose all the 25 patients with no-to-mild perceptual impairment (see feint upper curve in Figure 9.3 which we now describe in more details) recover then there will be 25 individual recovery times. These data can then be represented in a cumulative (recovery) survival curve as follows. First the individual recovery times are ordered from smallest to largest. Then beginning at time 0 (see Figure 9.3), and moving along horizontally, we reach the day of the patient with the shortest recovery time (approximately day 42). At that time we move upwards with a step equal to one patient. This step will be 1/25 or 0.04 on the probability scale. The horizontal move then recommences until day 44 when there is another step upwards at the time the next patient recovers, followed by a horizontal move until the next recovery time. This process continues until the very last (and longest) recovery time, to complete the survival curve. A similar process applies to the 20 patients with moderate-to-severe impairment of Figure 9.3.

It is clear from Figure 9.3, however, that the steps are not equal in height and neither does the curve reach completion at 1 (25 times the step of 0.04) of the vertical axis. The first may be explained by two (or more) patients having exactly the same recovery times and so there would be a double (or greater) step at that point. A second reason is the presence of patients with **censored** observations. These are patients who have had their stroke but have not (as yet) recovered sitting function. All we know for these patients is the date of the first event and the date of the last time they were assessed when they were observed not to be sitting independently. This time interval is known as the censored time. Figure 9.3 makes use of these censored times in those 25 patients with no to mild impairment and those 20 with moderate-to-severe impairment who have not achieved independence. Such patients account in part for the differing step sizes. Details of the precise method of calculating the (so called) **Kaplan–Meier** or **Product Limit** estimate of the survival curves are given in, for example, Parmar & Machin (1995).

Once calculated for the two groups (No-to-Mild and Moderate-to-Severe) comparisons can be made between them using the **logrank** test; however, the relationship between the rate of recovery of independency in the two groups may be summarised by the **Hazard Ratio (HR)**, which is similar to the OR

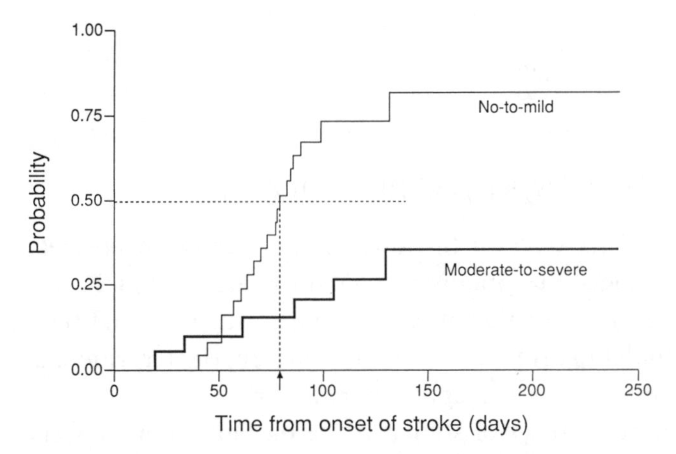

Figure 9.3. Probability of achieving independent sitting according to degreed of perceptual impairment. Reproduced from Mayo (1991).

introduced earlier. Many authors, including Mayo *et al.* (1991) use the term OR here also rather than distinguish this as a survival time context, by use of the HR as we have done.

To estimate the HR the total recovery times of all the patients with the two groups separately are first calculated. The observed total number of successes, i.e. patients who are now sitting independently, $O_{n-m} + O_{m-s}$, in both groups is calculated and then divided up in the ratio of the recovery time observed in each group. This leads to the expected number of successes, E_{n-m} and E_{m-s}, in each group. For this example the expected number of successes as 11.29 and 13.71, respectively. Note that there are some small discrepancies between the calculations quoted here and the original article as the authors used a different approach that we cannot reproduce exactly without reference to the raw data.

The ratios $O_{n-m}/E_{n-m} = 19/11.29 = 1.68$ and $O_{m-s}/E_{m-s} = 6/13.71 = 0.44$ compare the observed and expected recovery rates. Finally, the $HR = (O_{m-s}/E_{m-s})/(O_{n-m}/E_{n-m}) = 0.26$ which is given by Mayo *et al.* (1991) in their figure. A value of HR = 1 would indicate that the recovery rate in both impairment groups was the same. This is clearly not the case.

For technical reasons a CI for the HR is obtained first by obtaining a CI for $\log_e$ (HR) from

$$\log_e(\mathrm{HR}) - 1.96 \times \mathrm{SE}(\log_e \mathrm{HR}) \text{ to } \log_e(\mathrm{HR}) + 1.96 \times \mathrm{SE}(\log_e \mathrm{HR})$$

where $\log_e$(HR) replaces *d* in the general expression for a CI given earlier, and

$$\mathrm{SE}(\log_e \mathrm{HR}) = \sqrt{(1/E_{n-m} + 1/E_{m-s})}.$$

These data give

$$\log_e(\text{HR}) = \log_e 0.26 = 1.3471$$

and

$$\text{SE}\ (\log_e \text{HR}) = \surd[(1/11.29) + (1/13.71)] = 0.4019.$$

This calculation gives -2.13 to -0.56 for the lower and upper values, respectively, which are then antilogged to obtain 0.1 to 0.6 for the (95%) CI.

The interval does not include a value of HR = 1 and so suggests that those with no-or-mild perceptual impairment recover at a different (faster) rate than those who had moderate-to-severe perceptual impairment.

A useful summary figure in survival studies is the **median**, here recovery, time. This is calculated from the cumulative survival curve (Figure 9.3) by drawing a line parallel to the time axis and noting at which time(s) this cuts the survival curve(s). For the no-to-mild impairment group the line cuts the cumulative time to independence curve at approximately 80 days (11 weeks). We interpret this by saying that half the patients within this prognosis group have achieved independence within 11 weeks of their stroke. We cannot estimate the median time for the moderate-to-severe group as the recovery to independent sitting curve has not yet reached the required 50%. We can say, however, that only about 20% of this group have achieved independence in the first 11 weeks following their stroke (see vertical hatched line within Figure 9.3).

The results of survival type studies are often summarised in the format of Table 9.3. Formal comparisons between groups can be made using the logrank test (for details of this see Parmar & Machin, 1995).

Practical considerations

We have stressed the importance of good design but it is also important to consider how the data generated in any study are to be collected (perhaps on a paper form), collated and ultimately analysed. It is far better to enter data into a computer system as it is collected rather than leave it accumulating in a filing cabinet until the end of a study. Computer-based data entry allows for range (age must be between 18 and 65 years) and consistency (if male then pregnancy must be no) checks to be applied to the data. If a data value fails a test it is much easier to recheck the information obtained a few days after it was collected rather than several months or even years on. Studies involving follow-up of patients, i.e. repeated assessments over time, pose particular problems although specialised data management packages (COMPACT,

Table 9.3 *Summary of comparisons between patients with stroke who had non-mild or moderate-to-severe impairment*

		Number achieving Independent Sitting			
Prognostic Group	Number of patients *n*	Observed O	Expected E	Ratio O/E	HR
No or mild	25	19	11.29	1.68	0.26
Moderate-to-severe	20	6	13.71	0.44	
Total	45	25	25.00		

Source: calculations summarised in Mayo *et al.* (1991).

1990) are available. Computer software packages such as spreadsheets and databases may be used to organise the data; however it is important to check that the data can be transferred easily into the statistical package that will be used for the analysis. Good software will have transfer, or Import/Export, facilities that will enable files to be written and read in either ASCII (text), dBase or Lotus formats. Problems may occur here because of the way in which the data has been coded, for example, simple questions may be coded and entered onto a database as Y or N. Some statistical packages have problems handling this alphabetic data and prefer the data in a numeric format as 1 or 2. The ability to convert alphabetic data to numeric data is therefore a desirable feature of any statistical package. Dates routinely cause problems for statistical packages, databases and spreadsheet software handle dates well, but many statistical packages do not. Transferring duration information can cause problems. The solution to this may lie with the database or spreadsheet, by calculating time intervals between event dates, before transfer. Alternatively, dates may have to be stored as three items, day, month and year. This aspect should be considered at an early stage in the project before routine data collection has commenced.

It is important to identify a suitable statistical package, although specialists advice on this may have to be sought because some of the statistics that are required may not be offered, CIs are not generated by some packages for example. There are many packages available including SPSS, Minitab and Epi-Info. One of the dangers of using any statistical package is that the software will produce numbers and statistics in response to whatever data you enter and analysis you request. It is easy to be seduced into carrying out numerous analyses without considering whether the procedures chosen are appropriate or whether the statistics generated are correct. An understanding of the data being analysed is essential. One way to do this is to plot the data for visual inspection. Graphical display of data is offered in a variety of software including statistical, spreadsheet, database and graphical packages. It may be important, however, to distinguish whether the software can produce scientific plots as opposed to business charts. Not many packages will plot survival curves for example.

The range of statistical and data manipulation software available is enormous and there is overlap between these types of package. The functions needed for statistical analysis are available in varying degrees. When choosing software it is advisable to seek expert advice because despite the range available, some programs may be more appropriate for the study that you are about to undertake.

References

Campbell, M. J. & Machin, D. (1993). *Medical Statistics: A Commonsense Approach*, 2nd ed. Chichester: John Wiley.

COMPACT Steering Committee. (1990). Improving the quality of data in clinical trials in cancer. *British Journal of Cancer*, **63**, 412–15.

Gardner, M. J. & Altman, D. G. (1989). *Statistics with Confidence*. London: *British Medical Journal*.

Johannesen, T. (1991). Controlled trials in single subjects. 1. Value in clinical medicine. *British Medical Journal* , **303**, 173–4.

Lewis, J. A. (1991). Controlled trials in single subjects. 2. Limitations of use. *British Medical Journal*. **303**, 175–6.

Lundgren-Lindquist, B. & Jette, A. M. (1990). Mobility disability among elderly men and women in Sweden. *International Disability Studies*, **12**, 1–5.

Mayo, N. E., Korner-Bitensky, N. A. & Becker, R. (1991). Recovery time of independent function post-stroke. *American Journal of Physical Medicine and Rehabilitation*, **70**, 5–12.

Parmer, M. K. B. & Machin, D. (1995). *Survival Analysis : A Practical Approach*. Chichester: John Wiley.

Sackley, C. M. (1990). The relationship between weight-bearing asymmetry after stroke, motor function and activities of daily living. *Physiotherapy Theory and Practice*, **6**, 179–85.

Senn, S. (1993). *Cross-over Trials in Clinical Research*. Chichester: John Wiley.

Stowe, J., Thornley, G., Chamberlain, M. A. & Wright, V. (1992). Evaluation of aids and equipment for bathing : Survey II. *British Journal of Occupational Therapy*, **45**, 92–5.

Wigram, J. R., Lewith, G. T., Machin, D. & Church, J. J. (1986). Electroacupuncture for postoperative pain. *Physiotherapy Practice*, **2**, 83–8.

10

Social policy, disability and rehabilitation

CAROLINE GLENDINNING

Introduction: a historical and comparative framework

In most western societies, disabled people, their carers and all who provide treatment in one form or another find themselves faced with a bewildering array of provisions and services. These are likely to include specialised services directed towards people with specific disabling conditions (such as blindness or deafness); through general forms of provision that are restricted to certain social groups (such as older or retired people); to universally available services which benefit disabled people along with everybody else (such as access to free primary health care). The actual content of these various forms of provision will depend on a mixture of historic, social, political and economic influences; these are likely to vary from country to country and over time. The notion that there is a single social policy response to disability, even at one particular time and within the context of a single country, is both inaccurate and over-simplified. For example, policies towards people with learning disabilities and long-term mental illnesses have on the whole developed separately and been shaped by factors that are different from those which have shaped policies for people with physical disabilities. Policies for older disabled people may be different again (and, comparatively, in their infancy because longevity and hence disability in old age is a phenomenon that has only emerged gradually during this century in industrialised countries).

A single chapter cannot provide a detailed description of social welfare services and benefits for disabled people. Firstly, these will inevitably vary between different countries (and particularly between developed and developing societies); secondly, such a description would rapidly become out of date as new legislation is introduced and implemented. Above all, any 'official' accounts of services and other forms of help for disabled people are likely to be very different from the perceptions and evaluations of those services by disabled people themselves.

This chapter will therefore focus on the main issues and themes that shape both demands for services and the patterns and levels of services which are provided in response to those demands. It will outline the range of services that are particularly relevant to disabled people and will evaluate their effectiveness, both from a policy perspective and from the perspective of disabled people themselves.

Although this chapter focuses on the UK, many of the issues which it covers are common to other European and Scandinavian countries. Moreover, international self-advocacy movements and organisations of disabled people are likely to lead to rising expectations and increasing awareness of these issues among disabled people in other countries which do not yet enjoy the levels of economic development and public expenditure currently experienced by western societies. On the other hand, lower levels of preventative and primary health care services, combined with poor nutrition and legacies of civil unrest, are likely to create much higher needs for rehabilitation and supportive services for disabled people in developing countries. Thus although many issues and concerns will be common to disabled people in different societies at different times, there will inevitably be some variations according to the nature of the particular society.

The impact of industrialisation and technological change

A number of broad processes and trends have helped to shape both the circumstances of disabled people within different societies and the responses of those societies, as manifested in services and other forms of social welfare provision. One such factor is industrialisation and, more recently, technological change. These processes offer both a historical perspective on policy developments within the UK and also help to explain the different policy responses to disability between developed and developing countries today. For example Topliss (1979) has described how the process of industrialisation in late eighteenth-century Britain led to the exclusion of many disabled people from economic activities and their gradual segregation in separate institutions:

> the widespread incarceration of disabled people is directly attributable to the transition from agriculture and cottage-based industries to the large-scale factory-type system . . . Waged labour made the distinction between the able-bodied and the non-able-bodied poor crucially important.
> *(Barnes, 1991:15).*

On a more positive note, industrialisation also (eventually) led to the development in the UK of a system of compensation-based payments in respect of disabling injuries and diseases contracted in the course of employment (Baldwin *et al.*, 1981). Furthermore, some writers have argued that the development of new technologies in the contemporary developed world (and, eventually, in the developing world) should enable many barriers of exclusion and segregation to be broken down and lead to the gradual reintegration of disabled people into mainstream society as physical restrictions are overcome and disability comes to be perceived solely as a social restriction (Oliver, 1990).

The experience of war

Within the UK, the experience of war has also had major influence on the shaping of services for disabled people. For example, the very large numbers of soldiers injured during the 1914–18 war led to the establishment of a system of state war pensions which have remained considerably more generous than pensions for the 'civilian' disabled (Walker, 1981). Similarly, help with the extra costs of transport for people who have difficulty in walking has its origins in the 'motorised bath chairs' which were provided by the Red Cross for disabled ex-servicemen after the end of the 1914–18 war (Stokes, 1981).

Giving priority to employment and the labour market

Another important influence on the shape of social welfare provision in the UK is the greater priority given to supporting disabled people of working age or who are active members of the labour market compared with those who are, for reasons of age, severity of disability or ill health, economically inactive. It affects the provision of services, access to social security benefits and the levels of those benefits.

For example, in the UK principles of compensation derived from the legal concepts of tort and common law liability have underpinned and justified the much higher social security benefits that have been paid during much of this century to people disabled as the result of their employers' negligence (Walker, 1981). The principles of social insurance similarly justified higher levels of invalidity benefits for disabled people who had worked and therefore paid employment-related insurance contributions. In contrast, benefits for disabled school-leavers who never manage to establish adequate insurance records and for women whose employment and earnings are interrupted by caring for children and older relatives are both governed by more stringent eligibility criteria and are also paid at lower levels. For example, the Severe Disablement Allowance (SDA) is intended for disabled people who cannot work and have been unable to build up a record of insurance contributions. SDA claimants have to demonstrate not only that they are incapable of paid employment but also that they have a disability of at least 75%. Moreover, SDA is only 60% of the level of Invalidity Benefit, the main contributory benefit for disabled people until April 1995 (Lonsdale, 1990), and of Incapacity Benefit, which then replaced it.

This linking of disability benefit entitlement to employment records in the UK has historically reflected the principle that eligibility for benefits should depend on the disabled person having earned his or her entitlements through the payment of national insurance contributions while in paid employment. Such principles are becoming increasingly weak, as the entitlements that are derived from them exclude growing numbers of people (not only those with disabilities) who have difficulty sustaining continuous employment and contributions records (for an example, see Alcock, 1987, 1993). Moreover, differences between disabled people who have had some contact with the labour market and those who have not are continuing to diminish, as social security provision in the UK becomes more and more residual.

The changing demography of western societies

All western European and Scandinavian countries are characterised by growing populations of older people and by projected increases in the numbers of very elderly people. While disability and old age are by no means necessarily synonymous, nevertheless the risk of experiencing disability or infirmity does increase with advancing age and is particularly high for people aged 85 years and over. Since the beginning of the twentieth century the proportion of people in the UK aged 65 years and over has more than trebled, from 4.7% to 15.8% in 1991, and is expected to rise to over 20% by 2031. The proportion of over-85 year olds, currently 1.6% of the total population, is similarly expected to increase by half again, to 2.5%, by 2031. The incidence of disability for people aged 80 years and over is currently 59%, almost twice the rate for the over-60 age group as a whole (McGlone, 1992).

Concerns about the implications of rising numbers of frail older people has had two policy consequences. The first is the search throughout most industrialised nations for cheaper, for the state at any rate, ways than have hitherto been employed for meeting their health and social care needs. In the UK for example, working-age people have increasingly been encouraged to make financial provision for their old age through private and occupational pension schemes rather than through the state scheme (Department of Health and Social Security, 1985). Similarly, responsibility for the provision of personal and social care has increasingly been shifted from statutory health and social services authorities to the 'informal' sector, more often than not members of the immediate family (Department of Health, 1989; Glendinning, 1992*a*). How to pay for the anticipated growth in the amount of care needed by elderly and disabled people, in the context of declining birthrates and smaller proportions of economically active people, is now a common concern of most developed societies (Glendinning & McLaughlin, 1993).

A second consequence of this changing demographic profile has been the increasing tendency to ignore the particular needs associated with disability in older people: 'policy-makers have consistently tried to deny the existence of disability among this (older) group, arguing that it is a 'normal' part of the ageing process' (Walker, 1990:66). This is particularly evident in respect of state social security provision:

> . . . older people with disabilities face a double deprivation: on the one hand, as older people their incomes are lower than those of people below pension age (on average by 69%) and, on the other, they do not have access to additional income, above that received by non-disabled pensioners, to meet the extra costs of disability.
> *(Walker & Walker, 1991: 36)*

For example, in 1990 major changes were proposed to a number of UK social security benefits designed to help with the extra costs of disability (Department of Social Security, 1990). However, these changes failed to extend any help towards the costs of mobility to people who develop severe walking difficulties after the age of 65 years, or help with other disability costs to older people who have less severe personal care needs. It has been estimated that extending to older disabled people the financial benefits currently available to their younger counterparts would cost £1.5 billions a year (Berthoud *et al.*, 1993: 97).

Disability and rehabilitation in the UK : some current issues and themes in social policy

This section will briefly outline some of the major themes shaping the configurations of services and other forms of support for disabled people in the UK.

Although many services and other forms of social provisions, however, have been developed specifically for disabled people, disabled people are also substantially affected by the broader economic, political and policy trends that affect the country as a whole. Indeed, in many instances these broader trends outweigh the impact of 'special' measures designed specifically to enhance the quality of life of disabled people.

The changing meaning of 'community' care

The term 'community care' originally denoted the move from large-scale institutional care for physically and/or mentally disabled and chronically ill people, to the provision of domestic and personal care, educational and recreational services within a domiciliary setting. This notion of providing services in the community rather than institutions has seen a subtle shift in meaning over the past two decades; families, friends and neighbours have increasingly been viewed as the main providers of 'community care', rather than statutory or voluntary sector services. Thus care in the community has increasingly become care by the community (Parker, 1990: 10). Such assumptions underpinned the 1993 reorganisation of 'community care' in the UK, in which the role of statutory agencies was explicitly designated as one of giving support to informal carers in their role as the primary care-givers:

> . . . the great bulk of community care is provided by friends, family and neighbours . . . it is right they should be able to play their part in looking after those close to them . . . service providers (should) make practical support for carers a high priority'
> *(Department of Health, 1989:4–5).*

Official rhetoric about the central role of informal carers in the provision of social care has been helped to become a reality by successive restrictions on public sector expenditure. These restrictions have led to reductions or withdrawals in the provision of domiciliary services such as home helps and community nursing auxiliaries. Consequently disabled and elderly people who are living with someone else, particularly if this includes a non-elderly female relative, are much less likely to receive statutory services than disabled people who are living alone (Qureshi & Walker, 1989; Arber *et al.*, 1989; Parker, 1990). Moreover, as will be illustrated below, the financial and service supports which are available for informal care-givers are far from adequate.

Changes in the 'mix' of welfare services for disabled people

The shift from 'formal' to 'informal' sources of help is part of a broader change which reflects a wider political preoccupation with reducing the role of state services and state provision (McCarthy, 1989). No longer can disabled people in the UK expect to receive all the help they need from statutory social welfare and health services. Encouragement has been given instead to the development of a plurality of service providers, including both the private, commercial and the voluntary not-for-profit sectors as well as statutory authorities. The White Paper which preceded the 1993 'community care' changes exhorted local authorities to become 'arrangers and purchasers of care services, rather than monopolistic service providers . . . by developing their purchasing and contracting role' (Department of Health, 1989:17).

The shift in the 'mix' of service provision has a number of consequences for disabled people. Firstly, voluntary and non-governmental organisations have traditionally provided a range of specialist and innovative services for, among others, disabled and chronically ill people. It is likely that these organisations will become increasingly constrained by the formal contracts with statutory health and social services organisations into which they now have to enter. These contracts will seek to 'purchase' clearly specified services. The range of services available to disabled people is therefore likely to decrease rather than increase as a result (Common & Flynn, 1992; Lewis, 1993). Secondly, the increasingly contractual basis of the funding available to voluntary and non-governmental organisations is likely to reduce substantially the ability of these organisations to act as advocates on behalf of disabled people, whether by identifying new needs and campaigning for the development of services to meet those needs or by representing individual disabled people who may have complaints about current service provision. Thirdly, the increasing use of independent (both commercial and not-for-profit) service providers raises important issues of regulation and quality control for disabled people who, because of the personal nature of the help they often need, are likely to feel particularly vulnerable. These concerns about standards and quality arise whether personal care services are purchased by local authorities from private sector providers on behalf of disabled people, or are purchased directly by disabled people themselves using their own private resources or income from benefits. Disabled people whose personal and home care services are provided by independent organisations will need proper protection against the risk of exploitation and abuse and easy access to complaints and redress procedures if needed.

Education policies for disabled children

In line with the trends away from separate and segregated services and towards 'community' services for disabled people, steps have been taken over the past 15 years to integrate the education of disabled children more closely with that of children who do not have special needs (though whether those steps have gone far enough is a matter of some debate). The 1981 Education Act aimed to break down rigid distinctions between disabled and non-disabled children by creating a new concept, more of a continuum than a category, of 'special educational needs'. The 1981 Act was also intended to assist the integration of disabled children into 'mainstream' schools, by making the availability of extra help and resources dependent on the needs of the individual child rather than on the type of school they attend. Children who are assessed and subsequently receive a statement of their special educational needs are supposed then to have an entitlement to the educational support they have been assessed as needing.

Progress towards greater integration has been slow and has been further hampered by more recent developments in wider education policies. The assessment of needs has become severely constrained by financial restrictions on local education authorities, and by authorities' consequent anxiety about the risks of legal action by parents if they are unable to provide services that have been identified in a statement of educational needs. It is therefore now widely agreed that the issuing of statements by education authorities has fallen into disarray (Warnock, 1993). Figures on the proportions of children being educated in special, segregated schools show only a marginal drop between 1977 and 1989; indeed during that period a number of local authorities actually increased the proportions of children educated in segregated special schools (Swan, 1991).

Even greater threats to educational integration have been posed by the implementation of the 1988 Education Reform Act. This introduced a greater measure of financial autonomy to all individual schools; a standard national curriculum to be followed by all children in all schools; and a new ethos of competition, based on indicators such as public examination results, between schools. 'In such a climate, children with special educational needs may not be wanted and may well be singled out for exclusion or removal to segregated provision 'for their own good'. (Mittler, 1993:27).

Employment opportunities for disabled people

Disabled people experience disadvantage in both obtaining paid employment (Fry, 1986; Graham *et al*, 1990) and in achieving levels of earnings comparable to those of their non-disabled counterparts. Levels of unemployment among economically active disabled people are more than double those of non-disabled people (Martin *et al.*, 1989); among those who are in work, disabled adults earn significantly less than the working population in general (Martin & White, 1988).

Policies to end employment discrimination against disabled people have never been effective. The 1944 Disabled Persons Employment Act required all firms with 20 or more employees to ensure that at least 3% of these were registered disabled people. By the end of the 1970s two-thirds of private sector firms were failing to meet this quota and by 1990 no public sector employer was meeting its quota either (*Employment Gazette*, 1990). The fine for failing to comply with the quota has remained at £100 since 1944; up to 1989 only nine prosecutions had been brought against employers for failing to employ their quota of disabled people (Lonsdale, 1986). Instead, successive governments have pursued a strategy of persuasion, including 'good practice' awards to employers. Further legislation to outlaw discrimination against disabled people comes into force in 1996, but still only applies to businesses with over 20 employees; disabled people have again complained about the lack of rigorous enforcement mechanisms (see below).

Furthermore, the economic recessions and increasing unemployment of the 1980s and 1990s have hit disabled people much harder than their non-disabled counterparts. Arguably, these broader economic trends have had an impact on employment opportunities for disabled people which has far outweighed the potential benefits of any campaigns of persuasion:

> One of the effects of the economic recession of the 1980s is that disabled people who were regarded as 'essential manpower' forty years before are now increasingly seen as 'surplus labour'
> *(Gladstone, 1985: 103–104)*

For example, between 1979–80 and 1980–81, the number of disabled people placed in employment fell by 33%, compared with a fall of only 20% in overall employment placements during the same period.

Outcomes : policy evaluation

How successful are current social policies in enabling disabled people (and the families and households within which they live) to lead independent lives, enjoying the same risks, rights and living standards as non-disabled people? It will be argued that, particularly recently, wider social and economic policies have exerted very different, and ultimately far more powerful, influences on the quality of life of disabled people than have policies which have been 'targeted' specifically at them.

The risks of poverty

Extensive research carried out by both government and independent organisations in the UK over the past 30 years has established beyond any doubt that disabled people of all ages are at substantially greater risk of poverty than their non-disabled counterparts. This holds true regardless of whether an absolute measure of poverty is used (such as the numbers of people who fall below a specified income level), or a measure which is relative to the living standards enjoyed by the majority of people in the society.

The difficulties experienced by disabled people in gaining access to employment are one cause of this increased risk of poverty. The types of occupation, numbers of hours worked and rates of pay of disabled people are all less advantageous than in the general population (Martin *et al.*, 1989). In almost all categories of employees (men and women, manual and non-manual), disabled adults earn significantly less than the average for the working population as a whole (Martin & White, 1988). As a result, the loss of earnings potential associated with disability is as high as 85% for the most severely disabled men, compared with non-disabled men of similar ages and educational backgrounds (Berthoud *et al.*, 1993).

A second cause of the poverty experienced by disabled people is the low level of the social security benefits on which so many depend for most or all of their incomes. Eighty-nine per cent of disabled pensioners rely on state benefits, mainly the ordinary state retirement pension, as their main source of income. The single person's pension is barely one-fifth of average male earnings in the UK and less than one-third of the European Community's 'decency threshold' for the wages of full-time employees. 'Not surprisingly, therefore, the vast majority of older people with disabilities live in poverty' (Walker & Walker, 1991: 38–39). The gap between the incomes of disabled and non-disabled people below retirement age is also considerable. In 1985, the incomes of disabled people were less than three-quarters those of non-disabled people, after controlling for household size (Martin & White, 1988). Moreover, as the severity of disability increases, so do both financial need and dependence on state benefits (Martin & White, 1988). Consequently two-thirds of disabled people are reliant on one or both of the two main means-tested 'safety net' benefits (Berthoud *et al.*, 1993), which are widely regarded as signifying the UK's poverty 'threshold'.

A third cause of poverty among disabled people is the extra costs which their disabilities incur. These can be grouped into three main types: one-off, 'lump sum' spending on items such as house adaptations, special pieces of furniture and equipment; regular spending on special items required because of disability, such as special pharmacy items, the costs of hospital visits and the purchase of treatments and other services; and extra spending on items which most people buy but which disabled people need to spend more on: extra heating, special diets and extra laundry being among the most common. In 1985, a government national survey calculated that disabled people spent £6.10 extra on average each week on these two latter types of regular extra expenditure (Martin & White, 1988). This figure was vigorously challenged by organisations of disabled people as seriously misrepresenting the extra needs of very many severely disabled people (Large, 1991). Subsequent analysis of the 1985 survey data by government researchers confirmed that the single greatest factor affecting levels of extra spending by disabled people was their income level; many disabled people do not spend a great deal on the extra items that they need simply because they cannot afford to (Matthews & Truscott, 1990).

Since the early 1990s, the extra expenses incurred by disabled and frail older people have increased yet further because of the growing tendency of local authorities to impose charges for a wide range of domiciliary, day and respite care services. Although the levels of these charges vary very considerably across the UK, they can nevertheless create difficult choices for some disabled people about how to manage a range of extra demands on a limited income (National Consumer Council, 1995; Chetwynd *et al.*, 1996).

A fourth cause of poverty among disabled people is the complexity of social security benefits. This complexity leads to many disabled and frail elderly people failing to claim benefits to which they are entitled because they do not know about them, do not understand the eligibility criteria, or find the assessment process humiliating and stigmatising. During the 1980s, all the main political parties in the UK made explicit commitments to introducing a comprehensive and coherent system of social security benefits for disabled people. A much-heralded review of social security benefits for disabled people and their families (Department of Social Security, 1990), however, introduced only small extensions and rationalisations to existing benefits designed to meet the extra costs of disability, plus a new benefit (the Disability Working Allowance) to 'top up' the earnings of disabled people from low paid or part-time work.

These proposals were widely criticised for their piecemeal and limited scope, and especially for their failure to offer any additional financial help to the approximately 4.2 million disabled people over retirement age (Walker & Walker, 1991). The new Disability Working Allowance is likely to benefit only about 25 000 disabled people (Glendinning, 1991), while the 'rationalisation' of existing benefits for the extra costs of disability has in fact introduced no less than 11 different combinations of eligibility, involving nine different criteria, and an application form running to over 30 pages (Large, 1991: 117).

A fifth cause of poverty among disabled people stems from the impact of other, wider changes that have been made to the social security system. Here, despite rhetoric to the contrary, attempts to 'protect' the living standards of disabled people have been rendered nugatory (Glendinning, 1992*b*). For example, both the scope and the value of national insurance benefits, while never very satisfactory, have been systematically reduced and replaced by residual, means-tested social assistance as the mainstay of income maintenance provision in the UK. Similarly, major changes in 1988 to the means-tested social assistance scheme, on which so many disabled people had come to rely, resulted in between 80 000 (official government estimate) and one million (independent estimate) sick and disabled people being worse off (Glendinning, 1991). Also, in 1995 Invalidity Benefit was replaced by Incapacity Benefit. Eligibility for this is determined by a new, detailed medical test, not only of a claimant's incapacity in his/her normal occupation but for any work at all. Up to 250 000 people previously receiving Invalidity Benefit and a further 70 000 new claimants were estimated to be at risk of losing entitlement because of the new medical test (Welfare Rights Bulletin, April 1994, February 1995).

Moves to reduce the role of the state and increase the scope of private social security provision have also worsened the position of disabled people. During the 1980s, responsibility for sick pay and maternity pay was transferr-ed from the government to employers. Early monitoring of the new sick pay scheme revealed risks of discrimination by employers against employees with poor health records (Baloo *et al.*, 1986). Moreover, the occupational and personal pension schemes which have been increasingly promoted as alternatives to state provision rarely provide adequate cover for people whose earnings potential or capacity for work is interrupted by illness or disablement.

As well as failing to address the widespread risks of poverty experienced by disabled people, the criteria used to determine eligibility for social security benefits by disabled people frequently undermine their attempts to maintain and increase personal independence. Because entitlements are based on assessments of inability, functional impairment and the lack of independence, so training, marriage, employment or rehabilitation to increase personal mobility and self-care skills can all jeopardise a disabled person's entitlements to social security benefits, a deterrent to attempts to lead a 'normal' life (Glendinning, 1991):

> The more a person becomes able to function in the community, the more he or she will become exposed to the harsh realities of the general benefit system and the greater therefore will be the pressure to slide backwards along the dependency continuum.
> *(Fimister, 1988: 29).*

The consequences for family carers

Within the family context, providing care for a disabled or elderly relative is often part of a complex mixture of affection, obligation and internalised 'public morality' (Finch, 1989). Nevertheless, the shift from institutional to 'community' care, and the growing prominence of family and informal sources of help within that community care framework, have led to increasingly heavy burdens being placed on many relatives who receive little or no support with the day-to-day work of care-giving. Three different aspects of care-giving will be illustrated; the relative importance of each will vary according to the age and disability of the person who is being helped and the age and circumstances of family helpers.

The first is the sheer physical work that may be involved (Parker & Lawton, 1994), both directly (lifting, carrying, helping someone out of bed and up and down stairs) and indirectly (doing the extra laundry caused by incontinence, repairing damage to the home caused by a wheelchair or by someone who is mentally confused):

> To go to the town centre, I will have lifted her about eight times: out of the shower into the wheelchair, into the car, out of the car, and four more times to come home.
> *(Hicks, 1988: 168)*

A second consequence of care-giving is its impact on carers' social and psychological health. Stress, anxiety, depression and acute social isolation are frequently reported by those caring for disabled children, disabled spouses and frail elderly relatives alike:

> Just of lately, I cry for nothing. I can't understand it, I ought to be used to things but the least little thing and I'm sitting crying my heart out.
> *(Glendinning, 1983: 80)*

> You don't go anywhere, you don't do anything . . . it's like being in service, I got one evening off, Wednesday evening and one afternoon a month, on Sunday.
> *(Lewis & Meredith, 1988: 93)*

A third problem experienced by many working age people who are providing very substantial amounts of help to a disabled or frail elderly relative is, as with disabled people themselves, a greatly increased risk of poverty. Providing 20 hours or more a week of informal care increases significantly the chances of having to reduce hours of paid work or to stop work altogether (Green, 1988). Invalid Care Allowance, the social security benefit specifically for carers, is below the level of the means-tested benefit minimum 'safety net', and is received by only about one in ten carers who are providing upwards of 35 hours a week care (McLaughlin, 1991). A comparison of different types of financial support for informal care concluded that:

> compared with the other countries studied, the UK provides a relatively low level of cash allowances in support of informal care and these are received by relatively low proportions of the relevant populations.
> *(Glendinning & McLaughlin, 1993: 142)*

Moreover, because the incomes of disabled and elderly people are themselves so low, informal and family care-givers are also likely to have to contribute to some of the extra costs of the disabled person, particularly if they live in the same household; higher food and fuel bills, extra wear and tear on furniture, and cars and taxis to enable them and the person they are looking after to get out and about (Glendinning, 1992*c*). Reduced opportunities to earn and contribute to a pension, combined with this extra spending, increase the chances that carers will experience poverty themselves, especially if there is no employed earner in the household. Moreover, these risks of poverty are also likely to persist long after care-giving has ceased (Glendinning, 1992*c*; McLaughlin & Ritchie, 1994; Hancock & Jarvis, 1995).

The adequacy of health and personal social services

In recent years, disabled people have become increasingly critical of the piecemeal and uncoordinated manner in which personal care services are provided. Responsibilities are fragmented between different professionals, each with her/his own area of expertise, such as doctors, social workers, case managers, community nurses, psychiatric nurses, bathing assistants, home helps and personal aides, working from an increasingly wide range of health and personal social services organisations across the statutory, independent 'not-for-profit' and private commercial sectors. Problems of coordination between services are compounded by failures of communication between professionals and by the difficulties they experience in working in partnership with disabled people (Beardshaw, 1988; Fiedler, 1988):

> Many services are organised round the needs of the provider rather than those of the user. Statutory provision is usually restricted to 'office hours', with coverage limited or non-existent in the early mornings, evenings, at weekends and during holidays. Service delivery tends to be structured around predetermined tasks instead of user preferences and is often unpredictably timed . . . Those receiving services are often subject to a succession of interventions from a variety of people. The result is that disabled people are denied the right to organise their daily lives in the same way as the rest of the population. They have little or no control over who enters their homes or what professional helpers do once they get inside.
> *(Barnes, 1991: 143–4)*

One recent study found that services were unable to respond either to the particular requirements of individual disabled people, or to changes in those requirements. Indeed, far from enhancing independence, the levels and types of services which were provided imposed major restrictions on the lives of their disabled users. Statutory services were not available to help people leave or do anything outside their own homes (such as help with getting into and out of a car); home care services were increasingly restricted to personal care only, leaving disabled people unable to get their housework, laundry or shopping done; and community nurses were increasingly restricted to carrying out 'nursing' tasks only. Consequently, disabled people were forced to 'medicalise' their problems in order to get the help they needed, and felt very vulnerable to services being withdrawn altogether if they complained about the occasionally patronising, abusive or racist behaviour of the people who came into their homes (Morris, 1993*a*):

> Disabled people generally pay a price for those services, for example, invasions of privacy by a veritable army of professionals and having to accept the services the state thinks they should have or can afford, rather than those they know they need.
> *(Oliver & Barnes, 1991: 9)*

These difficulties of coordination and quality are only likely to increase with the development of the 'mixed economy of care' described above. Moreover, from 1993 applicants for day care, domiciliary and residential services must now undergo a detailed scrutiny of their individual and family circumstances by social workers and other professionals, as a prerequisite for deciding that 'publicly funded care can and should be arranged' (Department of Health, 1989: 18–21). This new assessment procedure constitutes an additional screening and 'gatekeeping' hurdle through which disabled people have to pass to secure the assistance and support they need, but without increasing in any way their involvement in, or control over, the services that are essential for their personal independence (Glendinning, 1992*c*).

Movements for change

Rather than dwelling on the failings of current social policies and the barriers and disadvantages which they create for disabled and elderly people, this final section will draw attention to the growing strength of organisations of disabled people and their families. This strength is reflected in the increasing involvement of disabled people in the planning of services, in the development of autonomous organisations of (rather than for) disabled people, and in coherent sets of proposals and demands for change.

The campaign for anti-discrimination legislation

Heartened by the success of campaigners in the USA, pressure has also grown in the UK for legislation to outlaw discrimination on the grounds of disability. Ideally this would cover areas such as employment, housing, contracts, services and access to buildings, transport and communication systems. It would address all those situations in which a person's disability is considered a sufficient reason for less favourable treatment. It would therefore encompass all 'special' provision and programmes for disabled people, barriers to full participation in society, and dependence on special social security payments.

While such a programme might appear somewhat idealistic, it should be noted that 1990 saw the passing of the Americans with Disabilities Act (ADA) by a Republican President and in the context of a society which historically has had a far greater commitment to deregulation than the UK. The ADA extended earlier legislation, which had banned discrimination by federally funded schemes or organisations, to cover discrimination within parts of the private sector as well. Employers with more than 15 workers, 'services, programmes or activities of a public entity' (ADA s.202), private sector services such as ships, cinemas, restaurants and schools, and telecommunications companies and equipment are all covered by the new US legislation, which also sets out clear definitions of unlawful discrimination.

In the UK, there were no fewer than nine attempts during the 1980s to get anti-discrimination legislation onto the statute books (Bynoe, 1991). Finally the Disability Discrimination Act was passed in 1995. This legislation aims to remove discrimination in employment and in relation to goods, facilities, services and transport. From April 1996, employers are obliged to adjust their working policies and environments accordingly; transport services are also to become more accessible. A newly created National Disability Council will have an advisory role in implementing the legislation.

Disabled campaigners, however, are disappointed at the limited scope of the UK legislation. The new legislation will depend on legal actions by individual disabled people to demonstrate that discrimination has occurred, and any changes in employment practices or working environments will be in response to an individual's specific needs. There are no requirements or incentives to make environments more 'user-friendly' or accessible to disabled people as a whole. No resources are available to help employers carry out workplace adaptations, other than in relation to the needs of a specific disabled individual (Thornton & Lunt, 1995).

Campaigners argue that to be fully effective, anti-discrimination legislation needs to be accompanied by Codes of Practice illustrating how the statutory concepts are applied; by clear minimum standards governing access to the built environment and communications systems; and by freedom of information legislation to open up the unofficial 'notes of guidance', correspondence and 'policy guidelines' which can determine the actual allocation of services and facilities (Oliver, 1990). In addition, there are doubts about how effectively the legislation can be enforced without the help of an independent rights commission, which would represent the views of disabled people, carry out research, produce enforceable Codes of Practice, recommend amendments to other existing legislation and provide resources and expertise for individual litigants.

The campaign for direct payments

Criticism of services provided by statutory health and social care organisations have led many disabled people in the UK to argue that, instead of providing (or purchasing) personal and domiciliary services themselves, local authorities should instead make cash payments directly to individual disabled people. These payments would enable disabled people themselves to purchase the particular services they require, when they require them and in a manner which is acceptable to them:

> If disabled people do not have control over the very basic activities of daily living then they cannot hope even to begin to participate in society on an equal basis . . . rather than being cared for, those who employ personal assistants are paying for tasks to be done which enable them to assert control over their lives.
> *(Morris, 1993b*: 162)

Although such payments were officially illegal until 1996 almost two-thirds of local authorities have admitted to making direct or indirect (i.e. through a third party) payments of this kind to disabled people (Browne, 1990). Furthermore, in some areas, organisations of disabled people have established support systems to help their members recruit and employ personal assistants. Again in response to pressure from disabled people, in December 1995 the government published legislation to allow local authorities to make direct payments with which disabled people could purchase the personal care services they require. At the time of writing (March 1996), however, it seemed likely that this legislation would remain permissive rather than mandatory, so that disabled people in some areas might still be unable to access a direct payments scheme. Older disabled people are likely to be excluded from the direct payments scheme which will also be restricted to cover a narrow range of services.

Advocacy and participation in services

A further development is the increasing expectation among disabled people and their organisations that they will be involved in discussions about the planning and delivery of services. Under the 1990 National Health Service and Community Care Act, local authorities are required to draw up plans of their community care services, in consultation with service users and carers. Since the preparation of the first set of community care plans in 1992, extensive publicity exercises have been carried out to inform disabled individuals and their organisations about the services in their area: public consultation meetings have been held; draft documents sent out for comment; and disabled people are increasingly represented on the working parties and teams that are responsible for drawing up the local community care plans (Bewley & Glendinning, 1994).

Underlying these developments are challenges by disabled people to the power which is often exerted by professionals in defining their needs and deciding how those needs should be met. This power is being challenged not only in relation to statutory services but in the voluntary sector also, where disabled people are also criticising the traditional approaches of charities which have hitherto been run by non-disabled people. Instead they are either demanding more involvement in these traditional service-providing organisations, or are setting up separate organisations which they themselves can control instead. Through advocacy and self-advocacy movements, people with learning disabilities are also gaining the necessary confidence and experience to take part in meetings about the services that they use and about the planning of new services (Brechin & Swain, 1987).

Conclusions

In conclusion, disabled people are, both in the UK and elsewhere, increasingly critical of social policies that are based on notions such as 'need', 'care' and 'protection'. Instead they are asserting their entitlements to services that are based on rights and active citizenship, rather than relying on a residual safety net of provision for 'deserving' or 'vulnerable' people. Rights are increasingly seen as providing a far better basis for delivering the 'choice' and 'independence' which have infused the rhetoric of social policy in the UK over the past decade.

References

Alcock, P. (1987). *Poverty and State Support*. Essex: Longman.

Alcock, P. (1993). *Understanding Poverty*. Basingstoke: Macmillan.

Arber, S., Gilbert, N. & Evandrou, M. (1989). Gender, household composition and receipt of domiciliary services by the elderly disabled. *Journal of Social Policy*, **17**, 153–75.

Baldwin, S., Bradshaw, J., Cooke, K. & Glendinning, C. (1981). The disabled person and cash benefits. In *Disability: Legislation and Practice*. ed. D. Guthrie. London: Macmillan.

Baloo, S., McMaster, I. & Sutton, K. (1986). *Statutory Sick Pay*. London and Leicester: Disability Alliance and Leicester Rights Centre.

Barnes, C. (1991). *Disabled People in Britain and Discrimination*. London: Hurst.

Beardshaw, V. (1988). *Last on the List; Community Services for People with Physical Disabilities*. London: King's Fund Institute.

Berthoud, R., Lakey, J. & McKay, R. (1993). *The Economic Problems of Disabled People*. London: Policy Studies Institute.

Bewley, C. & Glendinning, C. (1994). *Involving Disabled People in Community Care Planning*. York: Joseph Rowntree Foundation.

Brechin, A. & Swain, J. (1987). *Changing Relationships: Shared Action Planning with People with a Mental Handicap.* London: Harper Row.

Brown, L. (1990). *Survey of Local Authorities Direct Payments*. London: RADAR.

Bynoe, I. (1991). The case for Anti-Discrimination Legislation. In *Equal Rights for Disabled People*, ed. I. Bynoe, M. Oliver & C. Barnes. London: Institute for Public Policy Research.

Chetwynd, M. & Ritchie, J. in collaboration with Reith, L. & Howard, M. (1996). *The Cost of Care*. Joseph Rowntree Foundation, Bristol: Policy Press.

Common, R. & Flynn, N. (1992). *Contracting for Care*. York: Joseph Rowntree Foundation.

Department of Health and Social Security. (1985). *Reform of Social Security*, vols 1 and 2, Cmnd 9517 and Cmnd 9518. London: HMSO.

Department of Health. (1989). *Caring for People: Community Care in the Next Decade and Beyond*, Cmd 849. London: HMSO.

Department of Social Security. (1990). *The Way Ahead: Benefits for Disabled People*, Cm 917. London: HMSO.

Employment Gazette. (1990). Disabled Employees in the Public Sector, **98** 79–83.

Fiedler, B. (1988). *Living Options Lottery*. London: Prince of Wales Advisory Group on Disability.

Fimister, G. (1988). Leaving hospital after a long stay: the role and limitations of social security. In *Social Security and Community Care* ed. S. Baldwin, G. Parker & R. Walker. Aldershot: Gower.

Finch, J. (1989). *Family Obligations and Social Change*. Cambridge: Polity Press.

Fry, E. (1986). *An Equal Chance for Disabled People*? London: Spastics Society.

Gladstone D. (1985). 'Disabled people and employment'. *Social Policy and Administration*, **19**, 101–111.

Glendinning, C. (1983). *Unshared Care: Parents and their Disabled Children*. London: Routledge & Kegan Paul.

Glendinning, C. (1991). 'Losing ground'; social policy and disabled people in Great Britain, 1980–1990. *Disability Handicap and Society* **6**, 3–19.

Glendinning, C. (1992*a*). 'Community care': the financial consequences for women. In *Women and Poverty in Britain: the 1990s*, ed. C. Glendinning & J. Millar. Hemel Hempstead: Harvester Wheatsheaf.

Glendinning, C. (1992*b*). 'Residualism vs rights: social policy and disabled people'. In *Social Policy Review 4* ed. N. Manning & R. Page. Canterbury, Kent: Social Policy Association.

Glendinning, C. (1992*c*). *The Costs of Informal Care: Looking Inside the Household*. London: HMSO.

Glendinning, C. & McLaughlin, E. (1993). *Paying for Care: Lessons from Europe*. Social Security Advisory Committee Research Report 5. London: HMSO.

Graham, P., Jordan, A. & Lamb, B. (1990). *An Equal Chance? Or No Chance?* London: Spastics Society.

Green, H. (1988). *Informal Carers: Report from the 1985 General Household Survey, OPCS*. London: HMSO.

Hancock R. & Jarvis, C. (1995). *The Long Term Effects of Being a Carer*. Age Concern Institute of Gerontology. London: HMSO.

Hicks, C. (1988). *Who Cares*. London: Virago Press.

Large, P. (1991). Paying for the extra costs of disability. In *Disability and Social Policy* ed. G. Dalley. London: Policy Studies Institute.

Lewis, J. (1993). Developing the mixed economy of care: emerging issues for voluntary organisations. *Journal of Social Policy*, **22**, 173–92.

Lewis, J. & Meredith, B. (1988). *Daughters Who Care*. London: Routledge.

Lonsdale, S. (1986). *Work and Inequality*. London: Longman.

Lonsdale, S. (1990). *Women and Disability*. Basingstoke: Macmillan.

Matthews, A. & Truscott, P. (1990). *Disability, Household Income and Expenditure*. DSS Research Report 2. London: HMSO.

Martin J., White, A. & Meltzer, H. (1989). *Disabled Adults: Services, Transport and Employment*. OPCS. London: HMSO.

Martin, J. & White, A. (1988). *The Financial Circumstances of Disabled Adults living in Private Households*. OPCS. London: HMSO.

McCarthy, M. (1989). *The New Politics of Welfare*. Basingstoke: Macmillan.

McGlone, F. (1992). *Disability and Dependency in Old Age*. London: Family Policy Studies Centre.

McLaughlin E. (1991). *Social Security and Community Care: the Case of the Invalid Care Allowance*. DSS Research Report 4. London: HMSO.

McLaughlin, E. & Ritchie, J. (1994). Legacies of caring: the experience and circumstances of ex-carers. *Health and Social Care in the Community*, **2**, 241–54.

Mittler, P. (1993). Special needs at the crossroads. In *Special Education in Britain after Warnock* ed. J. Visser and G. Upton. London: David Fulton Publishers.

Morris, J. (1993*a*). *Community Care or Independent Living?* York: Joseph Rowntree Foundation.

Morris, J. (1993*b*). *Independent Lives? Community Care and Disabled People*. Basingstoke: Macmillan.

National Consumer Council. (1995). *Charging Consumers for Social Services; Local Authority Policy and Practice*. London: NCC.

Oliver, M. (1990). *The Politics of Disablement*. Basingstoke: Macmillan.

Oliver, M. & Barnes, C. (1991). Discrimination, disability and welfare: from needs to rights. In *Equal Rights for Disabled People* ed. I. Bynoe, M. Oliver & C. Barnes. London: Institute for Public Policy Research.

Parker, G. (1990). *With Due Care and Attention*. London: Family Policy Studies Centre.

Parker, G. & Lawton D. (1994). *Different Types of Care; Different Types of Carer*. Social Policy Research Unit. London: HMSO.

Qureshi, H. & Walker, A. (1989). *The Caring Relationship*. Basingstoke: Macmillan.

Stokes, A. (1981). The disabled person's mobility. In *Disability: Legislation and Practice* ed. D. Guthrie. London: Macmillan.

Swan, W. (1991). *Variations between LEAs in Levels of Segregation in Special Schools 1981–1990: Preliminary Report*. London: Centre for Studies on Integration in Education.

Thornton, P. & Lunt N. (1995). Working to rule. *Community Care*, **1080**, 21.

Topliss, E. (1979). *Provision for the Disabled*. Oxford: Blackwell & Robertson.

Walker, A. (1981). Disability and income. In *Disability in Britain* ed. A. Walker & P. Townsend. Oxford: Martin Robertson.

Walker, A. (1990). The benefits of old age? In *Age: The Unrecognised Discrimination* ed. E. McEwan. London: Age Concern England.

Walker, A. & Walker, L. (1991). Disability and financial need: the failure of the social security system. In *Disability and Social Policy* ed. G. Dalley. London: Policy Studies Institute.

Warnock, M. (1993). Foreword. In *Special Education in Britain after Warnock* ed. G. Upton & J. Visser. London: David Fulton Publishers.

Welfare Rights Bulletin April 1994; February 1995. London: Child Poverty Action Group.

11

Principles of the acquisition of sensorimotor skills

D. LINDSAY McLELLAN

Introduction

Learning, the acquisition of cognitive skills and the acquisition of sensorimotor skills are all functions of the brain. Although it is convenient to separate them when discussing the range of activities encountered in rehabilitation, the mechanisms involved are likely to have many similarities and to overlap with each other. The term 'sensorimotor' has been chosen rather than 'motor' to emphasise the importance of the integration of sensory and motor activity in all motor skills. All require feedback of performance detected through sensory mechanisms such as touch, pressure, joint position, velocity of movement, muscle tension, vision and hearing. Even at a neuronal level, there are individual neurones which fire under a range of such highly specific conditions that their function cannot be categorised as exclusively motor or exclusively sensory (Jeannerod, 1994).

This chapter will concentrate on sensorimotor skill as a practical and clinical phenomenon in rehabilitation, and a priority for rehabilitation research. Schmidt's '*Motor Control and Learning*' (1988) is recommended reading for those wishing to pursue this topic in more depth; further suggestions will be found in the bibliography at the end of the chapter.

The final common path of any movement is activation of motor neurones producing a particular pattern of muscular contraction and (as appropriate) movement of joints. Some aspects of motor performance will depend on the integrity and efficiency of these physiological and biomechanical processes. Many other factors that affect performance reside with the central nervous system (CNS) and skill is only one of these. Separating fluctuations of **performance** from the presence or absence of **skill** is one of the fundamental conceptual and practical challenges of research into the acquisition of skill.

In all mammals, the nervous system continues to develop after birth and, in humans, the fully adult pattern of conductivity and myelination is not complete until approximately the age of 18 years. During this time, the range and complexity of motor functions progressively increases and many of these functions are 'innate', the neuronal connectivity that underpins them being largely preprogrammed genetically. Such programmed growth and reshaping of connectivity is susceptible to focal or diffuse brain damage. The experiences and sensory environment of the animal during development are also crucial to establishing a capacity for a normal range of activity in adult life. Clearly such development provides the mechanisms through which skills are developed, but changes in performance which reflect only such maturational processes are not normally regarded as evidence of an acquired skill.

Similarly, as the brain begins to age, performance in motor skills gradually deteriorates. Is such deterioration to be regarded as evidence of loss of **skill** or as loss of the basic physical capacity to **perform** at the previous level?

In addition to these broad and continuous changes that affect all of us, a wide range of individual factors operate to produce different levels of performance in each individual. Many of these appear to be genetically determined and are intrinsic 'givens' in the individual. Detailed study can identify a range of highly specific elements of cognitive, motor and sensory function underlying such differences. Other differences between individuals reflect the state of nutrition and experiences of the subject during growth. Yet others reflect the cognitive and emotional state of the individual at the time of performance, i.e. factors such as alertness, tiredness, concentration and motivation. As regards skill, the degree of skill that can be acquired for different tasks varies between individuals, apparently reflecting the combined effects of inherent individual characteristics and the nature of any practice that has been undertaken.

Different factors appear to become important and some subsequently decline in importance as higher levels of skill are progressively acquired. Given all these different individual starting points, the pathways and the strategies used by individuals as they acquire a skill are likely to reflect individual as well as species-specific characteristics.

Learning and skill

Schmidt (1988: 346) defined motor learning as 'A set of processes associated with practice or experience leading to relatively permanent changes in the capability for responding'. The events leading to this response may be external to the individual, such as an approaching cricket ball, or deriving from a willed act, such as playing a tune from memory. Clearly not all improvements in performance can be attributed to skills and as Schmidt conceded, the word 'relatively' in his definition is open to negotiation. He went on to illustrate the difference between performance and skill by comparing the process of freezing and reheating water (in which the water's performance changes but returns to baseline once it is reheated) with that of boiling and cooling an egg. Boiling produces a relatively permanent change in the egg : a boiled egg will not return to its baseline condition when it is cooled.

The word 'capability' is also important, emphasising the provisional nature of skilled performance, which remains to some extent susceptible to transient internal and external conditions. It is crucially important to control such conditions in any study of skill acquisition.

Motor performance improves with practice, although it may be difficult to define exactly what has been learnt. A proficient skater can travel at speeds and follow trajectories impossible for a novice. The activity, however, does not simply express a different pattern of motor activity, but also provides a completely different set of expectations and sensory experiences for the skilled skater. How important is the learning and recognition of aspects of this **sensory** experience (the lateral stability of the blade of the skate, the inward lean of the trunk on cornering, the pattern of visual feedback experienced, the irregularity of the ice's surface detected by vibration of the blade) as opposed to the marshalling of appropriate patterns of muscular activity? To go further, a skater who obtains a score of 10 for 'artistic expression' in a competition has performed differently from one who scored only six, but is this difference an expression of greater sensorimotor skill?

In most areas of rehabilitation, such high performance tasks are rarely on the agenda. It may be that what is being required is a fairly basic activity, being in fact a re-acquisition of a previously acquired function, such as standing up. Alternatively, the goal may be to acquire a new skill because the function cannot be performed in its original manner, such as walking with a stick. Components of activities such as walking are not normally monitored closely by conscious attention; indeed an activity such as walking is so complex that it is impossible to monitor consciously more than a small proportion of what is going on at any one time. Other tasks such as tracking tasks (popular with experimenters because of the ease with which experimental conditions can be controlled) may involve a comparatively restricted repertoire of motor and sensory activity and highly focused degree of attention to motor aspects of the task.

The way a task is formulated and the selection of performance goals will inevitably influence the identity of the skills that are actually acquired.

Predicting skill acquisition

Although the capacity to acquire a sensorimotor skill will depend on intrinsic attributes of the subject's CNS, it is obvious that physical and biomechanical constraints may place a lower ceiling on this possible range of performance. In doing so, such restraints might of course alter the nature of the task. This greatly complicates the design of studies in which groups of impaired subjects are compared with normal subjects.

In normal subjects, the capacity to acquire a skill cannot reliably be predicted from aptitude tests even when a battery of tests is used (Schmidt 1988: 464–466); however, performance after training in complex psychomotor tasks that are selected on the basis of logical similarities with a criterion task may improve the accuracy of prediction. In other words, the best predictor of learning ability on a complex task may be the capacity to learn a battery of simpler but relevant tasks.

In rehabilitation, it would be very helpful to be able to predict the outcome of a course of training for individual patients or indeed for groups of patients. To date, such attempts have tended to concentrate on biological predictors of natural recovery of the CNS or biomechanical function (see D. Lindsay McLellan, Chapter 1) and have not drawn on the empirical insights and skills of the therapists, still less on some of the more sophisticated motor and sensory training tasks that have been explored, for example, in attempts to predict suitability for training as a pilot (Adams, 1953).

Performance curves and phases of skill acquisition

A reliable characteristic of sensorimotor skill acquisition is the shape of the performance curve during learning (Figure 11.1). After a variable period in which the subject 'settles in' and learns an initial understanding of the task, practice is accompanied by progressive improvement in performance. Rapid at first, it slows exponentially so that when performance is plotted against the number of practice sessions on a log-log axis, the result approximates to a straight line. For most practice purposes a ceiling is reached, but close inspection shows that in normal subjects, for some tasks, very small increments in performance continue to be possible after years of practice involving millions of repetitions (Crossman, 1959). It is quite possible that similar findings would be demonstrated in pathological conditions if sufficiently critical observations were made.

That is not to say, of course, that such changes would be of much practical relevance in either case. An operative who makes a cigar in 6.9 seconds is in the

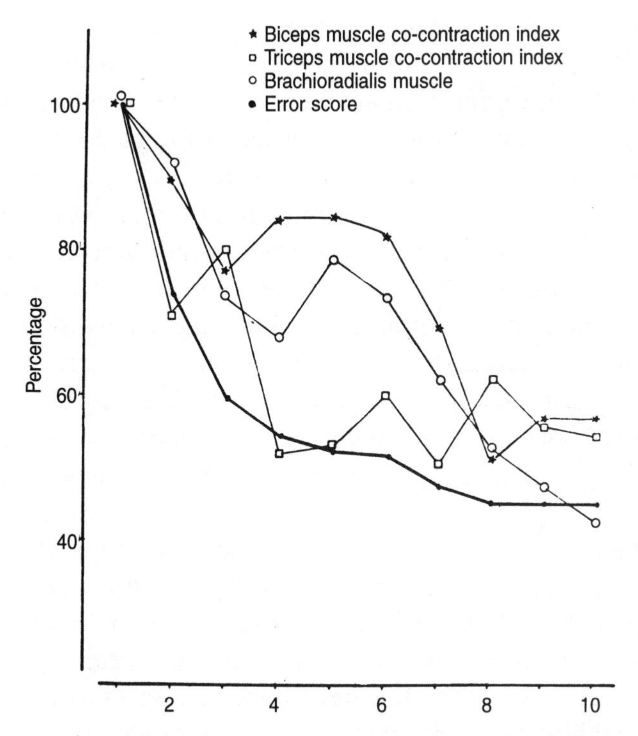

Figure 11.1. Accuracy and indices of coactivation in normal subjects performing an upper limb tracking task (*y* axis) over a period of ten trials (*x* axis) after a brief familiarisation phase. Accuracy (integrated distance from target) increased progressively. Initially this was achieved by increased levels of coactivation but then coactivation progressively declined, so that towards the end of the sequence of training, both the biochemical and metabolic cost factors were becoming optimised. The target moved sinusoidally at 0.64 Hz. The mean data from 12 normal subjects has been normalised to a percentage of the levels obtained in the first recording session. Reproduced from Hassan (1987).

same performance bracket as one who takes 7.2 seconds, even though it may have taken three years practice with 50 million cigars to achieve the faster rate. In all activities there will inevitably be a trade-off between the cost of practice (including opportunity costs) and the practical value of the resulting improvement in performance.

Studies of the process by which a skill continues to develop suggested that the process occurs in three stages (Fitts, 1964; Fitts & Posner, 1967). These phases have been termed the cognitive, associative and autonomous phases (Schmidt, 1988: 460–461). They overlap each other but are important because they may require different intrinsic attributes and probably call for different approaches from the teacher or trainer.

The first or cognitive phase is one of erratic but rapid progress in which the task and the basic cognitive and biomechanical strategies necessary to achieve it are tried out and understood. Training techniques such as demonstration, watching video tapes, verbal rehearsal, cognitive processing and guidance are likely to be helpful.

In the associative phase, the subject has established the most effective general strategy of doing the task and starts to make more subtle adjustments so that performance is more consistent. The rate of improvement is less than in the cognitive phase. The combination of reliability with being some distance from the ceiling of performance makes this stage a popular one to study. It is during the associative stage that most progress is made towards the reduction of redundant coactivation between antagonist muscles, allowing the movement to be achieved with lower levels of expenditure of energy and thus reduced fatigue. (Figure 11.1).

Some level of cognitive monitoring is still necessary, so that performance falls off if the subject's attention is distracted by a secondary task. A commentary on the manner with which the task is being undertaken and advice about performance and targets may be helpful, together with advice and training on the early and precise detection of error and deviation from the target, so improving the subject's ability to monitor their own performance. Some cognitive monitoring is still necessary because the performance falls off if the subjects' attention is distracted by a secondary task. Being fully familiar with the nature of the sensory feedback that is anticipated appears to be helpful. It may be held as an internalised memory or template serving both as a continuous target and a 'comparator' for monitoring performance. This principle is used by musical soloists in memorising the pieces that are to be played. Memorising the performance of the more advanced player may not only help to monitor ones own performance but accelerate the development of skill, as in the Suzuki method of learning to play the violin.

In the autonomous phase, the skill itself occupies less cognitive attention and monitoring; many of the sensory and motor components are delegated to subconscious levels of integration. For example, an experienced but preoccupied driver may find that he has driven to work without any recollection of having attended to road conditions or of his response to them. Extreme examples of this type of delegation are quoted by Schmidt, notably the reported ability of a concert pianist to do mental arithmetic while sight reading and playing piano music (Schmidt, 1988:461). Teaching to refine this level of skill still further may involve appealing to some cognitive experience or sense of effort related, perhaps, to the emotional or aesthetic qualities of the task. Clearly this is likely to be very demanding on the teacher and will need a well-developed sensitivity to the nature of the subjective experiences that are being encountered while undertaking the task. The latter requirement creates obvious difficulties in rehabilitation, where a therapist may have to instruct a patient with, for example, a congenital disorder of movement, in the absence of any direct personal experience of the pattern of sensations or cognitive modelling that is forming the patient's experience.

Transfer of skills

To what extent are motor skills transferable to other activities? The answer appears to be disappointingly little. Some highly skilled activities such as playing a musical instrument may involve basic sequences such as current and fast repeated flexion and extension of adjacent digits (trilling) or precise temporal coordination between the two hands at a range of different speeds or frequencies. As a general rule, however, each element of a task must be practised in a specific context and time frame before there is a reliable 'increase in the capacity to respond'.

When studying the acquisition of easier skills, it may be impossible to find out whether elements within a task are actually fragments of previously acquired skills or related sensory, motor or integrated components of the new task.

Factors influencing the effectiveness of practice

'Shadowing' or guidance

The studies of the effects of different conditions of practice are complicated by the need to separate a change in performance from a change in skill. Although intuitively it may seem obvious that establishing optimal performance during practice would provide a better springboard for further increments in skill, this is not always the case. For example, 'guidance', involving shadowing or support of the target movement by an instructor, can improve performance but resuming the task without guidance after an interval may show that less skill has been acquired than under unguided or 'discovery' (trial and error) conditions (Singer & Pease, 1976). On the other hand, such guidance may be essential early in the acquisition of a skill in order to provide reassurance and reduce the level of anxiety in a subject. This often applies in rehabilitation where, for example, a subject may feel at risk of falling. This underlies the importance of careful analysis of what the task involves or means to the subject.

Understanding and motivation

It is essential that the subject understands both which aspects of performance are desirable or 'right' and which are undesirable or 'wrong' and also how performance will be measured. The tasks should have a meaning and value to the subject and the performance of it must not appear impossibly out of reach. In rehabilitation a leap of faith is often demanded of a subject who may be frightened, confused or angry and find it difficult to accept the need to attempt the task or to undertake the activity in the manner desired by the therapist. Time has to be spent in gauging these factors and establishing trust and understanding before training starts, and continuing into the early stages of training. Behaviour modification techniques may help here, especially through the mechanisms of suggestion and personal support provided by peers tackling similar problems.

Feedback of performance

In describing the overlapping phases of skill acquisition (see earlier) attention is drawn to the need for preparatory information and feedback that is both timely and appropriate to the understanding and experiences of the subject and to the degree of skill that has been acquired. As with the acquisition of cognitive skills (see Chapter 12), feedback that requires processing by the subject appears to be more effective in enhancing performance than feedback that is received passively. When tasks are practised in clusters of short sessions, the subject may acquire a superficial facility based on an immediate 'memory' of what has just been carried out and the performance is then repeated, as it were, without thinking, without any deeper processing by the subject. This is not dissimilar to very short-term or 'echoic' memory for words or numbers. After a short break from practice, such superficial facility will be lost. This is probably not the same phenomenon as the improvement that occurs in the 'warm up' period of a few minutes that is often needed after a break in practice (and after the interpolation of different tasks) to attune skilled subjects to resume a familiar task.

Self-monitoring

The overall aim is for subjects to acquire: (a) the means to monitor their own performance, and (b) an internal concept or comparator against which such feedback can be judged. 'General encouragement' is likely to be helpful at all stages of skill acquisition in raising motivation and lessening anxiety. It is important, however, to combine this with clarity and precision of feedback on performance. For example, a patient learning to walk again after a stroke might find it difficult to interpret 'well done!' and even associate it with an unwanted component such as effort-related spasm of the attempt to walk unless the praise is specifically linked to relevant feedback, for example 'Well done, you've put weight on your left foot'. It is likely that the specific abilities of the patient will influence the ease with which various modalities of feedback can be processed, for example vision, hearing, touch or sense of movement. The same probably applies to mental imaging. Providing optimal feedback to an individual thus calls for considerable perceptiveness and sustained motivation on the part of the therapist.

Goal setting

Many studies have demonstrated the effectiveness of goal setting and enhancing both performance and the acquisition of skill. Goal setting probably involves two factors: focusing of attention on outcome, and the strength and belief of the possibility of success. It may also of course improve the focus of effort for the therapist as well. For goal setting to have these effects, it must be a mutual and negotiated process that has the active assent of the subject. In addition, it is essential that the goal is formulated in terms that define precisely the point at which it will have been reached. In rehabilitation, the difficulty in predicting outcome is sometimes used as a pretext for failing to set precise goals. Instead, vague aims are espoused such as 'to improve standing balance' or 'to enhance communication'. The impossibility of identifying the point at which vague aims have been reached is likely to result in: (a) suboptimal expectations and performance in the subject, and (b) stagnation in the development of skills in the therapist.

Evidence of the importance of this in training children with cerebral palsy is presented in Chapter 15, describing a study in which the setting of precise goals rather than vague aims was almost as powerful a determinant of progress as quadrupling the number of physiotherapy sessions (Bower *et al.*, 1996). Performance in activities that could be incorporated into the child's daily life continued to improve when therapy was withdrawn. By contrast, activities that were dependent on active participation by the therapist declined as soon as therapy was withdrawn.

Quantity and distribution (patterns) of practice sessions

Many studies of normal subjects have shown that performance curves are steeper when practice is distributed, i.e. when periods of non-practice time lasting hours or days are inserted between the practice sessions. This suggests that crowding practice sessions together makes them less effective; however, the relatively better performance in the last practice session of a programme of distributed practice is not in itself proof that a greater skill has been acquired. There does appear to be an element of fatigue when practice takes place in blocks rather than being distributed, and this fatigue could mask the degree of skill that has been acquired.

The time over which the whole sequence of practice sessions occurs may itself be an important factor in skill acquisition. Thus when two subjects, whose performance has diverged because one had continuous and the other had distributed practice sessions, are given a break and the task resumed a set period of time after the first practice session, their performance may become much closer, although distributed practice will always tend to be associated with a slightly better result.

There does not appear to be a general rule or principle that can predict the optimal duration, repetition rate or number of practice sessions for all subjects during any particular task or for any one subject doing all tasks. There may well be optimal patterns of practice for individuals in relation to specific tasks. Unfortunately it is often the case in rehabilitation practice (at least in the UK) that the pattern of practice offered to the patient is a pragmatic compromise between what the patient is expected to benefit from, what is available, and custom and habit among members of the rehabilitation team. Yet we should be aiming for a logical selection of practice patterns similar to the spacing of doses of drugs which is (ideally at least) based on a knowledge of the pharmacokinetics of the drug in the individual patient.

In the laboratory it is easy to study single tasks but in rehabilitation it would be unusual for a patient's therapy to be restricted to a single task. Studies of subjects without cognitive impairment learning more than one task suggests that having to switch attention and readjust to different tasks makes practice in each task more rather than less effective. This may be because the process of changing from one to another increases the degree of processing involved. 'Random practice' in which different tasks are practised in random order is more effective than practising each task in separate blocks, even when the number of sessions and overall duration of practice are controlled. Such considerations might not necessarily apply to subjects with disorders of memory or attention.

Observation and mental rehearsal

Humans, like other animals, can acquire a degree of sensorimotor skill by watching others perform a task. Much of this is probably concerned with understanding and reflecting on the nature of the task. Exactly what is learnt is likely to reflect the current level of skill in the person who is watching, and the skill of the performer. A novice may miss much of the 'message' that the moderately skilled person would acquire from watching a highly skilled one. A highly skilled performer, on the other hand, may obtain little or no benefit from watching a novice.

In recent years the phenomenon of 'mental rehearsal' has received increasing attention, especially in relation to professional sport where it is claimed that mental rehearsal enhances performance and can offset much of the decline in the performance that would otherwise occur during periods of abstinence, such as incapacity after injury. The mental rehearsal has to be precise to be effective and also has to be conducted in 'real time' and with the full concentration of the subject. For example, mentally rehearsing in real time a standard training programme that is very familiar to the subject (such as a professional footballer's daily training regime) involves imagining running a particular distance or performing a set of particular exercises occupying as nearly as possible the same time in the imagination as the task itself would take in reality. Attempts to invoke the flexibility of dreaming, when two miles can either be covered in a few seconds or appear to take all night, renders the practice ineffective. Some reports present evidence of a reduction in the amount of muscle wasting and enhanced metabolic efficiency of muscles that are relevant to such mental rehearsal in the absence of any electromyographic activity in the muscles during rehearsal (Yue & Cole, 1992; Decety *et al.*, 1993).

Some athletes have claimed particularly striking results from this technique and while a degree of scepticism may be justified, the evidence that mental rehearsal can accelerate the development of skill is now incontrovertible. This raises the intriguing possibility that one reason why some performers excel in an activity is that they spend much more time (or are much more efficient) than others in mental rehearsal.

These phenomena have received indirect support from recent neurophysiological work showing that individual neurones may be highly task specific and fire when an animal does a task with the eyes closed or when seeing another animal perform the task, but in no other condition (Jeannerod, 1994). If it is the case that the same neuronal network is activated in physical practice as in mental rehearsal, then hypotheses could be developed with which to test and link biological theory with rehabilitation practice in the same framework.

Clinical implications for skill acquisition in people with physical and cognitive impairments

An understanding of learning and skill acquisition is fundamental to the conceptual basis of rehabilitation. As we have seen, it has direct relevance to practice in the way that subjects are assessed, interacted with and monitored. As with learning and memory generally, patients with conceptual and perceptive impairments as well as physical or motor ones are at a double disadvantage when attempting to acquire a skill. If they cannot remember the stimulus of random practice, it may lead (as in other memory tasks in amnesic subjects) to consolidation of errors. 'Errorless learning' or guidance strategies may have to be adopted instead (Chapter 12). Slower acquisition of skills would be better than failing to learn at all, or learning an erroneous strategy.

A patient who cannot attend or is distracted, or lacks the ability to think, will lack the ability to process feedback or to make full use of the practice time and will not be able to engage in effective mental rehearsal. A lack of sensation or awareness of part of the body makes it impossible to 'imagine' the affected part so that mental rehearsal might be very difficult if not impossible. Perceptual difficulties may also impair the subject's ability to monitor performance and its results, and alternative less effective strategies may have to be developed.

These factors are exemplified by the recovery of motor function that occurs in patients with acquired hemiparesis from a lesion affecting the non-dominant parietal lobe. Recovery is slower than in patients with a comparable lesion of the dominant hemisphere. Recovery does occur and a similar level of skill is eventually acquired, but it takes longer.

Disorders of the motor system

What implications do these phenomena have for those with CNS disorders affecting the 'motor' system such as parkinsonism, dystonia or spasticity? It is certainly the case that people with parkinsonism can acquire new motor skills, improving their level of performance in simple manual tasks by a percentage similar to that of normal subjects doing the same amount of practice (Table 11.1). Whether they can re-acquire by practice a skill that has been lost (such as turning over in bed) because of a disease is less certain. It may be that a strategy has to be learned for doing this that is different from that intuitively employed, much as strategies for those with specific cognitive impairments usually involve working round the impairment rather than reversing it.

Table 11.1 *Percentage impairments in performance in a complex manual tracking task using an instrumented pen giving an auditory feedback of downward pressure against the paper.*

	Mean percentage improvement in measures of:		
	Accuracy	Pressure	Speed
Cases	55.3	65.6	17.9
Controls	56.5	71.0	20.1
Outcome of paired '*t*'-test	NS	NS	NS

Eight subjects with parkinsonism compared with eight normal controls (the spouses of the subjects). Although the absolute levels of function were at least twice as good in the controls throughout the four sessions of training, the differences in percentage improvement were not statistically different.
NS, not significant.
Source: Martin (1990).

Can practice be harmful?

Apart from 'wear and tear' on peripheral nerves and musculoskeletal structures, practice is rarely harmful. A possible exception to this general rule are the focal dystonias, especially the occupational dystonic cramps such as writer's cramp. They are of exceptional interest because of the apparent breakdown of the normal sequence of motor events that occur in affected individuals when a skill is regularly practised. Focal occupational dystonias tend to occur in individuals who have undergone considerable amounts of skilled practice over long periods of time, after which the usual pattern of minimal muscular coactivation with optimal biomechanical efficiency is gradually replaced by increasing and inappropriate muscular coactivation. Initially this is restricted to the muscles involved in this specific index task, but later it extends to involve adjacent muscle groups and starts to occur in tasks other than index tasks (Hughes & McLellan, 1985). What is the sequence of events that causes such a maladaptive response? It certainly appears to be irreversible, for the only way that function can be preserved in occupational focal dystonias is to adopt an obviously different movement strategy for performing the task or even to abstain from undertaking the task at all.

It is of interest that the most sensitive simple test of dexterity in suspected disorders of the basal ganglia or central motor pathways is to drum the middle and index fingers so that one finger extends and the other flexes simultaneously and then rapidly reverses. This is likely to involve the cerebral cortex maximally activating one set of highly localised motor neurones and simultaneously inhibiting another immediately adjacent set. At other times these two sets will often be coactivated in a range of different combinations as in writing, using tools or grasping and releasing the hand. This implies a very complex range of interactions between inhibition and facilitation neurones adjacent to each other both in the brain and in the spinal cord.

Personal and emotional barriers to skill acquisition

In conclusion, the complexities of sensorimotor skill acquisition bring home the importance of understanding a patient's psychological and philosophical situation when rehabilitation is attempted. A patient who is in a state of psychological shock, fear and denial will not be able to identify or work constructively to reasonable objectives, will not be able to give high-quality sustained attention to therapy, and will be most unlikely to spend free waking hours reflecting on goals and performance, or engaging in mental rehearsal. The 'late start' that some individuals show in their recovery from an acutely disabling illness such as stroke is likely to reflect the operation of at least some of these very human experiences.

References

Adams, J. A. (1953). The prediction of performance at advanced stages of training on a complex psychomotor task (Research Bulletin 53–49). Texas Lackland Air Force Base: Human Resources Research Center (Quoted by Schmidt, 1988).

Bower, E., McLellan, D. L., Arney, J. & Campbell, M.J. (1996). A randomised controlled trial of different intensities of physiotherapy and different goal-setting procedures in 44 children with cerebral palsy. *Developmental Medicine and Child Neurology*, **38**, 226–37.

Crossman, E. R. F. W. (1959). A theory of the acquisition of speed skill. *Ergonomics*, **2**, 153–66.

Decety, J., Jeannerod, M., Durozard, D. & Bavaret, G. (1993). Central activation of autonomic effectors during mental simulation of motor actions. *Journal of Physiology*, **461**, 549–63.

Fitts, P. M. (1964). Perceptual motor skills learning. In *Categories of Human Learning* ed. A. W. Melton. (pp. 243–85). New York: Academic Press.

Fitts, P. M. & Posner, M. I. (1967). *Human Performance*. Belmont CA: Brooks and Cole.

Hassan, N. H. (1987). *Muscle activation during repetitive movements in normal and spastic man*. PhD thesis, University of Southampton.

Hughes, M. & McLellan, D. L. (1985). Increased coactivation of the upper limb muscles in writer's cramp. *Journal of Neurology, Neurosurgery and Psychiatry*, **48**, 782–7.

Jeannerod, M. (1994). The representing brain : neural correlates of motor intention and imagery. *Behavioural and Brain Sciences*, **17**, 187–245.
Martin, M. (1990). *Acquiring a Skill in Parkinson's Disease*. Fourth year undergraduate student's project dissertation, University of Southampton.
Schmidt, R. A. (1988). *Motor Control and Learning. A Behavioural Emphasis*, 2nd edn. Champaign, IL: Human Kinetics Publishers.
Singer, R. N. & Pease, D. (1976). Effects of guided versus discovery learning strategies on learning, retention and transfer of a social motor task. *Research Quarterly*, **47**, 788–96.
Yue, G. & Cole, K. J. (1992). Strength increases from the motor program. Comparison of training with maximal voluntary and imagined muscle contractions. *Journal of Neurophysiology*, **67**, 1114–23.

Further reading

Catania, A. C. (1992). *Learning*, 3rd edn. London: Prentice Hall.
Delwaide, P. J. & Young, R. R. (ed) (1985). *Clinical Neurophysiology in Spasticity*. Amsterdam: Elsevier (Biomedical Division).
Rothwell, J. (1994). *Control of Human Voluntary Movement*, 2nd edn. London: Chapman and Hall.
Waxman, S. G. (ed) (1988). *Functional Recovery in Neurological Disease. Advances in Neurology, Vol. 47*. New York: Raven Press.

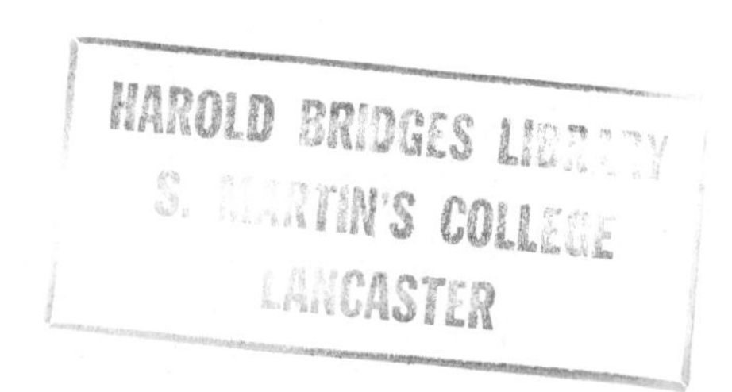

12

Management of acquired cognitive disorders

BARBARA A. WILSON

What is cognition?

Cognition refers to processes involved in knowing, understanding, learning, perceiving, remembering, judging and thinking. These can be contrasted with physical, behavioural or emotional processes although it is not always easy to separate them, particularly when they may in some circumstances interact with each other. Judging whether a person is exercising a cognitive or some other process, simply by observing behaviour, is not at all easy. For example, memory-impaired people who keep repeating the same question may be doing so because of anxiety (an emotional problem), or because they have forgotten they have already asked the question (a cognitive problem), or because they see that it is annoying for those around them and find this rewarding (a behavioural problem).

It is not easy to see beyond the physical manifestations of problems in order to recognise underlying cognitive failures. Consider, for example, apraxia which is a disorder of movement not resulting from paralysis, weakness or a failure to understand what is required. Hence a patient with apraxia may be unable to carry out a movement or a sequence of movements despite having the necessary strength and range of motion to do so. The failure is in fact at the level of organising, planning or sequencing of movements, and to determine whether someone has apraxia it is necessary to exclude paralysis, weakness and poor comprehension as explanations. An accurate diagnosis is made even more complicated in the case of brain-injured people who may have all of these processes impaired in combination with the apraxia.

Even when we are clear that a patient has a cognitive problem it may require further investigation to determine its exact nature. Suppose a patient fails to complete a block design task accurately after being given four blocks and asked to copy a design. We know the patient understands what is required, can see adequately and has no motor deficits. The failure could have many causes, such as visual perceptual deficit (failure to interpret the visual stimulus adequately), a planning deficit, a difficulty localising objects in space, a spatial orientation problem (an inability to orient the blocks in the same direction as those in the stimulus), or to a number of other things. The cognitive deficit responsible for the impaired performance on the block design task can best be determined by neuropsychological assessment.

Cognitive deficits after brain injury

To a large extent the part(s) of the brain affected by a particular accident, illness, infection or insult will determine the nature of the cognitive deficits. Cognitive functions tend to be located mainly on one or other side of the brain. In most people the left side is more important for language skills and the right side more important for spatial and perceptual skills. This is unlike movement where both the left and right sides of the brain are equally important for contralateral movements.

In addition to differences between the left and right cerebral hemispheres, there are differences within hemispheres. People with anterior lesions of the left hemisphere will have different language problems from those with more posterior lesions.

For brain-damaged people with unilateral, focal lesions the cognitive problems may be restricted to one particular skill or set of skills such as difficulty with expressive speech or impairment in face recognition. For many brain-injured people, however, and particularly those with a severe head injury or anoxia, the damage will be diffuse, resulting in a number of different problems. Head-injured people, for example, frequently have attention, planning and organisation problems resulting from frontal lobe damage. Memory functioning is also frequently impaired.

Some of the rare visuoperceptual and visuospatial difficulties are likely to result from anoxia following carbon monoxide poisoning or an anaesthetic accident, although they may also be seen after encephalitis, stroke or head injury.

Some of the major cognitive deficits are described below.

Language problems

Aphasia (or **dysphasia**) is the term used for a language disorder. A language disorder may be classified in several ways but there are two main types known as disorders of production (**expressive dysphasia**) and disorders of comprehension (**receptive dysphasia**). In expressive dysphasia the person has difficulty in producing speech. If the injury has affected the speech mechanisms themselves (for example the tongue or voice box) the condition is known as **dysarthria**. If it affects the area in the brain that is responsible for producing the correct sounds it is sometimes known as **Broca's aphasia**.

Another expressive disorder is caused by difficulty in choosing the correct word. This is often known as **anomia**. Word finding problems are seen in most language-impaired people. Another common problem is the production of an unintended word, phrase or sound when attempting to speak. For example, 'My little girl' for 'Her little boy', or 'trubs' instead of 'shrubs'. This condition is known as **paraphasia**.

Dysphasic patients often have difficulty with grammar or the structure of language, and may say something like 'My speech no sense' instead of 'My speech makes no sense'. This problem is known as **agrammaticism**. A less common problem occurs when a person cannot repeat words or numbers although in other ways that person can understand language and communicate normally. This repetition deficit is called **conduction aphasia**.

When the disorder affects understanding rather than expression of language then there is a problem in attaching meaning to words. This condition is known as **Wernicke's aphasia**. People with this problem may speak at great length but much of what they say does not make sense. They may also have difficulty in writing correctly.

If the problem of understanding speech is the result of **word deafness** (a rare condition in which speech does not sound like language at all but sounds like a meaningless noise) then reading and writing will not be affected and speech will be normal or nearly normal. In practice most language-impaired people will have both expressive and receptive deficits to some extent.

Reading and writing problems

People who have problems understanding or producing speech usually have problems with reading, writing and calculating. These latter conditions are known as **alexia** (or **dyslexia**) **agraphia** (or **dysgraphia**) and **acalculia** (or **discalculia**). Sometimes they will be unable to read whole words but will be able to read individual letters of a word and so can *understand* the printed word. Because they have to read letter-by-letter their reading is very slow. This condition is known as **letter-by-letter reading** or **alexia without agraphia** (i.e. absence of reading without absence of writing). People with this difficulty can write reasonably well although they are unable to read back what they have written.

Another kind of dyslexia occurs when people are able to read regularly spelled words such as 'mint' and 'beak' but not words spelled irregularly like 'pint' or 'steak'. 'Pint' will be read as it rhymes with 'mint' and 'steak' with 'beak'. This condition is known as **surface dyslexia** (words are read according to their surface structure or read phonetically). The spelling of people with surface dyslexia is usually even more phonetic than their reading. The following example of the spelling of one person with surface dyslexia shows that the writing is intelligible despite being incorrectly spelled: 'I told my farther I whase onle werking in the stors and not doin enything danerouse whitch carmed him down'.

Other people have an inability to read non-words such as 'wig' or 'plag', or words they have never met before. They tend to read non-words as if they were real words, (for example 'plag' might be read as 'plague'). This condition is known as **phonological dyslexia**. Writing is usually unaffected, at least for familiar words.

Another reading difficulty is called **deep dyslexia**. People with this condition find nouns much easier to read than verbs, prepositions or adjectives. They also tend to make errors of meaning (for example they might read 'boat' as 'train' or 'uncle' as 'aunt'). Visual errors are also common. The word 'posture', for example, might be read as 'postage' and 'choir' read as 'chord'. People with deep dyslexia also show a tendency to combine errors of meaning with visual errors. One man read 'generosity' as 'really old' ('geriatrics') and 'deny' as 'jeans' ('denims'). The writing ability of people with this condition is also similarly affected and so nouns are easier to write than verbs, and errors of meaning or visual errors are common.

People with very severe language problems may be unable to read and write at all. This condition is called **alexia** (loss of reading ability) and **agraphia** (loss of writing ability).

Perceptual problems

Perception is the process of making sense of what we see (visual perception), or of what we hear (auditory perception), or what we touch (tactile perception). Visual perceptual problems are common after damage in the right half of the brain. These problems should not be confused with poor eyesight. The eyes may be unaffected but the messages relayed back to the brain are not being dealt with properly. Adequate eyesight is of course necessary for visual perceptual functioning but absence of sight does not cause a perceptual problem. We would not, for example, regard a blind person as having visual perceptual problems or a deaf person as having auditory perceptual problems.

Some of the main visuoperceptual and visuospatial disorders are listed below:

1. *Visual object agnosia* or loss of ability to recognise what is seen despite the ability to see and the absence of word finding problems. This condition is rare.
2. *Prosopagnosia* or loss of ability to recognise familiar faces. In severe cases the person will not recognise his or her own face in the mirror or in a photograph. Family members can usually be recognised by their voices or their walk or other cues. Again this is a rare condition.
3. *Colour agnosia* or loss of ability to recognise colours.
4. *Unilateral neglect* or failure to attend to one side of space or one side of the body. People with unilateral neglect may bump into things on one side (usually the left), may fail to see food on the left side of a plate placed in front of them, may comb half their hair, shave or make up one side of their face. People with this condition are likely to have a number of accidents, experience problems manoeuvring their wheelchairs, and have difficulty getting from a wheelchair to the lavatory or other places. Unilateral neglect is seen in about 40% of right hemisphere stroke patients. Left hemisphere stroke patients may also show neglect but it is usually not so severe and it clears up more quickly.
5. *Difficulty judging depth, distance or space.* For example, a car may seem to be about to crash into the car in which the affected person is sitting although the oncoming car is in fact on the other side of the road.
6. *Constructional and dressing apraxia.* This refers to problems in constructing things such as jigsaw puzzles or model kits, and difficulties in dressing. Problems may be experienced in judging whether a garment to be worn is the right way round. Such difficulties may be missed or misunderstood, and may be put down to a need for new spectacles or even stupidity when in fact they are caused by perceptual impairments.

Memory problems

Memory is the ability to take in, store and retrieve information. Problems with memory occur frequently after brain injury. Usually, verbal memory is more impaired after left hemisphere damage and there will be greater difficulty remembering names, stories and other language-related information. Visual memory is usually more impaired after right hemisphere damage and there will be greater problems remembering faces, shapes, routes, and other non-language material. Any brain injury may however result in a generally poorer memory which will lead to failure to remember to do things such as taking tablets, watering plants or making telephone calls.

Although it is common to talk of memory as though it were one thing or one skill, something that is either 'good' or 'bad', there are in fact a number of memory systems working together. After any kind of brain injury it is usual to find immediate memory is relatively spared so that the affected person is able to repeat back a new name or telephone number. Problems remembering that same information may occur, however, if there is a delay or distraction. If memory is severely affected but all other cognitive skills are intact then the person is said to have amnesia or the amnesic syndrome. It is possible to have a pure amnesia after brain injury but it is more usual to find less severe memory problems together with other problems such as poor attention or poor word finding, or slowness in thinking. In such cases it is preferable to refer to the person as having memory impairment or memory problems rather than amnesia.

Memory-impaired people have difficulty learning new information and this is often more of a handicap than forgetting episodes from the past. It is usual to find that events which happened some years or months prior to the injury are remembered more easily than events that happened a short time before.

Attention problems

While awake we are constantly receiving information and signals from the environment through our five senses. For much of the time we are unaware of many of these signals because of our ability to exclude them from our attention. Attention is the ability to select which signals we want to enter our awareness and which we want to keep at bay. When driving, for example, we can usually attend to the traffic on the road and carry on a conversation with a passenger. If an unexpectedly tricky situation arises we stop talking to concentrate on the traffic. Following brain injury the ability to attend selectively to important information may be lost. The ability to shut out unimportant information may also be lost so that the affected person becomes distracted very easily.

Some of the other everyday problems that may result from impaired attention are irritability, poor memory, fatigue, impulsiveness, inability to plan ahead, or to do more than one thing at a time.

There are a number of ways of classifying attention disorders. The following method considers five types of attention:

1. *Focused attention* is the ability to attend to important aspects of the environment, such as the person who is speaking to you, or the traffic on the road. Some brain-injured patients, particularly in the early days, may be restricted so that they can respond only to internal messages such as pain or fear, and cannot focus on important external factors.
2. *Sustained attention* is the ability to keep one's awareness on the task in hand (i.e. not to switch off during a conversation or to stop attending to the traffic

on the road). Many brain-injured patients are unable to stop themselves from having lapses of attention.

3. *Selective attention* is the ability to exclude distracting information. For example, when listening to the radio we can,to a limited extent, exclude the noise of traffic outside, and when we are at a party we attend selectively to the person to whom we are talking while excluding conversations going on around us. Again, this is not always easy for brain-injured patients who might be unable to exclude what is unimportant.
4. *Alternating attention* is the ability to shift from one task or activity to another when it is important to do so. For example, to stop talking when driving if it is necessary to deal with a complex situation, and then to return to the conversation again when the difficulty has been overcome. Some brain-injured patients find that once they 'have got going' on a task they are unable to switch to another.
5. *Divided attention* is the ability to respond simultaneously to two or more things at the same time, such as talking while walking, or listening to a conversation while watching television. All of us will, of course, show attention problems on some occasions. If we have toothache or are very tired we may find our attention wandering. We can usually overcome this with an effort of will but many brain injured patients are unable to do this.

There are many other cognitive difficulties that may arise because of brain injury. These include impairments of **problem solving**, **reasoning**, **judgement**, **slow thinking**, and **apraxia**.

Cognitive rehabilitation: restoration of function or amelioration of deficit?

Cognitive rehabilitation is concerned with the remediation, amelioration and alleviation of cognitive deficits acquired as a result of brain injury. In practice it is similar to neuropsychological rehabilitation, which is also concerned with the treatment of cognitive deficits, the difference being that neuropsychological rehabilitation also encompasses the treatment of emotional, behavioural, personality and motor deficits.

Wood (1990:3) says 'Cognitive or neuropsychological rehabilitation utilises an assortment of procedures to improve or restore a diverse collection of abilities and skills'. Is it possible to restore lost cognitive functions? Miller (1984) and Wilson (1989*a*) believe there is little evidence that cognitive functions can be fully restored through cognitive rehabilitation. Of course, damaged cognitive skills do improve after brain injury, i.e. some natural recovery occurs. The question is does cognitive rehabilitation improve on natural recovery? It seems likely that we can inhibit or decrease the amount of natural recovery through lack of stimulation or through placing people in deprived environments (Stein, 1988), so it seems likely that stimulating and enriched environments can enhance natural recovery (Stein *et al.*, 1994). Even so, there is still relatively little evidence that lost cognitive functions can be restored through rehabilitation. What evidence there is suggests that partial restoration of *some* cognitive functions may be achieved through rehabilitation. Wilson (1994) describes two people who became almost totally alexic after head injury and who were taught to read again. Single case experimental designs (see Wilson, Chapter 8) showed that the restoration of reading resulted from the treatment programmes and not as a result of natural recovery. Nevertheless, neither of the subjects read normally. They both changed from being alexic (unable to read) to letter-by-letter readers. Furthermore, they both read and spelled phonetically, i.e they became surface dyslexics who were impaired on the reading and writing of irregularly spelled words.

Similarly successful programmes can be found for people with language disturbances (Byng, 1988), reading problems (Coltheart & Byng, 1989), and unilateral neglect (Robertson & North, 1992). In each case, however, the subjects learned some skills but did not return to their premorbid levels of cognitive functioning so it cannot be said that, in any of these cases, *restoration* of function occurred.

Perhaps one skill where it might be possible to restore functioning is in the area of attention (Robertson, 1990). Even here though the evidence is tentative and, once again, it is more likely that partial rather than complete restoration has taken place. In the field of memory we can be reasonably certain that rehabilitation does not restore functioning (Schacter & Glisky, 1986; Wilson, 1987). Instead we have to concentrate on amelioration of the deficit or compensatory strategies. Such approaches are frequently employed when treating other cognitive problems. As we shall see, there is mounting evidence to suggest that brain-injured people can be taught to compensate for their difficulties or to use their residual skills more efficiently.

Before leaving this section it is worth pointing out that although exercise, practice and stimulation of various cognitive abilities will probably not restore lost functioning, they can be useful in keeping people aroused and motivated as well as preventing them from getting stale and lethargic. Children raised in unstimulating environments are less likely to develop intellectual curiosity. Old people sitting around doing nothing may lose some of their intellectual capacity. So it is probably safe to assume that brain-injured people need intellectual exercise to allow the maximum recovery to take place and to keep their intellect from deteriorating once the injury has taken place.

Approaches to the management of acquired cognitive disorders

If we turn from stimulation, practice and exercise of cognitive skills to consider ways of compensating for cognitive disorders, there are at least three approaches to consider (Wilson, 1989*a*). These are

1. Bypassing or avoiding problem areas by changing or restructuring the environment.
2. Functional adaptation or finding another way to achieve a goal.
3. Using residual skills more efficiently.

Bypassing or avoiding problems

One of the simplest ways to help people with cognitive problems is to arrange the environment so as to reduce the need for cognition. Norman (1988), discussing environmental designs for those who are cognitively and neurologically intact, argues for knowledge to be in the world rather than in the head. By this he means that the correct use of any object should be so obvious that it is almost impossible to make a mistake. How to open doors, turn on showers and use the correct knob for each hotplate on the cooker are just some of the many examples provided by Norman in his thought-provoking book. We could extend Norman's ideas to help those with impaired cognitive functioning. For example, Wilkins *et al.* (1989) described how some environmental adjustments helped a stroke patient with visual perceptual difficulties. The woman had difficulty discriminating the inside from the outside of a cup. She also had problems walking, partly because she could not tell where her legs ended and her feet began. Wilkins *et al.* provided her with cups that were brightly coloured on the outside and white inside. This contrast enabled her to manage her drinking better. The same principle was used with the second problem. She was encouraged to wear dark trousers with light coloured socks (or vice versa).

Stroke patients with unilateral neglect are often helped if a bright red strip is placed to the left of the telephone or reading material and other equipment that may be neglected. People with planning problems may be helped by arranging the environment so that the planning is done for them: if they cannot, for example, sort their clothes out for dressing then garments could be put out one at a time.

Brain-injured patients with impaired judgement might be helped by organising rooms to reduce risks, by removing, for example, all medicines from the bathroom cupboard, locking up cleaning fluids, car keys and important papers.

For memory-impaired people who cannot remember which room is which or where things are kept, it may be helpful to label rooms and cupboards or make them very distinctive. Alternatively a line drawn on the floor may help someone find the way from the bedroom to the toilet. Another tip is to position things so they cannot be missed or forgotten (for example tying a front door key to a waist belt). It may be possible to reduce or eliminate repetitive behaviour by identifying situations, questions or statements which trigger these and then avoiding the triggers.

For people with very severe intellectual handicap or those with progressive deterioration, environmental adaptations may be the best we can do to enable people to cope with and reduce some of the confusion and frustration. Few studies have discussed ways in which environments can be designed to help people with severe cognitive impairment although it would seem a fruitful area for therapists, psychologists, engineers, architects and designers to join forces.

Functional adaptations or finding another way to achieve a goal

Just as occupational therapists provide equipment for people with physical disability to enable them to cope with activities of daily living so we can use similar methods to help people with cognitive disability. Providing a long-handled picking up stick or replacing buttons with Velcro for people with rheumatoid arthritis are analogous to the provision of 'talking books' for people who are blind or electronic personal organisers for those unable to remember without help. The general principle to adopt in these matters is to look for another way if the original way is no longer possible.

People who are dysarthric, i.e. unable to speak because of a problem controlling the muscles involved in articulation, can use cannon communicators (calculator-sized machines on which a message can be typed, the message then appearing on a piece of ticker tape) or other communication aids. People with dysphasia may be taught to communicate with visual symbols (Gardner *et al.*, 1976; Wilson, 1990).

People who have memory problems may be taught to use external memory aids. These help people remember by using systems to access or record information. Harris (1992) points out that there are two major kinds of external memory aids. The first are those which enable us to access internally stored information such as a timer to remind us to check something in the oven. These are not very helpful for people with memory impairment as they cannot remember what it is they need to remember when the cue sounds.

The second kind are those that record information externally and these are much more useful for memory-impaired people. This second group of external aids includes diaries, notebooks, lists, alarm clocks, watches, kitchen timers, wall charts, calendars and tape recorders. Some people with memory problems are reluctant to use such aids, claiming they do not want to become dependent on them, or they want to encourage the return of their previous memory capacity. Such resistance should be discouraged. It should be pointed out that everybody, including people with good memories, uses external aids and there is no evidence to suggest that using external aids prevents or slows down the recovery of memory. In fact the opposite is true. Furthermore, Wilson (1991) showed that memory-impaired people using six or more memory aids or strategies were significantly more likely to be independent than those using less than six aids or strategies.

Despite the importance of external aids for memory-impaired people, it is often a difficult and time consuming task to teach efficient use of them. People forget to use the aids, or do not recognise the need to use them, or find them too difficult, or the aids get used in an inefficient or disorganised way. For a discussion on how to teach the use of such aids see Sohlberg & Mateer (1989) and Wilson (1992).

Using residual skills more efficiently

Whatever the degree of cognitive impairment, there is usually some residual, albeit malfunctioning ability left. The most densely amnesic person will have some language skills and the most perceptually-impaired person will retain a certain level of perceptual ability.

Some rehabilitation programmes attempt to capitalise on these residual skills and help people use them more efficiently. Von Cramon *et al.* (1991), for example, taught people with problem solving deficits to deal with practical situations through applying specific problem solving techniques. Alderman & Ward (1991) also described a treatment for helping a behaviourally and cognitively disturbed woman control her own behaviour. Koning-Haanstra *et al.* (1990) and Berg *et al.* (1991) taught memory-impaired people how to make better use of their residual memory functioning through a number of principles including: (a) acceptance of the problem, (b) use of external aids, (c) focusing attention, (d) allowing extra time, (e) repeating information, (f) making associations or links with other, known material, (g) organising, and (h) anticipating, (i) being systematic. These general principles are similar to those described in Wilson (1992) when she described ways to improve encoding (getting information in, storage and retrieval).

Mnemonics and certain kinds of rehearsal and study techniques can also help people make better use of residual skills. These are described in Moffat (1992) and Wilson (1987, 1992).

Many of the programmes described for the treatment of patients with unilateral neglect are based on the principle of encouraging better use of residual abilities through, for example, self-instruction (Meichenbaum, 1977), finding an anchor point before scanning (Weinberg *et al.*, 1979) and moving the affected limb before scanning (Robertson, 1988).

The three approaches described above are not mutually exclusive. A memory-impaired person may, for example, be helped by (a) using signposts and labels, i.e. restructuring the environment; (b) learning efficient use of a diary and notebook, i.e. remembering in a different way, or (c) learning more efficient use of residual skills through rehearsal strategies and mnemonics (Wilson, 1992).

Computers in rehabilitation

A few years ago there was considerable excitement about the possible uses of microcomputers in rehabilitation. People hoped and indeed seemed to expect that computer-based cognitive training programmes would revolutionise rehabilitation and improve the functioning of brain-injured people. Skilbeck (1984), for example, believed that microcomputers could assist in the management of cognitive disorders by being applied to assessment, the monitoring of treatment effectiveness and re-training procedures themselves. Numerous software programmes have appeared in the 1980s. As Robertson (1990) points out, however, the role of microcomputers in cognitive rehabilitation has not been subjected to controlled investigation until recently. Skilbeck & Robertson (1992) and Glisky (1995) provide a more up to date review of computers in rehabilitation.

There have been a few encouraging reports about the use of computers in cognitive rehabilitation. Sohlberg & Mateer (1987, 1989) demonstrated improved attention functioning in head-injured people, and three patients described by Robertson (1988) showed less visual neglect after a computer training programme. Given the huge increase in the use of computers in rehabilitation centres around the world, demonstrations of their effectiveness have been negligible. Even the few success stories tend to report changes in test scores rather than improvements in everyday living. Furthermore, several studies have reported the non-effectiveness of computer programmes (for example, see Ponsford & Kinsella, 1988; Robertson, 1988).

Maybe we should not, at this stage, expect computers to have much effect on cognitive rehabilitation programmes. If we consider memory for a moment,

Harris & Sunderland (1981) point out that it is not like a muscle that improves or strengthens with exercise. Practice at a task may well improve performance on that particular activity but will not necessarily improve functioning in other areas. Practice at a memory exercise will not improve general memory functioning. The classic experiments by Ericsson *et al.* (1980) demonstrated that students could increase their digit span from the normal 7 (plus or minus 2) to a phenomenal 80 or more with constant drilling and practice; however, post training assessment on a similar letter span task revealed normal scores of 7 (plus or minus 2). Thus no improvement of memory functioning per se had occurred.

As far as other cognitive skills are concerned, Robertson (1990) points out that some highly specific disorders of language may improve with particular training programmes, but in general there is no clear evidence of the general effectiveness of computer-based language rehabilitation. The same is true with visuoperceptual remediation programmes. This situation in attention training is slightly different with some studies showing positive results (Sohlberg & Mateer, 1987, 1989; Robertson *et al.*, 1988; Sturm & Willmes, 1991) while others (Ponsford & Kinsella, 1988; Robertson, 1988) showed negative results. None of the cognitive rehabilitation programmes, however, showed generalisation to real life.

Computers can of course be of great assistance in the field of rehabilitation. They can save much time and lead to greater efficiency in certain assessment procedures, and they can provide immediate and effective feedback (see Mackey, 1989). Training in the use of computers has led to some exciting results from Schacter & Glisky (1986) and Glisky & Schacter (1987). The Glisky & Schacter studies are probably the best to date in the field of computers in memory rehabilitation. The authors taught a number of amnesic patients computer technology using their 'Method of Vanishing Cues' (identical to the forward and backward chaining used in behaviour modification). One of their patients was able to obtain employment as a computer programmer following several months of training.

Finally, computers may prove to be important as prosthetic aids. Bergman (1991) and Bergman & Kemmerer (1991), for example, describe how a head-injured woman with numerous cognitive problems was taught to control her financial affairs and other aspects of her life through a computer programme designed specifically for her needs. Hersh & Treadgold (1994) describe a very simple to operate prosthetic memory device called a 'NeuroPage'. This is a small pager with a screen linked to a central computer. Each subject's requirements are programmed so that the computer will relay messages to the NeuroPage at the appropriate time. For example, one memory-impaired person might receive the following messages:

9.00 am	take medication
9.15 am	prepare packed lunch
9.30 am	leave for work
10.00 am	phone bank
etc., etc.	

The message appears on the screen at the specified time, an alarm sounds and the subject is required to call a telephone number to confirm the message has been received. If this is not carried out, the message will be transmitted again (up to four times or more depending on how the computer has been programmed). One advantage of the NeuroPage is that the user controls everything with a single button, avoiding many of the difficulties inherent in using electronic organisers and other microcomputers. Another advantage is the acceptability of the machine. To most people having a pager is status enhancing.

The potential uses of NeuroPage are many, not only for memory-impaired people but also for people with other cognitive problems such as planning and organisation difficulties as well as for people with schizophrenia and people with age-related memory impairment.

Rehabilitation for everyday life

In the rehabilitation of patients with cognitive deficits our concern is to minimise the disruption to their everyday lives. We do not wish to teach them how to complete a particular laboratory task or to improve scores on standardised tests. It is possible, of course, that teaching a particular set of tasks in occupational, physio or speech therapy or clinical psychology will generalise to real life skills. Teaching people how to do block design tasks, for example, might result in an improvement in dressing (Diller & Gordon, 1981) but as we have seen in computer-based rehabilitation above, there is usually very little evidence of generalisation from these kinds of task to real life activities. Lincoln *et al.* (1985) showed, for example, that practice in perceptual tasks in occupational therapy did not result in greater improvement in everyday skills.

Some of the strategies described above, i.e. environmental adaptations, functional adaptations and helping people to use their residual skills more efficiently, can be applied to help reduce everyday problems caused by cognitive impairment. In addition, brain-injured people and their families may cope better with their difficulties if they are provided with information about the nature of the cognitive problems and how these relate to real life. For example, carers of someone with unilateral neglect will be able to change a home environment for that person if they are informed about how such a disability may lead to accidents involving bumping into walls, trapping a hemiplegic arm in wheelchair spokes, having difficulty getting on and off the toilet and so on.

Information about self-help and support groups such as Headway, The Alzheimer Disease Society, Action for Disabled Adults should be readily available. In addition, working together in groups (Evans & Wilson, 1992) may help reduce some of the anxiety and depression among those experiencing cognitive difficulties resulting from impairment to memory or some other process.

We can also apply principles of behavioural assessment and behaviour modification to the design of treatment programmes for people with cognitive impairment, thus virtually guaranteeing a focus on real life problems. It is also a useful structure to follow when unclear or uncertain about how to proceed with a particular patient.

Basically, a behavioural assessment should:

1. *Identify the problem to be worked on as unambiguously as possible.* We should avoid saying, for example, 'perceptual impairment' or 'planning problems' as these are too vague and non-specific. 'Bumping into walls' or 'inability to dress' are more appropriate.
2. *Clearly state goals or aims.* Again these should be as specific as possible, such as 'The goal is for Mrs Smith to wheel herself down the corridor from her bedroom to the dayroom without touching the walls on either side on six consecutive occasions'. It may be necessary to state long-term and short-term goals.
3. *Measure the deficit or obtain a baseline.* This may require counting how often (or how rarely) a behaviour occurs over a period of time. Alternatively, it might be more appropriate to measure how long some movement or task takes (e.g. 'How long does it take Mrs. Smith to wheel herself down the corridor?' or 'How many prompts are needed to achieve the desired behaviour'. Baselines will need to be taken until a clear pattern emerges.
4. *Plan the treatment*, e.g. 'Which strategy will be used?' 'How will it be implemented?' 'When and where should the treatment be carried out and by whom?'
5. *Begin treatment.*
6. *Monitor ongoing treatment*, i.e. keep records.
7. *Adjust, alter or extend the treatment as necessary.*

Clinical examples of how this structure has been used for the remediation of memory and reading problems can be found in Wilson (1989*b*, 1990, 1992). These references also consider how to identify problems, how to be selective in choosing problems to tackle, and advises on how many to tackle at any one time.

Evaluation of cognitive rehabilitation problems

To know whether cognitive rehabilitation programmes are effective, systematic evaluation is essential. Group studies are often unhelpful in such situations as they provide little guidance as to which individuals benefit or fail to benefit from a particular technique. The behavioural guidelines outlined above provide a built-in monitoring and evaluation device. Provided adequate baselines have been taken, it is possible to see whether there has been any change after the introduction of treatment. To make evaluation more sophisticated we can combine this with one of the single case experimental designs described by Wilson (Chapter 8). So, for example, if the plan is to tackle four problems faced by a single patient, four separate treatment programmes could be designed following the steps described above while actual treatment would focus on one problem at a time. If we stagger the introduction of treatments for problems 2, 3 and 4, i.e. use a multiple baseline across behaviours design, we will have a pretty good idea whether it is our treatment that is responsible for any change. Bryant & Machin (Chapter 9) and Horn (Chapter 14) provide further discussion on evaluation of rehabilitation.

References

Alderman, N. & Ward, A. (1991). Behavioural treatment of the dysexecutive syndrome: reduction of repetitive speech using response cost and cognitive overlearning. *Neuropsychological Rehabilitation*, **1**, 65–80.

Berg, I. J., Koning-Haanstra, M. & Deelman, B. G. (1991). Long-term effects of memory rehabilitation: a controlled study. *Neuropsychological Rehabilitation*, **1**, 97–111.

Bergman, M. M. (1991). Computer-enhanced self sufficiency: Part 1. Creation and implementation of a text writer for an individual with traumatic brain injury. *Neuropsychology*, **5**, 17–24.

Bergman, M. M. & Kemmerer, A. G. (1991). Computer-enhanced self-sufficiency: Part 2. Uses and subjective benefits of a text writer for an individual with traumatic brain injury. *Neuropsychology*, **5**, 25–8.

Byng, S. (1988). Sentence processing deficits: theory and therapy. *Cognitive Neuropsychology*, **5**, 629–76.

Coltheart, M. & Byng, S. (1989). A treatment for surface dyslexia. In *Cognitive Approaches in Neuropsychological Rehabilitation* ed. X. Seron & G. Deloche. Hillsdale, NJ: Lawrence Erlbaum Associates.

Diller, L. & Gordon, W. A. (1981). Rehabilitation and clinical neuropsychology. In *Handbook of Clinical Neuropsychology* ed. S. B. Filskov & T. J. Boll. New York: John Wiley.

Ericsson, K. A., Chase, W. G. & Falcon, S. (1980). Acquisition of a memory skill. *Science*, **208**, 1181–82.
Evans, J. J. & Wilson, B. A. (1992). A memory group for individuals with brain injury. *Clinical Rehabilitation*, **6**, 75–81.
Gardner, H., Zurif, E. B., Berry, T. & Baker, E. (1976). Visual communication in aphasia. *Neuropsychologia*, **14**, 275–92.
Glisky, E. (1995). Computers in memory rehabilitation. In *Handbook of Memory Disorders* ed. A. D. Baddeley, F. Watts & B. A. Wilson, pp. 557–75. Chichester: John Wiley.
Glisky, E. L. & Schacter, D. L. (1987). Acquisition of domain-specific knowledge in organic amnesia: training for computer-related work. *Neuropsychologia*, **25**, 893–906.
Harris, J. (1992). Ways to help memory. In *Clinical Management of Memory Problems* ed. B. A. Wilson & N. Moffat, 2nd edn. pp. 59–85. London: Chapman & Hall.
Harris, J. E. & Sunderland, A. (1981). A brief survey of the management of memory disorders in rehabilitation units in Britain. *International Rehabilitation Medicine*, **3**, 206–9.
Hersh, N. A. & Treadgold, L. G. (1994). NeuroPage: the rehabilitation of memory dysfunction by prosthetic memory and cueing. *Neurorehabilitation*, **4**, 187–97.
Koning-Haanstra, M., Berg, I. J. & Deelman, B. G. (1990). In *Traumatic Brain Injury* ed. B. G. Deelman, R. J. Saan & A. H. van Zomeren. pp. 145–68. Lisse, Netherlands: Swets & Zeitlinger.
Lincoln, N. B., Whiting, S., Cockburn, J. & Bhavnani, G. (1985). An evaluation of perceptual retraining. *International Rehabilitation Medicine*, **7**, 98–101.
Mackey, S. (1989). The use of computer-assisted feedback in a motor-control task for cerebral palsied children. *Physiotherapy*, **75**, 143–8.
Meichenbaum, D. (1977). *Cognitive-Behaviour Modification: An Integrative Approach*. New York: Plenum Press.
Miller, E. (1984). *Recovery and Management of Neuropsychological Impairments*. Chichester: John Wiley.
Moffat, N. (1992). Strategies of memory therapy. In *Clinical Management of Memory Problems* 2nd edn, B. A. Wilson & N. Moffat ed. pp. 86–119. London: Chapman & Hall.
Norman, D. (1988). *The Psychology of Everyday Things*. New York: Basic Books.
Ponsford, J. L. & Kinsella, G. (1988). Evaluation of a remedial programme for attentional deficits following closed head injury. *Journal of Clinical and Experimental Neuropsychology*, **10**, 693–708.
Robertson, I. H. (1988). *Unilateral Visual Neglect*. PhD thesis, University of London.
Robertson, I. (1990). Does computerised cognitive rehabilitation work? A review. *Aphasiology*, **4**, 381–405.
Robertson, I. H. & North, N. (1992). Spatio-motor cueing in unilateral left neglect: the role of hemispace, hand and motor activation. *Neuropsychologia*, **30**, 553–63.
Robertson, I., Gray, J. & McKenzie, S. (1988). Microcomputer-based cognitive rehabilitation of visual neglect. 3 multiple-baseline single-case studies. *Brain Injury*, **2**, 151–63.
Schacter, D. L. & Glisky, E. L. (1986). Memory remediation: restoration, alleviation and the acquisition of domain-specific knowledge. In *Clinical*

Neuropsychology of Intervention ed. B. P. Uzzell & Y. Gross., pp. 257–82. Boston: Martinus Nijhoff.

Skilbeck, C. (1984). Computer assistance in the management of memory and cognitive impairment. In. *Clinical Management of Memory Problems* 1st edn. ed. B. A. Wilson & N. Moffat. London: Croom Helm.

Skilbeck, C. & Robertson, I. H. (1992). Computer assistance in the management of memory and cognitive impairment. In *Clinical Management of Memory Problems* 2nd end, ed. B. A. Wilson & N. Moffat, pp.155–88. London: Chapman & Hall.

Sohlberg, M. M. & Mateer, C. A. (1987). Effectiveness of an attention training programme. *Journal of Clinical and Experimental Neuropsychology*, **9**, 117–30.

Sohlberg, M. & Mateer, C. (1989). Training use of compensatory memory books: a three-stage behavioral approach. *Journal of Clinical and Experimental Neuropsychology*, **11**, 871–91.

Stein, D. (1988). Contextual factors in recovery from brain damage. In *Neuropsychological Rehabilitation* ed. A. -L. Christensen & B. Uzzell, pp.1–18. Boston: Kluwer Academic Publishers.

Stein, D., Glasier, M. M. & Hoffman, S. W. (1994). Pharmacological and anatomical changes underlying recovery from brain injury. In *Brain Injury and Neuropsychological Rehabilitation: An International Perspective* ed. A. -L. Christensen & B. Uzzell, pp. 17–40. Hillsdale, NJ: Lawrence Erlbaum Associates.

Sturm, W. & Willmes, K. (1991). Efficacy of a reaction training on various attentional and cognitive functions in stroke patients. *Neuropsychological Rehabilitation*, **1**, 259–80.

Von Cramon, D. Y., Matthes-von Cramon, G. & Mai, N. (1991). Problem solving deficits in brain injured patients: a therapeutic approach. *Neuropsychological Rehabilitation*, **1**, 45–64.

Weinberg, J., Diller, L., Gordon, W., Gerstman, L., Lieberman, A., Lakin, P., Hodges, G. & Ezrachi, O. (1979). Training sensory awareness and spatial organization in people with right brain damage. *Archives of Physical and Medical Rehabilitation*, **60**, 491–6.

Wilkins, A. J., Plant, G. & Huddy, A. (1989). Neuropsychological principles applied to rehabilitation of a stroke patient. *Lancet*, **1**, 54.

Wilson, B. A. (1987). *Rehabilitation of Memory*. New York: Guilford Press.

Wilson, B. A. (1989*a*). Models of cognitive rehabilitation. In *Models of Brain Injury Rehabilitation* ed. R. L. Wood & P. Eames, pp. 117–41.

Wilson, B. A. (1989*b*). Designing memory therapy programmes. In *Everyday Cognition in Adulthood and Late Life* ed. L. W. Poon, D. C. Rubin & B. A. Wilson, pp. 615–38. Cambridge: Cambridge University Press.

Wilson, B. A. (1990). Cognitive rehabilitation for brain injured adults. In *Traumatic Brain Injury* ed. B. G. Deelman, R. J. Saan & A. H. van Zomeren, pp. 121–44. Lisse, Netherlands: Swets & Zeitlinger.

Wilson, B. A. (1991). Long-term prognosis of patients with severe memory disorders. *Neuropsychological Rehabilitation*, **1**, 117–34.

Wilson, B. A. (1992). Memory therapy in practice. In *Clinical Management of Memory Problems* 2nd edn, ed. B. A. Wilson & N. Moffat, pp. 120–53. London: Chapman & Hall.

Wilson, B. A. (1994). Syndromes of acquired dyslexia and patterns of recovery: a 6–10 year follow-up study of seven injured people. *Journal of Clinical and*

Experimental Neuropsychology.
Wood, R. Ll. (1990). Towards a model of cognitive rehabilitation. In *Cognitive Rehabilitation in Perspective* ed. R. Ll. Wood & I. Fussey, pp. 3–25. London: Taylor and Francis.

13

Challenging behaviour: helping people with severe brain damage

ALLAN READ

Introduction

Roget's Thesaurus mentions the following in association with 'behaviour': posture, appearance, motion, action, gesticulation, gesture, manner, habit, line of action, tactics, manoeuvre, behave towards, treat, deal with, manage. This all sounds very physical as well it might because when we talk of studying or changing animal behaviour, we are focusing on the things on which natural sciences focus attention, the physical world of matter.

An animal is a physical thing that can be studied like other physical things. We can try to detect events in various modalities, for example, can we see it move and if so, what can we see it do, what changes does it bring to its environment? For example, does it move things about, perhaps throw things? Also the modality of sound, does it growl, can you infer that it is striking something by the sounds that you hear? If it belongs to a gregarious species, what effect does its behaviour have on other members who are nearby? Other animals are part of the physical environment as well as inanimate things but, within a gregarious species, we may then call other animals the social environment.

When psychologists use the behavioural model, problems or issues are operationalised in a similar way to the procedures of other natural sciences. Animal behaviour becomes matter in motion and these phenomena are counted in units that are standard and absolute. Combinations of these basic units can be combined to describe additional more complex phenomena (Hersen & Bellack, 1981).

It should be emphasised that models are theoretical constructs, i.e. they are systematic ways of thinking about, describing and formulating issues. A model might be useful because it seems to explain many aspects of a problem. A model might also be useful because it helps us to choose a course of action, which leads to a solution or at least an improvement. The model may even supply us with a vision of what a solution might be, i.e. an idea of what we will have when the problem is solved. As we will see later, people often think that they know what the problem is but have no vision of how they will know when the problem is solved.

A successful model helps us to explore a problem, formulate it, choose an intervention and evaluate whether this has been a success. The behavioural model can often do this for us and in addition, by taking a natural science perspective, achieves this in a publicly verifiable way.

Using this approach does not mean the denial of things that are not observable, for example feelings or cognition, only that our measures will be of observable things which might well be fair measures of other things that we cannot see, for example learning.

Finally, it can be used side by side with other models and with non-behavioural treatments, for example to study the effect of a drug. It can be good practice to use several different types of measure that may indeed reflect the use of more than one model, for example measuring or studying the sequences of unusual behaviour but also taking samples of blood, measuring body weight, etc.

When the behavioural model is being applied, its use should follow a systematic experimental plan. A characteristic approach would be:

1. Define the problem and desired solution in publicly verifiable terms.
2. Study/measure it.
3. Develop a hypothesis about it (your best guess).
4. Decide on a goal and an action plan.
5. Implement this while continuing to observe. Measure possible changes predicted by the hypothesis.
6. Evaluate.

Defining the problem

Operationalising a problem into behavioural terms is most easily accomplished by asking the question 'What does he or she do to show there is a problem', or 'What will he or she do to show that the problem has been solved?'

Some examples of problem behaviours could be:

> 'Screams when I try to pull his shoes on'.
> 'Bangs his spoon on the table repeatedly while the meal is being served'.
> 'Slaps his forehead'.
> 'Grabs hold of people's shoulders when he talks to them'.

A very simple criterion for successful outcome might be the negation of the above problems, for example 'He no longer screams when I put his shoes on'. It is possible to generate more inspiring visions of problem resolution, but these often come later at the stage of producing hypotheses.

This exercise of operationalising a problem in behavioural terms can be fruitful in helping us to realise the assumptions we make about our physical world. Defining a problem as 'Fred is aggressive' is perhaps premature.

Studying and measuring the problem

Crucial aspects of measurement are: accuracy, i.e. how faithful a representation of reality is the measure; reliability, for example if two observers see the same behaviour do they get the same result (inter-rater reliability) or if the same behaviour is measured repeatedly during a period when it is not changing do you get the same result (test-retest reliability); and validity, i.e. are you measuring what you think you are measuring, for example you may have an accurate and reliable measure of the number of scrambled egg sandwiches eaten, but is this a valid measure of verbal reasoning? Probably not.

Accuracy can be best secured by using the most direct observation available. Indirect measures can also be used, for example the presence or absence of faeces in an inappropriate place or damage to property. To be valid of course, one must ensure that these behavioural by-products are specific to the behaviour being studied (Nelson, 1981).

Antecedents

This term denotes the context in which the behaviours occur and the events that lead up to it or precede it. This will require careful monitoring of the subject and the environment including the behaviours of other people, even when they are not intentionally reacting with the subject. For example, a subject might have developed a pattern of violent outbursts associated with a dislike of being ignored or excluded. An innocent whispered conversation or exchange of glances between people at the opposite end of the room could trigger outbursts that might superficially appear to have occurred 'spontaneously'.

Antecedents can also include unmet needs, for example needing to have a warmer environment or to be subjected to less noise.

Consequences

This term denotes the sequence of events following the problem behaviour, and their outcome. What is required is an exact description of what happens, not a hypothesis about causation.

Many issues to do with reliability can be solved by writing a clear set of instructions to the observers regarding the behaviour that is being studied, when this should be studied and what method to use. Altman (1974) gives detailed consideration to the advantages and disadvantages of a variety of procedures for observing and recording behaviour.

Validity is more difficult. When helping people with brain damage we may well know about the cause and location of the damage and its likely effects on sensation, perception, cognition and behaviour to formulate initial ideas about what the problem is. What we choose to observe will be guided by this, plus information obtained from others about the likely relevance of brain damage effects interacting with the current environment.

Often when we are concerned about reported behavioural events, for example shouting, damaging property, it is useful to record the sequence: Antecedents, Behavioural event and Consequences. All should be written in a style that describes publicly verifiable features and without attempts at interpretation at this stage. One particular aspect of behavioural sequencing is that of skill.

Skill

Fitts & Posner (1973) define skill as 'an organised sequence of behaviour towards a goal, performed with consistent quality and accuracy'. Clearly the sequence can be one involving reciprocity of behaviour between two or more animals or a stream of behaviour from one animal, for example picking up and cracking a nut then eating the kernel. With respect to consistency, it is one of life's realities that an amount of variation occurs in the behaviour of any individual animal, thus consistency relates to the trend in behaviour over time, allowing for this variation.

When the sequence of behaviour under consideration is a skill, a number of options are available. The quality of the completed (or not completed) task can be described, for example half chin shaved, milk omitted from tea, etc., but more constructively the sequence of skilled behaviour can be analysed in terms of the resources that have to be added to enable the person to complete the task properly. Resource can be the type of artificial signal that needs to be supplied.

The word prompt is usually used to describe these artificial signals. When the prompts come directly from another person (rather than for example a flashing light or painted label) they can easily be escalated in the following way: no prompt, a verbal prompt, a verbal prompt plus a gesture, and finally a verbal prompt combined with a physical prompt. Each of these can be broken down into a scale of more or less help, for example a hand on hand physical prompt combined with the verbal prompt. 'Now we shave your left cheek' constitutes a lot of physical prompt where the helper replaces the motor programme that is not happening. Touching the hand briefly could constitute a milder physical prompt.

It is obvious that this interactive form of skills assessment is also a therapeutic intervention and, as we see later, when combined with reinforcement procedures constitutes a highly effective and flexible form of skills teaching. It also provides a publicly verifiable record of skill acquisition in the form of trend in the level of prompt needed over time as in the example reported by Wilson (1991) when teaching an apraxic patient to drink from a cup.

This form of assessment, however, need not only apply to a sequence of motor acts to achieve a state of, for example, being fully dressed. Social skills can be studied in exactly the same way. The STEP (Skills Teaching Education Programme Planning) social skills training manual (Chamberlain, 1985) encourages the writing of task breakdowns for activities that require social skill, for example using a shop might begin as checking keys, money and shopping list and continue through steps such as walking to the bus, waiting for the bus, embarking, etc. A true baseline assessment (assessment before intervention) can be difficult when the duty of care could be compromised, but within ethical bounds this should be attempted. A baseline will require more than one assessment so that consistency of problems can be assessed. Data will consist of a list of behavioural assets and deficits judged by community standards.

Finally, it should be emphasised that any form of assessment based on escalated prompts is an intervention by definition. Like other forms of practical skill assessment it may also constitute an intervention by raising questions of the form: why is there not a vacuum cleaner, why is the kitchen locked, why does she never travel out of the hospital?

The difference between 'Can do' and 'Does do'

In everyday rehabilitation work the word skill is used to describe 'things people can do'. There are several reasons why a skill may not show. The concepts of damage, disability and handicap are of use here. **Damage** can literally mean 'What got broken' for example eyes in an acid attack. **Disability** can mean the function for which the person is disabled, for example not having vision. **Handicap** is the effect on the person's life style, i.e. an exhaustive list of things they cannot do because they are disabled for seeing. Disability is not, however, the only source of handicap.

If a person's life style is under the control of others, these others are potential sources of handicap. A person may have a normal skill but never be allowed to use it either formally 'We won't let you' or by other means 'We don't have the resources though it would be nice . . . '.

Often when people have received damage and lost a function they will use other strategies so that they minimise their handicap. Sometimes strategies will be mixed, for example if people have lost much of their ability to speak, they will sometimes try to speak, sometimes use gestures, etc. They will learn to use methods that are most effective or least costly in terms of effort.

People with severe brain damage often appear to the lay person as being impossible to communicate with because superficially they cannot send information nor do they act as if they can receive and act on information. Communication disability of any sort can handicap people by distorting how easily they can interact with others and thereby making them more effortful for intact people to be with. This often leads to people being avoided as, to others, they have become painful. Others learn the most effective methods of avoidance and which are least costly to *them*.

Just as skill can be seen as 'things people can do in a physical environment' so social skill can be seen as things people can do with/in their social environment'. If individual others' avoid contact with a brain-damaged person, so can collections of others who make up social systems, for example the family, the people in a nursing home or on a hospital ward. Other pressures on those who run systems of care may lead to their unintentionally aggravating the effects of a disability by making choices which ensure that the daily round of life on such units is least aversive to those running them. Such systems can actually develop around disability to such an extent that the disability seems to be essential to the system, which functions as if it has a life or purpose of its own (Goffman, 1961).

An objective study of the behaviour of a person with brain damage must, at some stage therefore take account of, and investigate the costs and gains to the surrounding social system of both 'problem behaviour' and its resolution. This takes us into the realms of systems theory which is beyond the scope of this chapter, but the interested reader is referred to Campbell & Draper (1985) and Haley (1978).

The ecology of a patient's behaviour (physical and social) will become apparent when behaviour or skill is systematically studied *in situ*. This will give the observer clues as to the way sequences of behaviour unfold, and what the function of the observed behaviour might be. Behavioural events/incidents will be watched over time and invariance noted, for example what generally tends to happen. Recording can be of the Antecedents, Behaviour, and Consequences type.

The message function of behaviour

La Vigna (1986) notes that the literature on the use of behavioural procedures has surprisingly little evidence of ecological analysis even when very intrusive procedures are being considered. La Vigna emphasises the communicative function of behaviour even when that behaviour is 'bizarre' or apparently destructive, and recommends that an analysis of behaviour should begin with the 'assumption that all behaviour has message value'. This approach 'acknowledges the legitimacy of attention seeking'.

In terms of social ecology it is interesting to note the frequency with which behaviour is dismissed or even punished because carers label it as attention seeking. The apparent message from the social system is 'We do not wish to receive your communication'. A benevolent system should study the method of communication used, consider the message, try to meet the needs conveyed by the message and where desirable, alter the method of communication to make it more normal and therefore more valuable for the sender. It is clearly not benevolent to deprive a person of (or punish a person for) the only form of communication they have. The principle of beneficence is supposed to be the meta principle of all health care work.

Donnellan *et al.* (1984) provide a useful matrix of functions and behaviours. The broad categories of function are: (a) **interactive**, for example requests, negations, comments, declarations about feelings and (b) **non-interactive**, for example self-regulation, rehearsal, habitual and tension release.

Donnellan's matrix requires regular observation over time, in a variety of environments and then individual study to validate the conclusions drawn from the observation.

Cathy East (unpublished data), a communication therapist, has developed a complementary extension of this paradigm enabling experimental procedures to be used with individual clients to answer questions of the sort, 'What methods of communication does this person use, and what information are they sending'?

East first developed her approach in 1984 while studying people with learning difficulties but it is entirely applicable to people from any clinical population where the normal channels of communication are not used or not used in the usual way and where, using La Vigna's criteria, there is at least the possibility that the behaviour has a message function.

To assess the person's method of communication, and the likely intended message, experimental situations are arranged that require him or her to communicate if needs/desires are to be met swiftly, for example instead of pouring and giving a cup of coffee, the therapist waits until 'asked' to do so. The person may simply look at the coffee, or perhaps look from the coffee to the therapist, or may point, or may vocalise or any combination of these.

Each step of the experiment is recorded on video tape for analysis later. As the experiment proceeds different types of message from the person can be elicited. In addition to requesting objects or actions, the person may wish to protest, comment on actions or objects, summon, greet, close a communication, simply respond to call, respond to a question or acknowledge the presence of the observer.

A typical experimental sequence might be to require the person to request food or drink; to request information of the therapists by the therapists looking into a box at something the person can't see; ignore the person while reading a magazine to see how they respond; to get a colleague to knock on the door and call the therapist's name to see if the person either responds at all or draws the therapist's attention to the matter. Protest can be elicited by temporarily removing a source of pleasure, for example switching off music.

Video presentations to care staff enable them to watch the sequences of interaction between themselves and the person. In so doing they receive ideas about processes that may have been less apparent when the experiment was taking place. It is possible to spot the earliest sign of a message from the person and to note whether the carer began to respond at that point or whether messages were repeated or amplified. They may have been missed altogether. Amplified messages are often seen as challenging behaviour.

General discussion can follow when the experimenter may ask carers questions of the sort 'In your day to day dealings with him or her, how do you know he or she is hungry/needs the toilet/wants to be with somebody else'? This helps carers to compare the person's social ecology with the experimental situation.

Hazards of failure to observe and to communicate

Sometimes the obvious difference will be that in real life there is virtually no need for any communication. Lunch happens at lunch time. The person is wheeled into a dining room. Food is served, washed down by a drink.

Toileting may be more or less scheduled around previous experience of when the person was manifestly wet. Employees in a service based on task allocation for physical survival will sometimes challenge the relevance of stretching sequences so that people need to communicate. 'But why? We are busy enough as it is'. Some systems of care engender the illusion that there is a need to rush everything as opposed to only those things that are truly urgent. This is a vicious circle. The rush prevents communication other than the one way 'Come to the toilet now Fred' type. By definition, no communication means a loss of social intimacy, and thereby a loss of the chance to enjoy the person on more equal terms. The person may still be valued, but only in the sense of a sad story. The ultimate illusion results 'isn't it sad when they are so damaged that they have to live like this? If that ever happens to me . . . etc'.

Communication, severely challenging behaviour and learning theory

In discussing severely challenging behaviour and helping people who send messages this way, it is necessary to look briefly at **learning theory**, which has for many years been associated with the essentially atheoretical behavioural model.

Learning theory is a generic term for a collection of explanations that have been advanced as to why animals behave as they do, and in particular, why external changes, i.e. environmental changes, are associated with changes in behaviour.

Three broad areas of learning theory are:

1. Classical conditioning
2. Operant conditioning
3. Vicarious learning

Classical conditioning

Here, the behaviour of an animal is explained in terms of it learning that at least two stimuli tend to go together, for example the sight of a bowl associated with the taste of food, sight of a particular room associated with pain, etc.

Pavlov (1927) demonstrated that a hungry dog could, as a result of experimental procedure, salivate on the sole presentation of an arbitrary stimulus such as a bell or a light if, on a number of previous occasions, this stimulus has closely preceded the presentation of meat powder. The bell or light was described by Pavlov as a **Conditional Stimulus** if it had this effect, and salivation, under this procedure has become a **Conditioned Response**.

Repeated pairings of this sort strengthen the association between the two as manifest by the animal's behaviour and conversely, the association can be broken if the conditional stimulus is presented continually without what Pavlov called the unconditional stimulus, for example in the case of the dog, frequent use of the bell not being followed by meat powder. Breaking the association in this way is called **extinction**.

Finally, the association can generalise so that other stimuli similar to the conditional stimulus have the same or similar behavioural effects, for example salivating to a bell of different pitch.

Operant conditioning

Here animal behaviour is explained in terms of learning from the consequences of its behaviour. Skinner (1938) who invented the term operant conditioning demonstrated experimentally that the probability of a behaviour could increase if it were immediately followed by an event that was useful to the individual concerned, for example pushing a lever down and then receiving food, drink, etc. As with classical conditioning, extinction can be achieved, this time by no longer making the behaviour positively useful, for example no longer presenting food when a lever is pressed, thus breaking the learned association between the two. The event that makes a behaviour useful is called a **reinforcer**, although it has to be said that careful scrutiny of behaviour is needed to explain why some events are reinforcers, i.e. not all reinforcers are what most people would call 'nice' rewards! A **punisher** is something that makes a behaviour costly and this is also judged by the effect it has on behaviour.

There is a vast literature on operant conditioning, often called behaviour modification, which is too detailed to discuss in this chapter but one aspect which is relevant is a procedure called **shaping**.

When a behaviour is desirable but does not occur, a behaviour that is similar can be selected and reinforced. Strictly speaking this is proven by the behaviour becoming more probable. Once this has been achieved, the reinforcer is only presented when the behaviour becomes a little closer in form to what is desired. By selecting a series of steps from the behaviour that exists, to that which is desired, behaviour can be shaped.

Observational or vicarious learning

Here the behaviour of one animal in the context of its reinforced behaviour, and the signals that also seem to affect its behaviour, is observed by another animal, which learns contingency this way.

A child might learn not to assert himself against a playground bully because he has seen what happens to others who try. Thus he learns from observing the contingencies that affect other children's behaviour. A child might learn to be fearful of certain stimuli simply because he has seen his parents react in a fearful way, etc.

This 'Cook's Tour' of Learning Theory helps us to consider severely challenging behaviour in terms of the signals, reinforcers and punishers that operate in the person's social ecology.

Previously the study of Antecedents, Behaviours and Consequences was mentioned. This method of studying a sequence of events enables us to identify what might be Pavlovian stimuli or signals and those consequences which might be reinforcers, with the person's behaviour the operant between the two. Consequences may seem various and yet there may be a common theme linking all consequences. This theme may be the function of the behaviour. Antecedents are often signals that carry the message 'behave in a particular way *now*, and a certain consequence will result'.

Hypotheses concerning the function of a behaviour can be further tested by the use of benign interventions, for example the manipulation of consequences to see whether behaviour alters. Details of the setting and the presumed triggers or signals can also be manipulated to see how behaviour changes. Mostly we are concerned with a change of trend of behaviour and must therefore allow enough time for this to become apparent. Systematic change to reinforcement or signals is usually called a behavioural programme and comes under the rubric of Behaviour Modification (Kazdin, 1975).

Case study: Cindy

Earlier when discussing the work of East it was noted that messages which are not attended, i.e. where the target person behaves as though they have not received a message, can be amplified or altered by the sender to achieve the desired effect. Thus the function of some 'disturbed' behaviour is to amplify a message.

A good example of this is the behaviour of a woman we shall call Cindy who at the time of writing still lives on a ward for people who have acquired brain damage in adulthood. At 20 years of age Cindy acquired severe brain damage as a result of having too much insulin for her diabetic condition. The rest of this chapter will present a case study of Cindy to illustrate some of the principles outlined above.

Cindy has profound deficits in comprehension and no actual speech except briefly on awakening when she may speak quietly and simply about the content of a dream, for example 'I've been painting'. Her main vocalisations consist of extremely loud perseverations of the type 'Horeeareeareea' or 'solly solly solly' or 'de de de de'.

In addition she has acquired a condition called hyperphagia in which much of her unstructured time is spent looking for things to eat. This includes the dangerous phenomenon of **Pica**, i.e. the eating of non-foods such as furniture, dust, flakes of paint, etc.

She is capable of violence (velocity, ferocity and force) although there is almost no evidence of aggression (clear intent to harm). Frustration, for example having her path to the dining room blocked, can be followed by instant screaming and crying and on occasions lashing out although seldom making contact or harming anybody.

She has epilepsy and still has insulin-dependent diabetes.

This combination of hyperphagia, diabetes and profound comprehension deficits means that she is always looking for food, cannot be given large amounts of her favourite foods even at a ward party but lacks the comprehension to understand why and then becomes violently distressed.

When first under observation, naturalistic examples of message value in Cindy's behaviour abound. For example she would often stand by the (locked) dining room door, looking into the dining room, sometimes holding hands with people and leading them to the dining room door, even putting other people's hands onto the door handle. When people were thus led to the door she would vocalise at the door. If people clearly refused to open the door or pulled away roughly, she would sometimes scream or make crying noises. She generally avoided looking into people's faces and when spoken to often held her head down towards her stomach after a very brief orientation reflex.

She became unpopular with some people because she was noisy, difficult to control in the way that care staff wished and when unsupervised, damaged a lot of the ward fittings.

A typical incident would go as follows: the dining room door is accidentally left unlocked, Cindy walks in, nurses panic and grapple with her, Cindy throws herself to the ground, props herself up on one elbow and screams while looking at her hand, nurses grapple with her on the floor leading to mutual distress with Cindy crying. Attempts at pushing nurses away would be interpreted by some as bad behaviour. In fact some care staff labelled any patient who escalated their messages as bad. In psychodynamic terms this could represent a form of countertransference revealing something of their parenting style.

The case of Cindy is very appropriate for this chapter because it highlights the vulnerability and torment of profoundly mentally disabled people who send messages that others cannot or will not receive. It was Cindy who was defined as the problem, not the inflexibility of the service she received. She was viewed as hopeless and not rehabilitation material. Value judgements were made by some of those whose professional ethic should exclude judgmental behaviour.

Behavioural observations and reports from nurses showed that there were no structured events in her life beyond being bathed, toileted, fed, encouraged to bed, etc. Some nurses had tried to engage her in games or to look at pictures but a fundamental problem was the severe lack of comprehension and an apparent lack of any sort of social meshing or turn taking. She would sit on an armchair and make loud vocalisations. When nurses came up to attempt interaction the vocalisations continued but might get louder, she might grab at their arm then pull them (frontal grasp reflex), at which point she often began screaming. Thus, constructive behaviour by nurses had been punished, leading in some cases to a severe deterioration in relationships with Cindy.

A clinical psychologist took on the case, with the following objectives:

1. To find out how Cindy communicated and what her messages were.
2. To discover her preferences, desires, needs and torments.
3. To find ways of ameliorating her distress.
4. To set a series of realistic short-term skill goals from which communication and relationships could develop.
5. To design a lifestyle to meet her needs.
6. To use this design to advocate for her not only in the present service but in a future brain injury service that was being planned.
7. To help others to want to help her by improving her public image, for example to make her look more skilled and attractive. In particular to comfort her parents who, on rare traumatic visits, accumulated images of their screaming daughter being vigorously removed from places where nursing staff did not want her to be.

Once rudimentary relationships had been formed with Cindy, the intention to communicate paradigm (started by East) was to be a crucial element of all therapeutic goals.

The clinical psychologist and psychology assistant gave Cindy two clinical contacts a week, these always taking place in an empty room off of the ward in a disused part of the hospital. This facilitated the best experimental control in that there were no distractions and psychologists manipulated all stimuli.

A Latin square experimental design enabled pairwise comparisons of foods and drinks to see which were her favourites from an array that had no exchange value with respect to the diabetes. Her choice, i.e. which of two things she took was noted and rank ordered from most to least frequently chosen. She always chose carefully with no lunging at food hoppers.

A similar Latin square design was used to study her reactions to different types of music as it was rumoured that she liked music. Sequences of different types of music were played, for example one minute of rock music, one minute of jazz, one minute of choral music, etc. Music which was more often associated with Cindy looking calm and briefly looking at the therapists was judged more useful than music associated with pica-related behaviour.

So even at this early stage the mere presentation of choice enabled her to communicate. To begin with she was reluctant to choose, often looking down at her chest. It was noticed that she was actually scanning the floor by the male psychologist's feet. Experimentation showed that she would choose food in the company only of the female assistant so to begin with, the man stood outside the room and viewed Cindy's choices by the use of a mirror. Gradually she became used to both psychologists, choosing food and drink as required. She always took her time choosing and did not grab at food vigorously, unlike her behaviour on the ward.

When reinforcer assessment was complete, it was decided to embark on an open ended plan of intervention beginning with two programmes both of which were included in each session:

1. To teach her to feed herself at a normal speed. Nurses were feeding Cindy as on the ward she tended to lunge at food and force it into her mouth.
2. To help her to go for highly supervised walks outside the ward without pica.

The plan was to add modules of activity to each of these programmes as her skills developed. Thus programme one might develop into a sequence of structured activities indoors, while programme two would become the equivalent for outdoor activities.

Both initial programmes would enhance her public image by making her more competent and normal in appearance while being the basis for a structured day of activity for her as sequences developed.

A major factor in planning interventions was the long-term commitment required so that Cindy could, by repetition, learn to predict what was going to happen in the sessions and hopefully, therefore develop expectancy, i.e. look forward to the sessions and gradually anticipate each step so that reciprocity and communication might develop. It was hoped that from this, stimulus control of behaviour would also develop, and that problem behaviour would reduce or cease within therapy sessions.

The ground rules for psychology sessions are worth detailing:

1. All of her behaviour would be treated as having message value, and sessions were videoed for analysis later.
2. Therapists would model behavioural definitions of respect by ensuring that all therapist behaviour was gentle, calm, quiet and affectionate.
3. To marginalise the nuisance factor of hyperphagia, small pieces of vegetable would be available in sessions but would be earned by Cindy, who, with help from the therapists in the form of escalating prompts, would complete simple achievable goals. Thus a procedure which reduced hyperphagia served the purpose of a reinforcer.

Prompts were initially escalated from verbal only, then verbal plus a gesture and, if necessary, a very gentle physical prompt. This system of escalated prompts from least to most help, with food and praise as reinforcers can be seen as more or less errorless learning in that many behaviours targeted this way are guaranteed to occur, but with the trend towards fewer prompts or less powerful prompts as time goes by as in this way the person receives praise or tangible reward sooner. This practice was extended to all contact which the therapists had with her on therapy days including preparing her for the session, for example getting her to sit, to offer her feet one at a time so that her shoes could be put on, getting her to stand, walk to a door, sit at a table in the therapy room, etc.

Thus in all contact with her she got no more help than she needed at the particular moment and the programme could be evaluated in terms of changes in the level of prompt needed (Wilson, 1991).

It is important to emphasise the therapeutic and ethical stance that this treatment method reveals. It is basically this: identify what resources are needed to enable a patient to experience an ordinary life activity or event, and then provide it varying it as the requirement varies. This should be compared with more conventional approaches.

The approach chosen paid dividends not only in achieving specific goals but also the meshing of behaviour between Cindy and the therapists. The earliest sessions were associated with resistance to the unfamiliar with Cindy screaming or throwing herself on the floor when it was hoped that she would walk with the psychologists, or throwing herself down outside and engaging in pica. At no time did the psychologists struggle with her. When she threw herself on the ground (a behavioural event) therapists waited a few seconds until her posture could be described as a state (not an event) and then a reinforcer primer was given. She was simply given a piece of vegetable with the comment 'This is for you'. The therapists then said 'Cindy can you stand up' and gestured with their arms or, alternatively, opened a hand and quietly called her name. Thus primed with food she stood up and held the therapist's hand when another food reward was given to the comment 'well done'.

Using these procedures Cindy learned (within 10 sessions) to cooperate totally with the planned sequences of activity. When she saw the psychologist carrying her trainers she would hold hands and walk to a chair, offering her feet one at a time and stamping her foot down if the shoes were hard to put on. She learned to walk to the door at the same pace as the psychologist and would turn the handle when the door was unlocked. Her walking could be guided by holding her hand and also gesturing when a change of direction was planned. Pica on outside walks was suppressed by vegetable rewards for fixed periods of no pica. Stopping at kerbs was taught using a similar technique. Vocalisation on walks simply went to zero.

Indoors, Cindy swiftly learned to feed herself with a spoon or fork in her right hand and at an acceptable speed. The food on the plate was a natural reinforcer. The nursing team adopted this approach for ward-based meals.

Early sessions indoors were marked by less distress than the walks probably because food was served as meals but there was a marked lack of social meshing, with Cindy usually looking away from the psychologists, unless their backs were turned, when they were apparently scrutinised by her. She would avoid eye contact for some time to come. During the earliest sessions she sat at a table alone, with one psychologist serving meals and running the contingency programme and the other taking notes from afar. This was to ensure that she had the best chance of learning to feed herself with no human distraction.

As soon as possible, however, the two psychologists sat at the table with Cindy, one serving and the other also being served food. As she had learnt that food was assured, she was unconcerned about the food on her neighbour's plate and did not steal it or interfere with it in anyway. She began to take glances at her new friends as she raised her head between taking mouthfuls of food.

Messages were sent to her friends by noise and gesture. At the start of a meal she would sit looking at the bowl from which food was served and sometimes hold her hand out while giving loud and long vocal perseverations 'Ree or ree or ree', etc. These stopped as she began to eat.

To initiate turn taking and a simple form of social interaction, the feeding programme was followed by a new programme in which small pieces of vegetable were put in an array on a plate in the centre of the table. The goal was to get her to eat the pieces one at a time and to tolerate her friends sharing in the treat. When the plate was empty, it was refilled from a hopper to increase training opportunity. If she took two or more pieces at once, the plate was moved out of her reach for 15 seconds and then returned. She soon learned to carry out this activity.

When the plate had been emptied, she would either look at the plate, perhaps vocalising, or simply look down at the table or her chest. This was in association with the psychologist's habit of automatically replenishing the plate. This is worthy of comparison with a third programme in which she was given drinks in tiny amounts so that she could learn to hand back the cup for more. When required to communicate, and when given escalating prompts of the form 'please can I have the glass', then repeated with an open handed gesture, she soon learned to hand over the glass for more drink.

The psychologists, however, began to realise the fact that with respect to communication, Cindy was still not getting maximum therapeutic value from the sessions and it was feared that latent communication might be wasted. For example during session 31 (which for practical reasons was run by one psychologist only), she gave prolonged eye contact in response to a noise from outside of the room, and a questioning facial expression.

Meanwhile, as part of a staff development initiative, preparations were beginning for a staff workshop to teach East's intention to communicate paradigm. Other residents with profound communication disorders were being selected for video vignets and it was hoped that Cindy would be included. Much of the ground work had already been accomplished, for example her reinforcers were known and she was already used to video.

Figure 13.1 shows a detailed description of the results of the first few seconds of Cindy's video. She initiated most of her messages by looking. She also frequently anticipated events showing a lot of responsiveness, for example visual tracking of people, swivelling in her seat, changing body posture, holding out her hand with open palm (a gestural prompt to others), then escalating or amplifying the message with vocalisation. Eye contact now existed and was in the form of turn taking.

The main task set for her as a result of this exercise was to work on her non-verbal strengths to compensate for and even reduce her loud vocalisations which made her stand out as very abnormal in the company of strangers. To do this, sequences of interpersonal behaviour would be stretched to necessitate and encourage communication of the most valuing sort. Implicit in this was the desire to respond to her earliest communications and thus further reduce distress. The following changes were therefore made to her sessions:

1. Psychologists would watch for and immediately respond to the earliest non-verbal messages of the request object or repeated action form. This made these non-verbal messages useful to her. No food would be served or activity begun if long loud vocalisations were actually in progress.

TRANSCRIPTION

CLIENT'S NAME: **CINDY** DATE: SHEET No: **1** CODING COUNTER:

CHANNEL

Eye gaze to Person	-EGP
Eye gaze to Object	-EGO
Verbal	-Ve
Vocal	-Vo
Facial Expression	-FE
Physical Contact	-FC
Body Movement	-BM
Sign	-S
Point	-P
Nod	-N
Open/Palm	-OP
Push/Move Away	-P/MA
Idiosyncratic	-IDIOSYN

FUNCTION

Request Action	-RA
Request Object	-RO
Request Information	- RI
Direct Attention to Self	-DAS
Direct Attention for Communication	-DAC
Direct Attention to an Object	-DAO
Direct Attention to an Action	-DAA
Answer	-Ans
Protest	-Pro
Response to Person	-RTP
Response to Action	-RTA
Response to Event	-RTE

CODING		STAFF MEMBERS = J + A		Event No	Turn Tak-ing	CLIENT - CINDY		CODING	
Chann.	Int. Func.	Vocal/Verbal Events	Non-Verbal Events			Non-Verbal Events	Vocal/Verbal Events	Int. Func.	Chann.
				1		CINDY LOOKS TO J'S RIGHT AT CAN OF COLA DRINK		R T E	E G O
		J SAYS TO A "ARE WE UP AND RUNNING"		2					
				3		CINDY LOOKS AT A THEN AT DRINKS		R T A	E G O
		WOULD YOU LIKE A DRINK CINDY		4					
				5		CINDY LOOKS AT J EYES		R T P	E G P
				6		CINDY LOOKS AT TABLE NEAR J	HOREEA REA REA	R O	E V G O O
				7		LOOKS AT GLASSES AND DRINK	HOREEA REA REA	R O	E V G O O
			J POURS A DRINK FOR HERSELF	8					
				9		CINDY WATCHES LIFTS HER RIGHT ARM	LOUDER HOREEA REA	R R O A	E V G O P
				10		PULLS TABLE TOWARDS HER		R R O A	E V G O O
				11		VISUALLY FOL-LOWS GLASS TO J'S MOUTH		R R R I A O	E G O
				12		LOOKS INTO J'S EYES HAND STRET-CHED OUT	HORREA REA	R A	E G P

Figure 13.1. Details of the results of the first few seconds of Cindy's video.

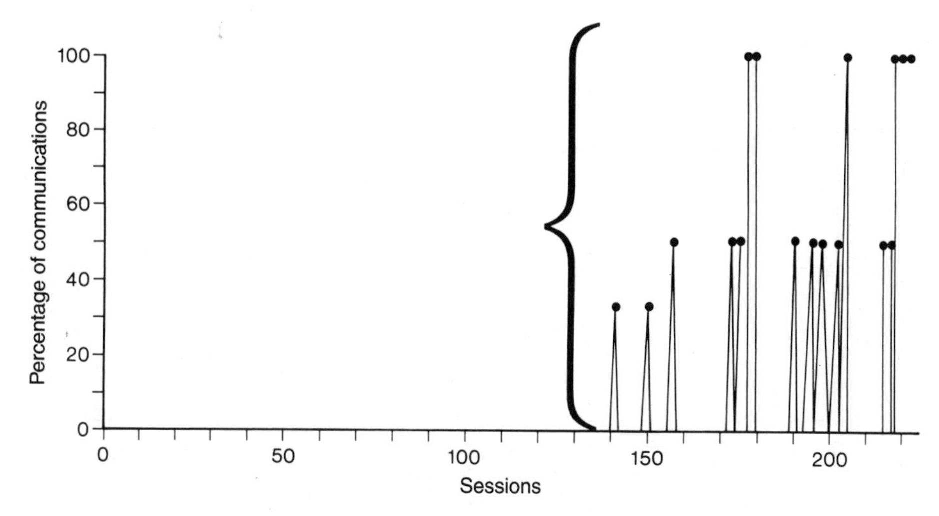

Figure 13.2. Mealtime communication: percentage of servings requested by eye to object communication. The bracket shows intention training from sessions 136 onwards.

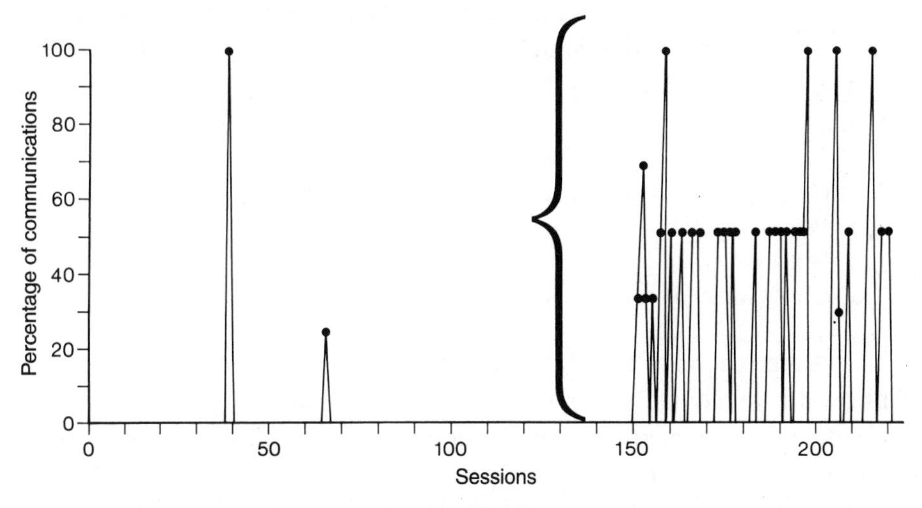

Figure 13.3. Mealtime communication: percentage of servings, including eye contact. Bracket shows intention training from session 136 onwards.

2. Cindy would be taught to play ball games to provide a continuous form of reciprocity between herself and others. This would also constitute comparatively normal activity.
3. She would be taught to choose music cassettes by pointing.

Figures 13.2–13.4 show some of the results of the programme for served meals and for food sharing. For served meals there was an immediate increase in

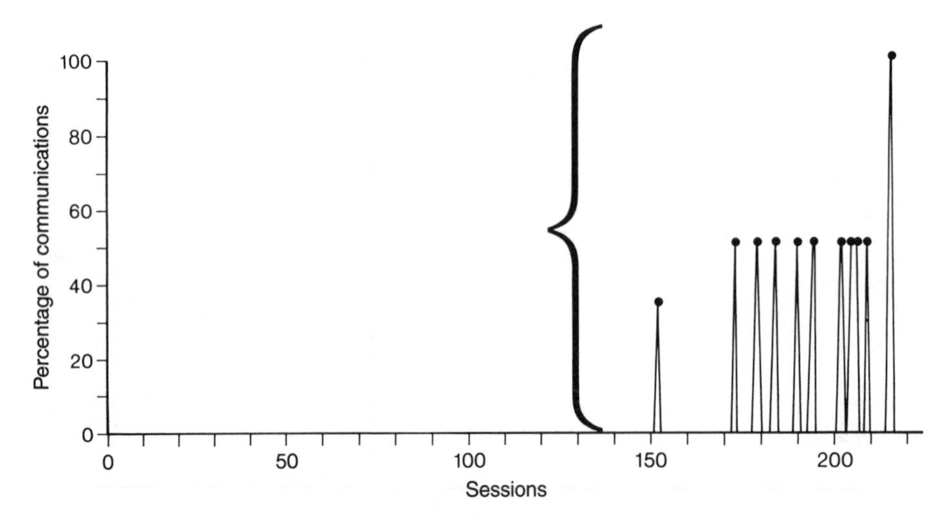

Figure 13.4. Mealtime communication: percentage of servings, including smiles or chuckles. Bracket shows intention training from session 136 onwards.

Cindy putting her fork down and also a tendency to push her fork and plate towards the person serving. Simultaneously eye contact and eye object behaviour increased, with smiling and chuckling also occurring in a turn taking way.

A typical sequence might be as follows:

a. Cindy puts her fork down and looks at the food hopper.
b. Psychologist says 'Yes let's have some more'.
c. Other psychologist says 'Is this nice'?
d. Cindy looks at speaker, smiles and chuckles.

Vocalisations tended to be briefer and again, turn taking in form, for example 'This food is lovely isn't it', Cindy quietly 'Solleeda'.

The data are similar for the application of these rules for sharing food from a plate in the centre of a table. Eye contact and eye object were particularly impressive in relation to this more socially intimate activity (Figure 13.5).

Ball games

The aim was to teach Cindy to roll a small ball along a table to her companions who were seated with her around the table. This could then become a simple method to be used by others to engage in a social activity with her. Ultimate plans were for her to learn to play skittles and also to kick a large football to her companions. This would give variety of activity and look a little more normal than table ball games.

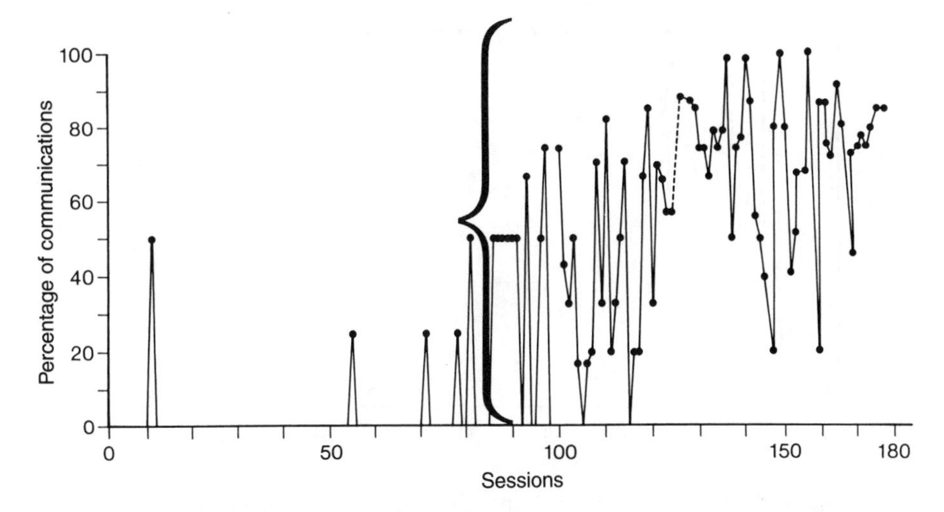

Figure 13.5. Shared foods communication: percentage of servings requested by eye–object communication. Bracket shows intention training from session 86 onwards.

As she did not possess the ability to roll a ball, simply holding it, biting it, or handing it to the psychologist, she was taught to roll it by a shaping procedure which progressed in the following stages: she touches the ball, the ball rolls irrespective of how this happens, she clearly tries to roll it, she rolls the ball down the length of the table, she rolls it to her companions. Her progress can be seen in Figure 13.6. Cindy would often smile or chuckle as she played.

Having learned the reciprocal nature of table ball play, Cindy soon learned to kick a large ball to her companions while seated on a chair. Kicking a ball while standing was more challenging for her as she is a little unsteady on her feet, but this was also achieved by the use of a companion to hold her hand, which steadied her and helped to prevent distractible behaviour which was always more probable when she was mobile (Figure 13.7).

Musical choice

Sessions were often finished off by listening to her favourite music. To enable her to choose the music, audio cassettes were placed in front of her in pairs with, for example, the comment, 'What shall we listen to Abba or Madonna'? This was accompanied by a gestural prompt of pointing to each cassette as it was named. Choosing behaviour was shaped by responding immediately to the earliest sign of intention, for example the cassette at which she looked, touched, moved or pointed.

The psychologist responses were of the form, 'Yes let's play Abba' or 'Yes you chose Abba well done'. The cassette was inserted into the player and as the

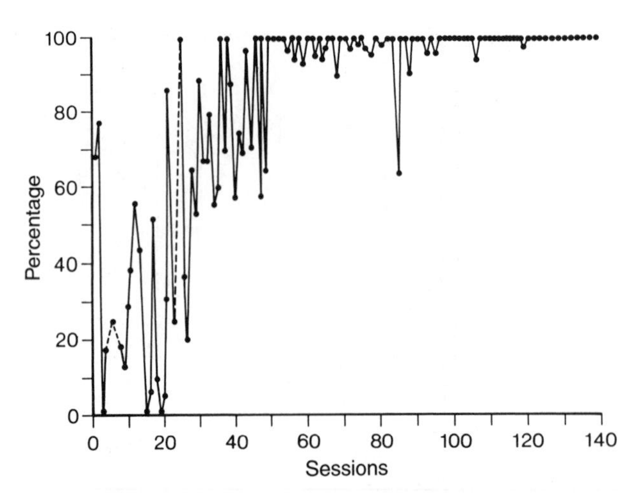

Figure 13.6. Percentage of events that were perfect ball rolls down the length of the table. ---, Missing data/no data.

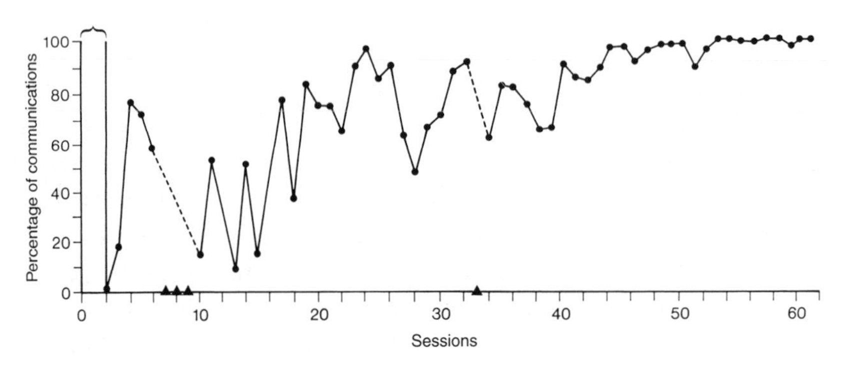

Figure 13.7. Percentage of kicks or hand rolls requiring no prompt while playing seated football. Bracket shows pilot project. ▲, no data; ---, no data.

music started Cindy was given three tiny sugar free jelly sweets to eat.

Figures 13.8–13.10 illustrate Cindy's progress. Again, there was smiling and chuckling, and also she began to initiate holding hands with her companions.

If as rarely happened she stood up from the table where music was being played, the psychologist would say 'Shall we stop'? or 'Shall we go back to the ward'? Cindy might walk to the door and stand there, which was taken as a desire to return to the ward.

So what does the work with Cindy tell us?

Her methods of communication were investigated then used experimentally to establish good warm, affectionate relationships with the psychologists and

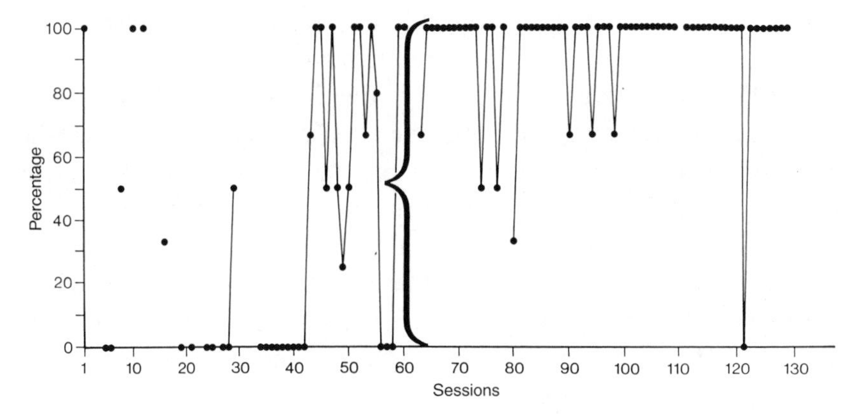

Figure 13.8. Percentage of played cassettes chosen by pointing or touching. Bracket shows contingency condition from session 61 onwards.

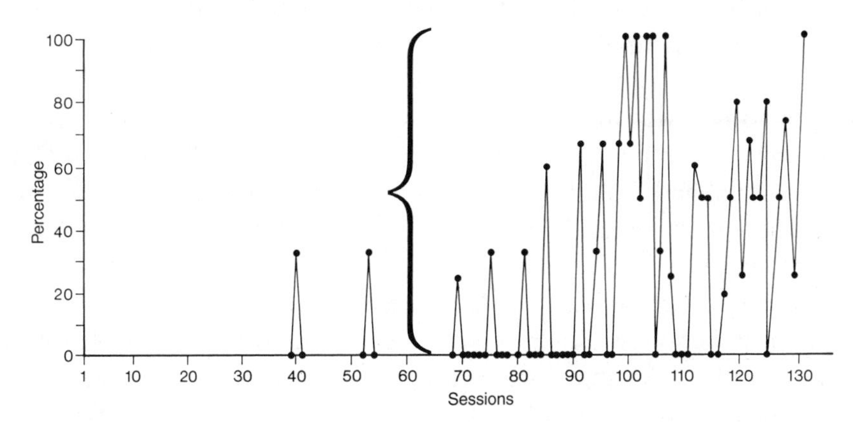

Figure 13.9. Percentage of musical cassette choices with hand holding. Bracket shows contingency condition from session 61 onwards.

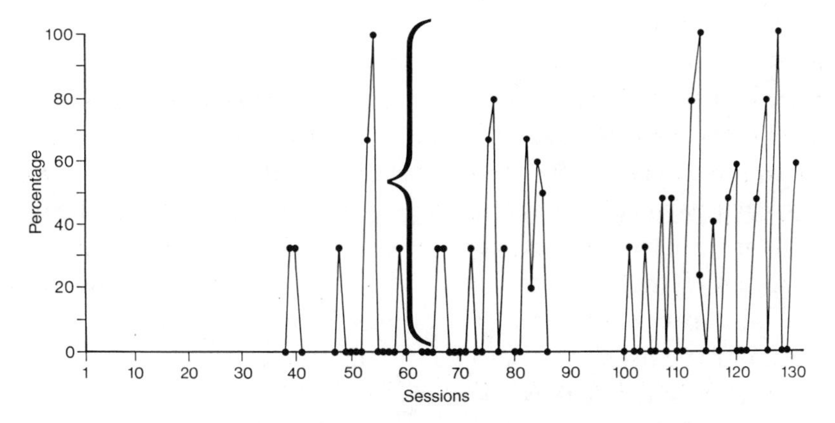

Figure 13.10. Percentage of musical cassette choices with smiles or chuckles. Bracket shows contingency condition from session 61 onwards.

others. The functions of her behaviour and the content of her messages were analysed and used immediately. For example throwing herself on the ground was a general purpose escape behaviour whether in the face of being manhandled or whether experiencing fear in the face of a strange situation, as when a physiotherapist bounced a huge inflated ball to her. Looking at her hand seemed to be a way of reducing arousal during periods of anticipation, as when waiting for food to be served.

A severe hyperphagic syndrome could be suppressed with structured activity, praise and small vegetable reinforcers. Distress went to zero during sessions, as did violent behaviour. Smiling began and increased.

Sessions which at their most intense accounted for less than 4% of her waking life were nonetheless highly effective at teaching valuing skills to a profoundly mentally disabled patient who had for years been seen as hopeless.

Photographs were taken to celebrate her achievements, for example choosing cassettes, playing football and even smiling. These were put into a photograph album which included photographs taken before her brain damage. The resulting album showed the interested viewer that life and hope continue after the most appalling brain damage. It was also testimony to the fact that Cindy was valued and had friends who found her attractive. Her parents now received different images of their daughter and proudly showed their relatives. 'We are proud of her' they said.

The work with Cindy also accrued simple resources for her, for example photographs of her out walking, playing ball and so forth were displayed in a photograph cabinet on the ward establishing 'social space' for her. Thus, Cindy was seen as somebody who sits holdings hands with her friends or her parents, a three-seater sofa being a pleasant 'social' piece of furniture instead of individual chairs.

She was seen as a person who goes out for walks, thus in need of attractive age and gender appropriate clothes and shoes.

It became known that she chooses cassettes to play so her own stereo radio and cassette player would be useful.

As she was financially very poor, her conscientious key worker nurse obtained special payments from the hospital manager to pay for Christmas and birthday presents to support the above activities. When people visited the ward, particularly if they came to meet her for the first time, these possessions could have an impact on the first impressions formed about her.

As the accoutrements of social space accumulate, it will be easier to demand more for her from future service planners.

The work with Cindy perhaps demonstrates the following:

1. Disruptive behaviour can have message value and it is proper for this aspect of the behaviour to be considered.
2. Simple but effective methods of studying communications from profoundly disabled people exist and should be used.
3. Behavioural procedures such as shaping can be applied effectively even in the severest cases and should be, given that medication and nursing care can help but do not have all the answers.
4. Effective goal setting requires vision and long-term commitment.
5. Skills do not have to be taught *in situ*, they can generalise.
6. People with the greatest disability can benefit from and deserve high levels of resources.
7. Such resourcing facilitates the use of the scientific case study approach which is most suited to this highly heterogeneous client group.

References

Altman, J. (1974). Observational study of behaviour: sampling methods. *Behaviour*, **49**, 227–67.
Campbell, D. & Draper, R. (1985). *Applications of Systemic Family Therapy, The Milan Approach*. London: Grune and Stratton.
Chamberlain, P. (1985). *STEP Social Skills Assessment Manual*. British Association of Applied Behavioural Psychotherapy. Birmingham: Plan Publications.
Donnellan, A. M., Mirenda, P., Mesaros, R. & Fassbender, L. (1984). A strategy for analysing the communicative functions of behaviour. *Journal of The Association for Persons with Severe Handicaps*. **11**, 201–12.
Fitts, P. M. & Posner, M. I. (1973). *Human Performance*. London: Prentice Hall International.
Goffman, E. (1961). *Asylums*. Harmondsworth, Middlesex, Britain: Penguin Books.
Haley, J. (1978). *Problem Solving Therapy*. New York, London: Harper & Row.
Hersen, M. & Bellack, A. S. (1981). *Behavioural Assessment: A Practical Handbook*, 2nd ed. New York, Oxford: Pergamon Press.
Kazdin, A. E. (1975). *Behaviour Modification in Applied Settings*. Homewood: Dorsey Press.
La Vigna, G. W. (1986). *Alternatives to Punishment: Solving Behavioural Problems using Non-Aversive Strategies*. New York: Irvington Publishers.
Nelson, R. O. (1981). Realistic dependent measures for clinical use. *Journal of Consulting and Clinical Psychology*, **49**, 168–82.
Pavlov, I. P. (1927). *Conditioned Reflexes*. New York: Oxford University Press.
Skinner, B. F. (1938). *The Behaviour of Organisms*. New York: Appleton-Century-Crofts.
Wilson, B. A. (1991). Behaviour therapy in the treatment of neurologically impaired adults. In *Handbook of Behaviour Therapy and Psychological Science* ed. P. R. Martin. New York: Pergamon Press.

14

Pain

SANDRA HORN

The nature of pain

Pain is an important issue for the rehabilitation practitioner, not only because it is so common among patients but because it has far-reaching effects on a variety of functions crucial to the rehabilitation process. Pain can affect emotional life, cognition, the level and pattern of activity, and relationships. It may be difficult or impossible for the patient in pain to attend to and remember instructions; irritability and depression associated with pain may affect motivation and cooperation. The relief of pain often dominates all other concerns. These difficulties arise not from neurosis on the part of the patient, but from the complex nature of pain itself: it is an unpleasant, urgent sensation that characteristically dominates one's thoughts. It is a primary drive like hunger and thirst, and at its root is the urge for survival.

The subjective experience of pain, however, is subject to wide individual variations. You and I both know what pain is, but I do not know your pain, and you cannot know mine. We may both use the same words to describe it, but may mean different things. Both the perception of pain, and the way it is reported or demonstrated by the sufferer, are moderated by many interweaving factors : 'a complex web of subjective, behavioural, physiological and pathological phenomena' as Steptoe & Pearce (1983) have written. Lewith & Kenyon (1984) have also commented on the fact that there are still many painful diseases whose pathology is poorly understood, and many clinically effective therapies whose physiology and pharmacology remain elusive. This is in large part because the interweaving factors that determine both the inner experience and outward manifestation of pain, cross many disciplines : neurophysiology and chemistry, anatomy, pharmacology, psychology (individual and social). There is also the problem that pain cannot be directly measured. It may be inferred from observation of gross behaviour patterns or from physiological measurements, or taken from self-report, or a mixture of these, but they will only yield analogues of the pain. How closely they approximate to the original experience cannot be known, but only guessed at from results which are sufficiently consistent.

Even the word 'pain' itself has proved difficult to define in a way that is universally accepted. Sternbach's (1968) attempt at a three-part definition demonstrates some of the problems:

1. Pain is a personal, private sensation of hurt.
2. Pain is a harmful stimulus which signals current of impending tissue damage.
3. Pain is a pattern of responses which operate to protect the organism from harm.

This definition links the elements of hurt (unpleasantness), harm and the generation of avoidance behaviour. The 'pattern of responses' referred to has the primary aim of harm avoidance.

The idea that a primary function of pain is to signal tissue damage is a problem, however. Many writers, among them Melzack & Wall (1982) have commented on the variable relationship between pain and tissue damage. In some cases of pain of the acute type, the relationship seems straightforward, but there are many others where the link between the site and severity of the damage and the experience of pain is variable or non-existent. For example, in referred pain the damage is in one place but the pain is experienced in another; there are also 'trigger zones', areas of the body that can, when stimulated, cause pain to be felt somewhere else. There are silent pathological changes, in which extensive damage to tissue takes place in the absence of pain. There is the severe intractable pain associated with damage to the thalamus and surrounding areas; the pain is perceived as arising from the body, but is generated centrally. There are the well-known phenomena of phantom limb pain after amputation, and causalgia, an intense burning sensation associated with peripheral nerve injury, which may be exacerbated by the lightest touch on the skin. Causalgia, like neuralgia (sharp shooting pain also associated with peripheral nerve damage such as that caused by shingles), characteristically comes on after the damage appears to have healed.

These examples show that the disease model of pain, i.e. the idea that the experience of acute pain may be defined by its relationship with an injury, is inadequate in many cases. Pain *may* be perceived as arising from the injury site or close by it, it *may* vary in intensity with the severity of the tissue damage, it *may* fade away as healing takes place. Each of these statements must be qualified with ifs and buts. When pain has become chronic, however, the relationship between the experience and any underlying tissue disturbance is even less clear.

Cervero & Laird (1991) postulate a three-phase model of pain from (a) 'normal nociception' (the processing of a brief noxious stimulus) to (b) 'normal nociceptive systems under prolonged noxious stimulation' (peripheral tissue damage and inflammation) to (c) 'abnormal neuropathic pain' (including peripheral neuropathies and central pain). Prolonged noxious stimulation changes the input to the CNS in two ways:

1. Nociceptors may be sensitised: i.e. show a lowered response threshold, so that they may be activated by innocuous stimuli.
2. Silent or 'sleepy' nociceptors that do not respond to noxious stimuli under normal conditions, but which become active when the tissue they innervate becomes inflamed, may be triggered.

These changes in the input to the central nervous system (CNS) lead to changes in the central component of pain perception; there is a move to a new, more excitable state, so that the direct relationship between peripheral input and pain perception is distorted. The puzzle of why phase three 'abnormal' pain is seen only in a minority of patients remains. Cervero & Laird comment that the development of phase three pain may involve genetic, cognitive or emotional factors which have yet to be identified.

Grzesiak (1984) offers a list of five ways of defining chronic pain:

1. Pain of more than six month's duration.
2. Pain that continues beyond the normal expected healing time.
3. Pain with no apparent pathophysiological basis.
4. Pain which has a demonstrable tissue origin, but which is disproportionate to the organic features.
5. Pain with a demonstrable non-neoplastic cause but no appropriate medical, surgical or pharmacological approach to control it (chronic benign pain).

Grzesiak's first category is another example of the problem described by Cervero & Laird; there are chronically painful conditions such as rheumatoid arthritis, in which pain can persist (albeit with variations in intensity) for a very long time, but that do not come in to the category of abnormal or chronic. As Brena & Chapman (1985) have said, 'the real question is not the experience of persistent pain, but why a percentage of those experiencing such pain become disabled and dependent in a maladaptive way'.

Calliet (1979) offers a theoretical model for the progression of events as follows:

1. Nociception (from tissue irritation).
2. Pain.
3. Suffering (affective response).
4. Pain behaviour.

Again, Calliet's scheme contains the hint that time scale might have a role to play, as he talks about the engram of pain becoming 'embossed' in the CNS with time. The gate control theory of Melzack & Wall (1965) also contains the notion of the 'memory' of pain. These ideas might explain why some pains become persistent, but do not account for why some people with persistent pain develop pain behaviour, or the chronic pain syndrome.

The search for explanations of the variability in pain experiences and behaviour has resulted in many lines of enquiry. These range from research into the underlying mechanisms of pain transmission to investigations of personality 'types' and other individual differences, social factors and the role of learning.

The major current lines of thinking will be described here, together with methods of measurement and treatment.

Pain and neurophysiology : specificity versus patterning

Early theories about the transmission of pain can be divided into those based on the idea that activity in specialised sensory nerve endings signals pain (**specificity theories**) and those based on the idea that any sensory nerve ending will signal pain if it receives excessive stimulation, i.e. stimuli coming very close together in space or over time (**pattern theories**). Pattern theorists (for an example see Weddell, 1955) argue that the same sensory nerve could, at different times, transmit touch, cold, warmth or pain. This approach takes no account of evidence for receptor specialisation, whereas specificity theory cannot account for the lack of correlation between tissue damage and pain.

The focus of both specificity and pattern theories is neurophysiological: which cell or group of cells does what, under what degrees of excitation.

The Gate Control Theory of pain (Melzack & Wall, 1965) incorporates elements of specificity and patterning. It is not without its critics, and still leaves many questions to be answered, but it is to date the only theory to integrate the psychological and neurological aspects of pain, and to stress the importance of the psychological component.

A conceptual leap was performed by Melzack & Wall when they described the gate control theory. It had already been demonstrated that certain cutaneous sensations are transmitted by different types of fibre which converge in the dorsal horn of the spinal cord. Large diameter myelinated ('A') fibres carry the sensation of light touch, and small diameter unmyelinated ('C') fibres transmit diffuse burning pain. An important aspect of the gate theory is that the transmission of pain depends on the balance of activity between these two types of afferent fibre. Low levels of activity in the 'C' fibres may be blocked by intense activity in the 'A' fibres, i.e. sufficient stimulation of the 'light touch' pathways can close the gate to pain transmission.

The other important aspect of the theory is that descending fibres from the brainstem reticular formation and the cerebral cortex also feed into the dorsal horn, and may facilitate or inhibit the activity of ascending pathways. Thus ascending information may be influenced by input from the limbic forebrain (motivational–affective system) via the brainstem reticular formation, and the somatosensory cortex (discriminative system).

Work by Melzack (1975) suggests that there is also a central biasing mechanism in the brainstem, which modulates the transmission of painful stimuli to the higher centres, and which acts as an inhibitory feedback system. Low levels of sensory input would weaken the inhibitory system, whereas increased sensory input would increase the inhibition of pain transmission. The analgesia produced by acupuncture, or by TENS (Transcutaneous Electrical Nerve Stimulation) may work by increasing the sensory input and thereby activating the inhibitory mechanism, but that does not explain why the analgesia outlasts the stimulation. Melzack & Wall further suggest that pain may persist because of self-exciting circuits, resulting in memory-like processes, and that brief intense input from acupuncture or TENS might disrupt the circuts. When pain is relieved, the increased physical activity permitted would lead to raised levels of sensory input, which would increase the inhibition of pain transmission, or would prevent the recurrence of the deviant neural activity.

The four key elements of the gate control theory of pain are:

1. The balance of inputs into the peripheral sensory nerves.
2. The brainstem central biasing mechanism.
3. The input from the descending pathways.
4. The memory-like process involved in persistent pain.

The resultant experience of pain is the sum of a complex series of interactions between peripheral and central (including higher cortical) activity. The central variables include a wide range of possible influences from perceptual, emotional and cognitive factors, such as other distracting stimuli, beliefs and expectations, and previous learning.

Some researchers have argued that pain sensation is not invariably linked to activity in specific types of nerve fibre (Dyck *et al.*, 1976; Iggo, 1972), and have called into question the existence of a gating mechanism such as that described by Melzack & Wall. It is clear that the pain-modulating mechanisms in the spinal cord and brain are not yet completely understood, and that some anatomical and physiological aspects of the theory might change as new technology permits more sophisticated investigations to be made. To date, however, the gate control theory, with its emphasis on the interplay between psychological variables and neurophysiological mechanisms, is still the most influential model of pain perception. As Weisenberg (1977) has said, 'It has had a profound influence on pain research and the clinical control of pain . . . stimulating a multidisciplinary view of pain for research and treatment'.

Pain and biochemistry

In 1969, Reynolds demonstrated that analgesia could be produced by electrical stimulation of certain areas of the brain. This finding prompted a search for the neurochemical basis for the effect. During the 1970s, the existence of naturally-occurring narcotic-like substances (opioids) was demonstrated in neural tissue in parts of the brain and spinal cord. These substances are proenkephalins, which have a widespread distribution in the nervous and endocrine systems, beta-endorphins, in the limbic system and brainstem among other places, and prodynorphin in the gut, posterior pituitary and brain (Akil *et al.*, 1984). Considerable numbers of studies have been undertaken into the part played by these naturally-occurring opiates in pain control, mood and behaviour. They have an analgesic action, and also produce feelings of calmness and well-being.

Enkephalins and narcotic receptors are concentrated in an area of the midbrain that produces analgesia when it is stimulated electrically. Experiments have shown that the midbrain generates impulses that descend into the spinal cord, and prevent the transmission of pain signals to the brain. Enkephalins and narcotic receptors are also found in the cord, particularly in the dorsal laminae close to the terminal points of the descending fibres from the midbrain. At these sites, injections of small amounts of narcotics produce inhibition of the transmission of impulses from an injured area. It is clear, however, that endorphins and enkephalins are not the only substances implicated in the production of analgesia, and there is not one but several descending control systems, some of which use these endogenous opiates as transmitters and some do not. Some descending fibres from the midbrain use serotonin, for example, and substance P is the main primary afferent neurotransmitter. Many other neurotransmitters, such as dopamine and noradrenaline, are also involved, and as yet the interactions between them and the endogenous opiates are not well understood. Indeed, the precise conditions under which enkephalins and endorphins are released have not yet been documented; they are part of a pain suppression system which is not always in operation. What triggers it? It is known that they are produced as a response to injury, and some other forms of stress including fear and prolonged strenuous exercise. Melzack & Wall have suggested that they may act so as to prevent the organism from being overwhelmed by pain.

Some studies have demonstrated a link between acupuncture analgesia and endorphin release, while others have failed to find any such relationship. It is likely that the production of these endogenous chemicals is under multifactorial control, and that as yet, only some of the factors have been documented.

Laboratory studies using standard noxious stimuli have demonstrated some individual variability in pain threshold (the point at which a strong stimulus is described as painful) and wide individual variation in pain tolerance (the point at which the subject finds the stimulus unbearable and asks for it to be terminated). Psychological, environmental and sociocultural factors have all been shown to influence reactions to standard painful stimuli, and if they influence the behavioural reactions, they may be influencing the body's neurochemistry as well.

Documenting pain

The subjective nature of pain is the first problem in the systematic documentation of the problem. Pain is a private experience, and its characteristics can only be inferred from observed behaviour, self-report and physiological changes. These are not direct measures of the pain itself, but merely analogues of it. There are difficulties inherent in the measurement of pain, both in laboratory and clinical settings, which will be described in the following section.

Pain thresholds and tolerance: social and environmental influences

In the laboratory, standard noxious stimuli such as ice-water, radiant heat, electric shock and pressure have been used to determine pain threshold and pain tolerance. Pain threshold is the point at which the strength of a stimulus or its duration causes the subject to describe it as painful rather than hot, cold, tingling or tight, for example. Pain tolerance is the point at which the subject describes the stimulus as unbearable, and requests its termination.

Studies have demonstrated wide individual variability. One example is described by Wardle (1985). It is an early attempt by Hardy *et al.* (1952) to investigate the relationship between stimulus magnitude and the subjects' responses. The results showed that consistency of response could only be achieved with constantly prevailing conditions and highly practised subjects. The responses were influenced by a number of factors such as environmental and psychological variables, including mood, fatigue, anxiety, concurrent sensory stimulation and suggestion.

Sociocultural effects on pain threshold and tolerance have also been demonstrated. For example, Clark & Clark (1980) showed the effects of cultural learning on groups of Nepalese Sherpas and the western mountaineers for whom they were working. Although both groups showed comparable levels of sensory discrimination to electric shock, the Nepalese required higher levels of stimulation before they described the shocks as painful. The fact that both groups demonstrated similar levels of sensory discrimination suggests that the differences were not simply physiological, and further evidence of the role of cultural learning in pain tolerance is provided by the study carried out by Lambert *et al.* (1960). They showed that by manipulating group identification, they could influence the pain tolerance limits of Jewish and Protestant women. In individual testing sessions, the amount of pain subjects could endure was determined by the use of a sphygmomanometer cuff with hard projections sewn into the inner surface. The cuff was placed on the subjects' upper arms, and inflated until the subject pronounced it intolerable. Subjects were told that a retest would take place in five minutes. Before retesting, half the Jewish subjects were told that Jews as a group can take less pain than Christians, and half the Protestant group were told that Christians can take less pain than Jews. On retesting, both the Jewish and Protestant experimental groups had increased their intolerable pain limits significantly, whereas neither control group showed any change. Lambert *et al.* suggested that the implied attack on the reference group was a pressure powerful enough to increase the willingness and capacity of the group members to suffer intense pain. Studies such as these show that even at the level of psychophysics, there are many subtle and powerful influences operating on pain perception and/or on the willingness of subjects to report pain.

Clinical methods of pain assessment

Clinically, pain may be assessed by observation of overt behaviour, by measuring its physiological concomitants, or by self-report; combinations of methods are sometimes used. Sternbach (1974) described a technique that borrows laboratory methodology; the Tourniquet Pain Ratio. Ischaemic pain is induced by means of a tourniquet on one arm, and the patient reports when the pain level is equivalent to the normal level of clinical pain. The technique has high test–retest reliability, and in some circumstances the tourniquet pain ratio score correlates well with a self-report pain estimate. It is not in wide use, however, and one reason for this is probably the danger inherent in the method, not to mention the ethics of inducing pain deliberately in order to obtain an estimate of another pain.

Observational methods have included recording variables such as time spent resting, demand for medication, verbal expressions of pain, and sleep patterns. They may be used as measures before and after pain-relieving medicine or other procedures. They are costly in terms of time and the need for trained staff, but may be the preferred option in cases where self-report is felt to be unreliable or impossible, as in pain assessment of small children, people with a severe learning difficulty, or any case where verbal communication is not appropriate. An example of such a measure is the Burns Treatment Distress Scale (BTDS) of Elliot & Olsen (1983) which consists of eight distressed behaviour items, all of which have operational definitions. The items are Groans and Screams, Verbal Fear, Verbal Pain, Emotional Support (verbal or non-verbal solicitation of hugs, physical comfort, expression of empathy), Muscular Rigidity, Verbal Resistance, Physical Resistance and Flailing.

While techniques such as the BTDS can provide objective and reliable data when carried out by trained observers, they cannot quantify pain directly, and the behaviour under observation might change for a number of reasons, not all of them to do with pain. Combining them with the subject's self-report is a means of relating the overt behaviour to the covert experience.

An imaginative example of a self-report technique which can be used with children is the Eland Colour Tool (Eland, 1985). It is used during an interview in which the child is asked about the kinds of things that have hurt him or her in the past. They are asked what was the worst, what was bad but not as bad as the worst hurt, what hurt a little, what did not hurt at all. They select coloured crayons to correspond to the four degrees of hurt they have identified, and colour in the appropriate areas on outline body shapes to show current of recent pain levels. They are asked if this pain is happening now, or was it felt earlier in the day; is it like that all the time, or on and off. The developmental stage of the child, particularly with regard to verbal and social skills, is crucial in determining the appropriateness of the technique, which can be helpful in giving early diagnostic clues, monitoring progress, and evaluating treatment.

There are also self-report scales on which pain is given an apparently objective (i.e. numerical) score, although there are problems with these numbers, which are discussed below. Among these measures are visual analogue scales of which the most simple is a ten-centimetre line with both endpoints identified. Subjects are invited to mark the line at the point most closely corresponding to their level of pain (Figure 14.1).

A variation of this method is to specify some of the divisions on the line so as to provide points of reference (Figure 14.2).

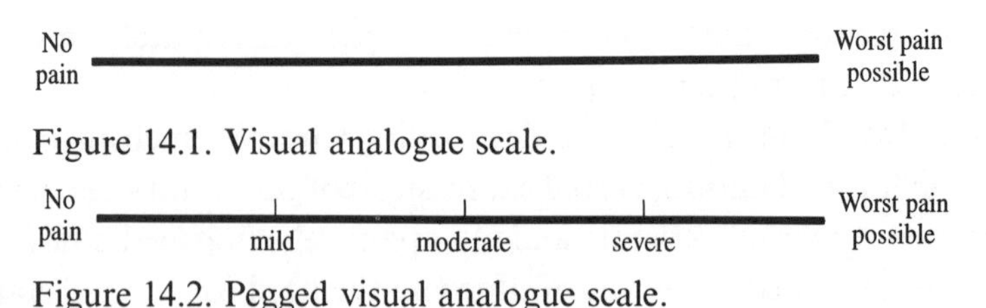

Figure 14.1. Visual analogue scale.

Figure 14.2. Pegged visual analogue scale.

Note that equal intervals between the points cannot be assumed. It is possible to obtain equal scale intervals in this and similar scales by having items such as 'minimal', 'little', 'moderate', 'severe', etc. ranked in order of increasing severity by a large number of subjects, who are also required to weight or score the items, and then construct the scale only from those items with good agreement for the numerical scores across subjects. When this preliminary scaling and weighting has not been carried out, these scales serve only to illustrate a subject's experience pictorially. They cannot be used to compare across subjects, and should not be assigned numerical scores.

There are also descriptive scales, on which the respondent is asked to indicate the statement that most closely corresponds to their current level of pain. The best-known of these is the McGill Pain Questionnaire (Melzack, 1975) which attempts to estimate both the intensity and quality of pain. The questionnaire was constructed by giving 102 pain descriptors to a group of subjects, who were asked to sort them into groups which described different aspects of pain. The preliminary sorting resulted in the identification of three major groups of pain descriptors; words concerning the sensory qualities of pain, words describing the affective qualities, and evaluative words concerned with the intensity of the experience. (Some later studies have cast doubt on the split between the affective and evaluative components, suggesting that they are one and the same.) In a second part of the study, groups of doctors, patients and students were asked to assign an intensity value to each of the words. The result was that there was no overall agreement on intensity values for the three groups, but adequate overall agreement for the relative positions of the words. The Pain Rating Index is computed; it is the sum of the ranked values of the words chosen as closest to the present pain experienced by the subject. The legitimacy of this statistic is questionable, as there is no agreement on intensity values across the three groups. Individual scores for each group may also be computed, and as the rank ordering of the words was shown to have agreement across subjects, some meaning might be attributed to the scores.

Another part of the questionnaire is the Present Pain Intensity (PPI) scale. Respondents are asked to indicate their level of pain from five statements: no pain (0), mild (1), discomforting (2), distressing (3), horrible (4) and excruciating (5). The descriptors are taken from a previously-determined ordering of pain evaluative words, and were chosen because they were approximately equally far apart on mean rankings, and thus 'represent equal scale intervals'. This is an argument of doubtful validity. Mean rankings, 'approximately equally far apart' do not represent equal scale intervals. Again, while there are grounds for accepting the rank ordering of the items, there are no grounds for adding numbers that imply equal intervals to the scale.

A scale that relates pain level to functional disability is the Oswestry Low Back Pain Disability Questionnaire (Fairbank *et al.*, 1980). The questionnaire consists of nine sections designed to sample a range of activities of daily living; personal care, lifting, walking, sitting, standing, sleeping, sex life, social life and travelling, and a section on the use of pain killers to obtain relief. Each section contains six simply-worded statements, graded from 1 to 5, with 1 representing no disability, and 5 the greatest disability. For example, in the section on sitting, 1 is 'I can sit in any chair as long as I like' and 5 is 'Pain prevents me from sitting at all'. Scores are summed and expressed as percentage disability, although summing scores where equal scale intervals have not been demonstrated is of doubtful validity. Nevertheless, internal consistency has been demonstrated, i.e. scores on each individual section show a relationship to the pain intensity section. For the purpose of planning a rehabilitation programme, however, the scores on individual sections would obviously be of more use than a crude overall score, and the dubious summing would be avoided.

The questionnaire has been standardised on low back pain patients only, but with further standardisation studies it could be a useful device for a range of pain patients where a short, simple, self-report scale is needed for monitoring progress.

All these scales are potentially useful in a clinical setting, where an individual's self-reported pain through time, or before and after intervention, needs to be recorded in a form that permits comparisons to be made. Their use as research tools, however, is questionable except perhaps in single case designs, because the data obtained are essentially subjective and 'soft'.

Emotional, motivational and cognitive factors

The simple view of pain, i.e. a sensation generated by tissue damage at a site of disease or injury (nociception), has proved to be inadequate even at a basic biological level. Many writers have drawn attention to the inadequacy inherent in describing pain merely as a sensation, among them Weisenberg (1977), who comments that in some respects pain is a sensation, and in others it is an emotional–motivational phenomenon leading to escape and avoidance behaviour. The sensation of pain is unpleasant, and it has other qualities too; it can be both urgent and insistent. It is hard to think about anything else when one is in pain. These qualities are part of the emotional–motivational component. They also relate to a common physiological accompaniment to the onset of pain: namely arousal in the sympathetic nervous system. Acute pain may cause arousal in the same way that any other threat to the organism does. This is demonstrated by the fact that painful stimuli raise blood pressure even in a sedated or lightly anaesthetised organism, and are also used routinely to stimulate respiration in the newborn. Pain prepares the body for intense physical activity so that the perceived threat can be avoided by running away, or overcome by fighting. Wall (1979) has suggested, however, that one function of pain is to encourage behaviour which will facilitate recuperation, i.e. rest and the avoidance of effort. This is clearly incompatible with a state of arousal, but it is suggested that pain is inhibited during arousal (while the major focus of activity is escape from danger) and reappears when the need for fight or flight is past. There is some anecdotal evidence to suggest that strong emotions such as fear can serve to block pain, and pharmacological studies have also shown that fear potentiates the release of the body's natural opiates. The line between levels of anxiety, which appear to exacerbate pain, and those which block it is far from clear. It may be influenced by environmental factors, such as other threats or sources of help, and personal factors such as previous experience. Wardle (1985) also draws a distinction between the effects of anxiety about the pain itself, and pain-irrelevant worries. Anxiety about the pain itself might be concerned with factors such as the possible cause, whether it will get worse, if it can be treated, whether it is fatal. Pain-irrelevant worries might be focused on escape from danger. Wardle suggests that pain-irrelevant fears might distract the sufferer from the pain, whereas pain-relevant fears might exacerbate it.

Cognitive factors

A constellation of variables concerned with beliefs about the self has been identified in several studies. They include Locus of Control (Rotter, 1966) and Self-efficacy (Bandura, 1977). An individual's locus of control is determined by the extent to which he perceives events as being a consequence of his own behaviour (internal locus of control) or the result of luck or the influence of powerful others (external locus of control). Craig (1984) has developed a scale to measure the locus of control that has been used in a number of studies of treatment outcome. For example, in a retrospective study of headache treated by biofeedback, Hudzinski & Levenson (1985) demonstrated a relationship between internal locus and good treatment outcome. Mizener *et al.* (1988) showed that a group of patients being treated for migraine changed their locus of control towards internality as treatment progressed and they learned to control some physiological processes.

Bandura has described self-efficacy, the belief that one is the sort of person who can accomplish one's goals, and argues that the strength of the belief will determine whether someone will emit and persist with a coping response. Self-efficacy is seen not as an unchangeable personal characteristic but as an attribute that can be manipulated (strengthened or weakened). Variables such as verbal persuasion, vicarious experience (modelling), level of arousal and performance accomplishment will have an effect on self-efficacy expectation, and thus on coping with pain. Dolce (1987) has reviewed a number of papers investigating the relationship between self-efficacy and the perception and management of pain, some based on clinical observation and some on experimental data. He concludes that behavioural interventions in pain management may be refined when self-efficacy is taken into account.

Other cognitive interventions, such as preparation for the painful experience by information giving (Egbert *et al.*, 1964; Auerbach, 1979; Staub & Kellett, 1972) have been shown to reduce pain and distress ratings. Expectations based on past experience (Savedra, 1977; Kelley, 1984) have also been shown to influence pain behaviour. The studies involved burned children undergoing repeated painful treatments. The children did not habituate, but rather tended to exhibit less and less tolerance of the painful stimuli, and to show marked increases in pain behaviour across treatment sessions. White (1986) has pointed out that the burned child encounters frequent pairings of environmental stimuli with pain (the same treatment room, nurses gowning up) and even very young children exhibit anticipatory fear and distress in the presence of a stimulus previously associated with a painful procedure. It is likely that the induction of anticipatory distress reduces pain tolerance, whereas the reduction of anticipatory distress facilitates tolerance. Another illustration of the power of cognitive factors is given by the well-known study by Beecher (1959) in which he compared the responses of soldiers wounded in battle with those of civilians with similar surgical lesions. In their complaints about the level of pain they were experiencing, and in their requests for morphine for pain relief, the two groups differed markedly. The civilians claimed to be in severe pain and requested morphine far more often than the soldiers. Beecher concluded that it was the *meaning* the pain had (relief from battle for the soldiers, the calamity of major surgery for the civilians) that was the major determining factor in the level of pain experienced. The significance of this and similar findings is that many of the factors which bear on the experience of pain can be manipulated, even at the level of acute pain. As Craig (1984: 835) comments:

> The substantial range of individual responses to comparable tissue damage has demanded explanation . . . considerable evidence now supports the view that each individual's experience of pain, and the manner of expression, can be explained only as a product of the sufferer's personal background, the interpersonal context in which pain is experienced, the meaning the experience has for the individual, as well as the sensory input provided by the noxious stimulus.

Pain and personality characteristics

The search for particular personality types in the chronic pain syndrome has been largely unproductive. A major difficulty occurs when studies are carried out on those who have current pain, and whose responses will therefore be affected by it. If a characteristic profile is obtained, is it a predisposing factor, or a consequence? Bond & Pearson (1969) used the Eysenck Personality Inventory (EPI) in a study of three groups of women with cancer. They looked at self-reported pain scores and the patterns of asking for and receiving analgesics. One group had no pain. They had low Neuroticism scores and high Extraversion scores. The two groups with pain had high Neuroticism scores. Those with pain who also had high Extraversion scores tended to ask for and receive more analgesics than those with low Extraversion scores. Bond & Pearson suggest that Neuroticism as measured by the EPI may be related to levels of arousal and therefore to sensitivity to pain, and Extraversion may be related to readiness to communicate about it. It may be that a high Neuroticism score is a reaction to pain, and not a cause. Some studies (for examples, see Cox *et al.*, 1978; Bond, 1979) have shown abnormal profiles on the Minnesota Multiphasic Personality Inventory (MMPI) in pain patients, with high scores on variables such as hypochondriasis, hysteria and depression. Sternbach (1974), Sternbach & Timmermans (1975) and Elton *et al.* (1978), however, have demonstrated that significant *decreases* on indices of psychological disturbance occurred in those whose persistent pain had been successfully treated.

Brena & Koch (1975) have taken yet another view of the relationship between pain and personal characteristics. They have not sought for predisposing factors, but have described pain patients in terms of the balance between tissue pathology and pain behaviour. Their Emory Pain Estimate Model (EPEM) provides operational definitions of chronic pain patients.

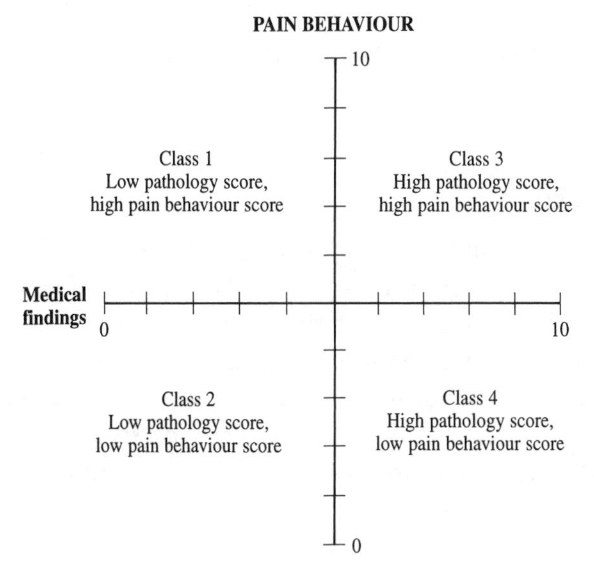

Figure 14.3. Emory pain estimate model.

Medical data, a mixture of functional assessment and pathology, are rated on a 1–10 horizontal scale of severity by a physician. Scoring guidelines are given. Behavioural scores are obtained from patient self-report on a paper and pencil test, and are a compound of estimated activity levels, drug usage and personality variables. They are also entered on a 1–10 scale, which crosses the midline of the horizontal scale, thus generating four cells (Figure 14.3).

Brena & Koch (1975) suggest that there are four classes of chronic pain patients:

1. High pain behaviour with low tissue pathology = Pain amplifiers.
2. Low pain behaviour with low tissue pathology = Pain verbalisers.
3. High pain behaviour with high tissue pathology = Chronic sufferers.
4. Low pain behaviour with high tissue pathology = Pain reducers.

The suggestion is that different treatment strategies should be used for the four types of patient identified by the EPEM. Although the aggregation of so much data of different types into single scale scores is questionable, and there is no evidence that the two scales are orthogonal, studies have demonstrated the validity of the EPEM in predicting the responses of chronic pain patients (Brena & Chapman, 1982; Hammonds & Brena, 1983). It is not widely used, however, and may be no more valuable than a clinical judgement based on carefully collected information in a standard interview. The tendency to name the patient as a 'pain amplifier' instead of describing someone as exhibiting pain-amplifying behaviour is also a problem with this model, as it tends to carry the suggestion of a 'personality type' rather than a reaction, and this is not the most helpful way to approach pain management.

Pain and learning

Brena & Chapman comment on the lack of success in finding the 'pain prone patient' in the research literature, and suggest that in any individual, once coping strategies have broken down under the weight of physical, social and emotional difficulties, distress may be somatised as illness behaviour (which may include pain). They use the term 'learned pain syndrome' to typify the state and to differentiate it from pain which is merely persistent. They have described the so-called 'Five Ds Syndrome': five groups of symptoms that can be found in the learned pain syndrome:

1. *Dramatisation of complaints*
   Patients with learned pain behaviour tend to use words with high emotional impact to describe their suffering.
2. *Disuse*
   Patients tend to become physically inactive, as they fear that activity will increase their pain.
3. *Drug misuse*
   The search for pain relief tends to lead to over use of drugs and often multiple drugs, the side-effects and cross-reactions of which cause extra psychological and physiological upset.
4. *Dependency*
   There is a drift from self-reliance to learned helplessness with the loss of competent coping skills.
5. *Disability*
   Secondary impairments caused by inactivity may be more distressing and disabling than the original pathological condition, and may be taken as evidence for further pathology.

It is important to stress that 'The 5 Ds' is a *descriptive* schema, i.e. based on clinical observation and not on research findings. Some of The 5 Ds are seen in some chronic pain patients, and all have a valid raison d'etre; they arise when strategies designed to achieve pain reduction fail. There is still no indication here as to why some people develop learned pain behaviour.

Fordyce (1984) has set out the argument for viewing pain in terms derived from behavioural science. He points out that an individual signals that pain is a problem by emitting pain behaviours. Pain behaviours are subject to the same influences as any other behaviours: they are vulnerable to learning/conditioning effects. They operate on the environment by eliciting consequences that may be reinforcing or aversive. Several factors operate together to determine the extent of conditioning. They include:

1. The persistence of the nociception, as the longer it lasts the more chances there are for conditioning to take place.
2. The previous experience of people with the pain problem, which may lead them to expect reinforcing or aversive consequences of their behaviour.
3. The extent to which the environment is arranged so as to reinforce pain behaviour directly, or indirectly by allowing the avoidance of aversive consequences.

This model, like the others, is descriptive, but it allows for precise behavioural analysis of pain behaviour, and thereby to treatment strategies, which will be described in the section on treatment.

Treatment of pain

Pharmacology

Wardle (1985) has commented on the advances in anaesthesia and analgesia in the treatment of acute pain, and the difficulties inherent in the pharmacological treatment of chronic pain, where the underlying pathology may be untreatable or unidentified.

The use of analgesics in the treatment of pain from mild to severe, from acute to chronic, is widespread and ranges from self-medication with aspirin for headache to the use of opiates by mouth or intravenously for pain associated with diseases such as cancer. Primary analgesics fall roughly into two types: non-steroidal anti-inflammatory drugs (NSAIDs) such as aspirin and paracetamol, and opiates such as morphine and its derivatives. Secondly analgesics include those which operate directly on nervous and muscular tissue, such as anticonvulsants and antispasmodics, and those with a more central mode of action, such as tranquillisers and antidepressants.

NSAIDs act locally. Substances known as prostaglandins are produced locally in response to tissue damage. They cause inflammation at the damage site, in a sense they amplify the signal 'damage'. NSAIDs block the production of prostaglandins and therefore inhibit inflammation. Pain which is not associated with inflammation will not be affected by NSAIDs. Nevertheless, they are widely used every day for the self-treatment of many types of pain, inflammatory or otherwise. The extent to which they give relief from pain across so broad a spectrum is a testimonial for the powers of belief. I have a pain. I take a tablet because I believe it will help. I can then relax and forget about it, and concentrate on something else. This sequence of events is as true for inflammatory pain as for any other kind; the effect of belief (or placebo) is an important part of *any* treatment.

Opiates, on the other hand, act on the central nervous system and have wide-ranging effects. They affect both the descending control system (midbrain) and the transmission of signals about tissue damage through the spinal cord. Like the natural opioids, they also produce feelings of calmness and well-being. Melzack & Wall (1982) have suggested that the role of the endogenous opioids is to prevent the organism from being overwhelmed by the pain by a combination of analgesia and mood changes that promote rest, and the opiates mimic these functions. They are most useful in treating severe pain with a rapid onset, as in some medical emergencies. Their long-term use is problematic because they produce nausea, cause constipation by their paralysing effect on smooth muscle, inhibit higher cortical functions, and tend to promote dependence and overuse because the mood enhancement which is experienced soon after taking a dose tends to be followed by irritability and depression as the levels in the bloodstream drop, but can be restored rapidly by taking another dose. In the management of very painful conditions such as some types of terminal cancer, 'cocktails' of opiates with other drugs may be used to counteract the undesirable side-effects, and self-administration by intravenous pump has been used successfully to deliver appropriate doses at need. The use of these strong analgesics for the treatment of the chronic pain syndrome tends to maintain maladaptive behaviour patterns such as reduced activity levels, drug dependency and depression.

Nerve blocks

The transmission of impulses through peripheral nerves may be disrupted by the use of local anaesthetics injected directly onto the nerve, or by the use of agents which destroy the nerve, such as alcohol, phenol, freezing, radiowaves, or surgical transection. While these techniques have their place in the treatment of severe intractable pain, they are not without problems, as nerves do not merely transmit pain; and the possibility of persistent numbness and other effects such as motor dysfunction, must be weighed against the potential benefit of pain relief. It is usual for a short-acting trial block to be performed first, sometimes more than once, so that an estimate of the benefit/deficit ratio can be obtained. Some of the problems have been overcome with the development of cryotherapy and radio frequency lesioning (Hughes, 1985). The use of these techniques, however, in the relief of chronic (learned) pain is minimal because of poor results.

Non-pharmacological treatment

Non-pharmacological treatment of pain may involve traditional methods such as the local application of energy in the form of vibration, heat, cold, infrared light, short-wave diathermy, microwave diathermy and ultrasound. Levi & Maikafer (1987) have described the range of application of these treatments in acute and subacute pain, or as adjunct therapy in a comprehensive approach to chronic pain. The local application of heat, cold, etc. will have specific effects such as reducing inflammation or muscular spasm, and may also serve to 'close the gate' by changing the balance of stimulation in the sensory neurones. Again, while the appropriate application of these techniques can be invaluable in the treatment of acute pain, it is unlikely that they will have an impact on chronic (learned) pain on their own. They may be helpful as part of a comprehensive treatment package for chronic pain, particularly if they are simple, do not require elaborate or prolonged application and can be self-administered. In other words, they are likely to be effective if they reduce pain without reinforcing pain behaviour.

Acupuncture and associated methods of treatment such as acupressure or transcutaneous electrical nerve stimulation (TENS) using the acupuncture points are widely used in treating pain of acute and/or persistent type, and may also be used as adjunct therapy in chronic pain treatment programmes. As with almost all treatments for pain, their exact mechanism of action is not known. The mode of action of acupuncture has spawned a range of possible explanations, from counter-irritation through gate control to endorphin release and hypnosis. Lewith & Kenyon (1984) have reviewed the various explanatory models. They comment that there is good evidence for the notion that acupuncture and TENS have an effect on sites in the CNS, and affect many central neurotransmitters. In common with all other methods of treatment, however, the success rate is variable and the influence of other intra- and inter personal factors must be acknowledged.

Psychological treatments are also widely used in the treatment of chronic pain syndrome, and in acute and persistent pain. They include the use of cognitive/behavioural interventions such as relaxation, biofeedback, distraction, hypnosis and the pain modification programmes that use a combination of techniques.

Relaxation and biofeedback

Relaxation training is essentially about teaching progressive relaxation of the skeletal muscles. It was first described by Jacobson (1938) as a means of treating a variety of psychosomatic complaints. Jacobson believed that uncomfortable subjective feelings of anxiety arose largely out of the muscle contractions accompanying increased tension, and that relaxation of the muscles reduced the emotional arousal. He noted that blood pressure and pulse rate dropped as muscle tension decreased. He recommended that people should focus their attention on muscle relaxation at times of stress; he was, in fact, teaching the learned self-control of physiological activity. In the treatment of pain, the use of relaxation training where increased muscle tension is contributing directly to the pain, has a common-sense validity. A direct relationship between pain and muscle tension has been hard to establish in many cases, even in the so-called tension headache (Harper & Steger, 1978). The effectiveness of relaxation training may have more to do with central effects, such as reducing arousal, than with changes in muscle tone alone. Relaxation has been shown to have beneficial effects on a range of painful conditions, from myofascial pain to migraine; in many of them, skeletal muscle tension is not implicated.

Biofeedback is the use of instrumentation to amplify and transform biological information, which is often imperceptible, into signals that can be perceived by the senses, and modified by learning. It should therefore enhance the effectiveness of relaxation training, and could also be used in painful conditions where skeletal muscle tension is not involved in the genesis of pain. For example, vasoconstriction and dilatation are implicated in the pain of Raynaud's syndrome and migraine. It has been shown that temperature feedback enhances vasodilation in those with Raynaud's syndrome (for example, see Yocum *et al*, 1985). On the other hand, Holmes & Burish (1983) concluded that there is no evidence that finger temperature biofeedback training is effective in migraine. There is, of course, no reason why it should be, as there is no evidence that increasing the blood flow to the fingers means that it is decreased in the extracranial vessels.

The range of application of the techniques of relaxation and biofeedback, and the variable success rates, raises a number of questions. Firstly, the question of what is being learned. Is it muscular relaxation, peripheral vasodilation, etc. or is it a more global process involving many autonomic processes? In other words, by sitting quietly and concentrating on muscle tension or on a pointer or a light, are people simply learning to reduce arousal? Secondly, there is the question of the appropriate use of the techniques. Why should relaxation of the skeletal muscles affect migraine? Why should peripheral vasodilation affect the flow in the extracranial vessels? The answer to both of these questions must be that there is no obvious reason why. In very few studies have specific effects been demonstrated. Where close attention has been paid to matching the technique with the underlying problem, results have tended to be promising, but there are many studies with poor or inexplicable results.

Turner & Chapman (1982) have reviewed relaxation training and biofeedback as psychological interventions for chronic pain. They comment on the disregard of cognitive factors in many studies, and on the oversimplification of the nature of chronic pain problems implied in the techniques. They make a plea for a reappraisal of these methods, to enable a better fit with the growing understanding of the psychological dimensions of chronic pain. For example, if relaxation is taught as a coping skill it may help the patient identify and respond to the stresses that trigger or exacerbate the pain, and be a truly useful therapeutic tool.

Distraction and other cognitive strategies

Many pain treatment techniques, including relaxation and biofeedback, contain elements of distraction, i.e. the attention is drawn away from the pain and engaged elsewhere. It is a technique used by mothers the world over to calm children who have suffered a minor hurt, or to enable procedures such as injections to be carried out with the least distress. Elliot & Olson (1983) and Kelly *et al.* (1984) have demonstrated the effectiveness of distraction techniques of dressing change and debridement. In Kelley's study, the effect of the distraction was enhanced by the use of a star chart to reward decreases in pain behaviour, whereas Elliot & Olson noted that the effect was only evident when the psychologist was present to coach the child. It did not generalise to other days. It should be noted that these children were in severe acute pain, and even so some benefit was achieved by simple methods. The benefit was enhanced by reinforcement in one case, and the presence of a calming adult on the other. Again, contextual and interpersonal factors were shown to be important moderators of learning.

Other cognitive interventions include the use of pleasant imagery and sensory transformation, during which the patient uses imaginative strategies to reinterpret the pain as a sensory stimulus without a noxious component. For example, the tight or throbbing nature of a pain might be attended to. Imagery may then be used to operate on that aspect of the stimulus; the tightness might be imagined as a steel band which is being progressively loosened. Linton (1982) has commented on the lack of properly controlled studies, and the confounding of cognitive with non-cognitive effects. He questions whether the effects of cognitive treatment are truly cognitive, or are related to a general relaxation response. The question of specific versus general effects hinders many of the psychological treatments for pain, including hypnosis.

Hypnosis

As Karle (1988) has pointed out, hypnosis is not a treatment but a way of administering a treatment. It uses the natural attribute we all possess to a greater or lesser extent, to daydream or fantasise. Although hypnosis usually begins with induction by the therapist, it is always essentially self-generated. The patient collaborates with suggestions designed to focus awareness away from extraneous factors, and attains a state of intense, narrowly-focused concentration together with deep relaxation. During the hypnotic state, suggestions designed to reinterpret the pain are readily accepted; the imaginative faculty is enhanced. Patients can be taught to self-hypnotise at will. There is a continuing debate about whether hypnotic induction is a necessary part of the process, or whether it can be dispensed with. Perhaps the conscious cooperation of the patient in accepting suggestions does not need a hypnotic induction. Certainly in the emergency treatment of pain, as Wallace (1987) puts it, 'the preliminaries are not necessary, as an authoritative and caring voice amidst the apparent chaos and pain is often sufficient for a patient to be prepared to follow any reasonable suggestion that will bring relief'. On the other hand, the tinge of mystery associated with hypnosis might act as a powerful enhancer of relaxation and suggestibility for some people. Barber & Adrian (1982) have provided a discussion of the place of hypnotherapy in the treatment of pain.

Behavioural management

Fordyce (1984) has argued that pain which exists for more than a few days or weeks is vulnerable to conditioning effects. Pain behaviour may be conditioned directly by being rewarded with attention, permission to rest, etc., or indirectly by being linked with the sanctioned avoidance of aversive events, such as heavy work or stressful social encounters. The outcome of persistent pain is determined by the persistence of the nociception; the previous experience of the person, which leads to anticipation of rewarding or aversive consequences to the expression of pain behaviour; and the way the environment responds to the pain behaviour. Fordyce-type pain management programmes centre around allowing pain behaviour to extinguish by non-reinforcement, while at the same time helping the patient to develop alternative behaviours. Patients and their families are involved in the treatment programme, so that the environmental component of pain behaviour can continue in the home. Typically, analgesic medication is changed to a time-contingent rather than a pain-contingent regimen. Where analgesics are being over-used, they may be given in the form of an elixir which stays constant in volume while the dose of the drug is reduced. Current toleration for a given exercise or activity is assessed, and a quota is assigned that starts with slightly low expectations and builds up over the days. Rest periods are contingent on the quota. This pattern helps to eliminate the common 'working to tolerance' mode commonly seen in pain behaviour, where patients tend to go on with an activity until pain forces them to stop. Attention and social feedback from the health care team and the family is focused on attainment, not on pain. Education about pain, particularly the gate theory, is often included for patients and relatives, and alternative methods of pain control such as relaxation may also be taught. The programmes usually run over six weeks, and the aim is for a full day's activity to be attained by the end, with medication at a stable low or eliminated altogether if appropriate. This type of pain behaviour management has become increasingly widely used in cases of persistent pain for which no medical intervention is appropriate, and which are causing significant disruption to normal functioning. Linton (1982) has reviewed a number of these programmes, and comments on the considerable improvements at discharge and follow-up in variables such as pain reports, mood, drug use and activity. He also points out the difficulty in judging the clinical significance of the improvements as a group, as there are wide variations in methodology and treatment, and actual data are often not reported. In addition, because the treatment packages use a variety of components, the efficacy of individual components is impossible to evaluate. The broad-based approach acknowledges, however, the complexity of the pain problem, and combines the most effective parts of other treatments. Controlled studies are now needed. The multifactorial nature of pain, which crosses disciplines and conceptual models, means that assessment and treatment are inevitably complex. Some advances in understanding have been made in recent years, but much remains elusive. There is a need for carefully-controlled studies of interventions for pain, so that reliable and valid data can be gathered and analysed. The general and specific effects of interventions need to be identified, so that treatments can be more precisely tailored to fit the underlying problem.

The management of pain still presents the rehabilitation practitioner with exciting challenges and opportunities for innovative thinking, in both clinical and research fields.

References

Akil, H., Watson, S. J., Young, E., Lewis, M. E., Khachaturian, H. & Walker, J. M. (1984). Endogenous opioids: biology and function. *Annual Review of Neuroscience*, **7**, 223–55.

Auerbach, S. M. (1979). Preoperative preparation for surgery. In *Research in Psychology and Medicine*, ed. D. J. Osborne. vol. 2. London: Academic Press.

Bandura, A. (1977). Self-efficacy: toward a unifying theory of behavioural change. *Psychological Review*, **84**, 191–215.

Barber, J. & Adrian, C. (1982). *Psychological Approaches to the Management of Pain*. New York: Brunner/Mazel.

Beecher, H. K. (1959). *Measurement of Subjective Responses*. New York: Oxford University Press.

Bond, M. R. (1979). *Pain: Its Nature, Analysis and Treatment*. New York: Longman.

Bond, M. R. & Pearson, I. B. (1969). Psychological aspects of pain in women with advanced cancer of the cervix. *Journal of Psychosomatic Research*, **13**, 13–19.

Brena, S. E. & Chapman, S. L. (1985). Acute versus chronic pain states: the 'Learned Pain Syndrome'. *Clinics in Anaesthesiology*, **3**, 41–55.

Brena, S. E. & Chapman, S. L. (1982). The validity of the Emory Pain Estimate Model. *Anaesthesiology Review*, **9**, 42–5.

Brena, S. E. & Koch, D. L. (1975). The 'Pain Estimate' model for quantification and classification of chronic pain states. *Anaesthesiology Review*, **2**, 8–13.

Calliet, R. (1979). Chronic pain: is it necessary? *Archives of Physical Medicine and Rehabilitation*, **60**, 4–7.

Cervero, F. & Laird, J. M. A. (1991). One pain or many pains? A new look at pain mechanisms. *News In Physiological Sciences*, **6**, 268–73.

Clark, W. C. & Clark, S. B. (1980). Pain responses in Nepalese porters. *Science*, **209**, 410–12.

Cox, G. B., Chapman, C. R. & Black, R. G. (1978). The MMPI and chronic pain: the diagnosis of psychogenic pain. *Journal of Behavioural Medicine*, **1**, 437–44.

Craig, K. D. (1984). Psychology of pain. *Postgraduate Medical Journal*, **60**, 835–40.

Dolce, J. J. (1987). Self-efficacy and disability beliefs in behavioural treatment of pain, *Behaviour Research and Therapy*, **25**, 289–99.

Dyck, P. J., Lambert, E. H. & O'Brien, P. C. (1976). Pain in peripheral neuropathy related to rate and kind of fibre degeneration. *Neurology*, **22**, 466–71.

Egbert, L. D., Battit, G. E., Welch, C. E. & Bartlett, M. K. (1964). Reduction of postoperative pain by encouragement and instruction of patients: a study of doctor-patient rapport. *New England Journal of Medicine*, **270**, 825–7.

Eland, J. (1985). *Nursing Now Series, Pain*. Springhouse PA: Springhouse Corporation, 108–19.

Elliott, C. H. & Olsen, R. A. (1983). The management of children's distress in response to painful medical treatment for burns injuries. *Behaviour Research and Therapy*, **21**, 675–83.

Elton, D., Stuart, G. V. & Burrows, G. D. (1978). Self-esteem and chronic pain. *Journal of Psychosomatic Research*, **22**, 25–30.

Fairbank, J. T., Couper, J., Davies, J. B. & O'Brien, J. P. (1980). The Oswestry

Low Back Pain Disability Questionnaire. *Physiotherapy*, **66**, 271–3.
Fordyce, W. E. (1984). Behavioural science and chronic pain. *Postgraduate Medical Journal*, **60**, 865–8.
Grzesiak, R. (1984). Rehabilitation of chronic pain syndromes. In *Current Topics in Rehabilitation Psychology* ed. C. J. Golden. Philadelphia, PA: Grune & Stratton.
Hammonds, W. & Brena, S. F. (1983). Pain classification and vocational evaluation of chronic pain states. In *Pain Measurement and Assessment* ed. R. Melzack. New York: Raven Press.
Hardy, J. D., Wolff, H. G. & Goodell, H. (1952). *Pain Sensations and Reactions*. New York: Haffner.
Harper, R. G. & Steger, J. C. (1978). Psychological correlates of frontalis EMG and pain in tension headache. *Headache*, **18**, 215–18.
Holmes, D. S. & Burish, T. G. (1983). Effectiveness of biofeedback for treating migraine and tension headache: a review of the evidence. *Journal of Psychosomatic Research*, **27**, 513–32.
Hudzinski, L. G. & Levenson, H. (1985). Biofeedback behavioural treatment of headache with locus of control pain analysis: a 20-month retrospective study. *Headache*, **25**, 380–6.
Hughes, T. J. (1985). Relief of pain: the role of the pain clinic. *Update*, 15 August, 263–73.
Iggo, A. (1972). Critical remarks on the gate control theory. In *Pain: Basic Principles, Pharmacology, Therapy* ed. R. Janzen, W. D. Keidel, A. Herz, C. Steichele, J. P. Payne & R. A. P. Burt. Stuttgart, West Germany: Georg Thieme.
Jacobson, E. (1938). *Progressive Relaxation*. Chicago: University of Chicago Press.
Kelly, M. L., Jarie, G. J., Middlebrook, J. L. McNeer, M. F. & Drabman, R. S. (1984). Decreasing burned children's pain behaviour: impacting the trauma of hydrotherapy. *Journal of Applied Behavioural Analysis*, **17**, 147–58.
Karle, H. W. A. (1988). *Hypnosis and Hypnotherapy: A Patient's Guide*. Wellingborough, Northants: Thorson's.
Lambert, W. E., Libman, E. & Poser, E. G. (1960). Effect of increased salience of membership group on pain tolerance. *Journal of Personality*. **28**, 350–7.
Levi, S. J. & Maikafer, G. C. (1987). Traditional approaches to pain. In *Pain* ed. J. C. Echternach. New York: Churchill Livingstone.
Lewith, G. T. & Kenyon, J. N. (1984). Physiological and psychological explanations for the mechanism of acupuncture as a treatment for chronic pain. *Social Science and Medicine*, **19**, 1367–78.
Linton, S. J. (1982). A critical review of behavioural treatments for chronic benign pain other than headache. *British Journal of Clinical Psychology*, **21**, 321–37.
Melzack, R. (1975). The McGill Pain Questionnaire: major properties and scoring methods. *Pain*, **1**, 277–99.
Melzack, R. & Wall, P. D. (1965). Pain mechanisms: a new theory. *Science*, **150**, 971–9.
Melzack, R. & Wall, P. D. (1982). *The Challenge of Pain*. Harmondsworth, England: Penguin Books.
Mizener, D., Thomas, M. & Billings, R. (1988). Cognitive changes in migraineurs receiving biofeedback training. *Headache*, **28**, 339–43.
Reynolds, D. V. (1969). Surgery in the rat during electrical analgesia induced by focal brain stimulation. *Science*, **164**, 444–5.

Rotter, J. B. (1966). Generalized expectancies for internal versus external control of reinforcement. *Psychological Monographs*, **80** (whole no. 609, 1).
Savedra, M. (1977). Coping with pain. Strategies of severely burned children. *Maternal–Child Nursing Journal*, **5**, 197–203.
Staub, E. & Kellet, D. S. (1972). Increasing pain tolerance by information about aversive stimuli. *Journal of Personality and Social Psychology*, **21**, 198.
Steptoe, A. & Pearce, S. (1983). Common ground in pain and stress research. *Journal of Psychosomatic Research*, **27**, 337–8.
Sternbach, R. A. (1968). *Pain: a Psychophysiological Analysis*. New York: Academic Press.
Sternbach, R. A. (1974). *Pain Patients: Traits and Treatment*. New York: Academic Press.
Sternbach, R. A. & Timmermans, G. (1975). Personality changes associated with the reduction of pain. *Pain*, **1**, 177–81.
Turner, J. A. & Chapman, C. R. (1982). Psychological interventions for chronic pain: a critical review. 1. Relaxation training and biofeedback. *Pain*, **12**, 1–21.
Wall, P. D. (1979). On the relation of injury to pain. The John J. Bonica Lecture. *Pain*, **6**, 253–64.
Wallace, L. M. (1987). Hypnosis and pain control on an English burns unit. *Intensive Care Nursing*, **3**, 50–55.
Wardle, J. (1985). Pain. In *New Developments in Clinical Psychology*, ed. F. Watts. BPS in association with John Wiley, Chichester, England.
Weddell, G. (1955). Somesthesis and the chemical senses. *Annual Review of Psychology*, **6**, 119–36.
Weisenberg, M. (1977). Pain and pain control. *Psychological Bulletin*, **84**, 1008–44.
White, J. (1986). *An exploratory study of paediatric pain. The assessment and modification of the pain behaviour of burned children*. Dissertation submitted for the British Psychological Society Diploma in Clinical Psychology, Autumn 1986, unpublished.
Yocum, D. E., Hodes, R., Sundstrom, W. R. & Cleeland, C. S. (1985). Use of biofeedback training in treatment of Raynaud's disease and phenomenon. *Journal of Rheumatology*, **12**, 90–3.

15

The multiply handicapped child

EVA BOWER

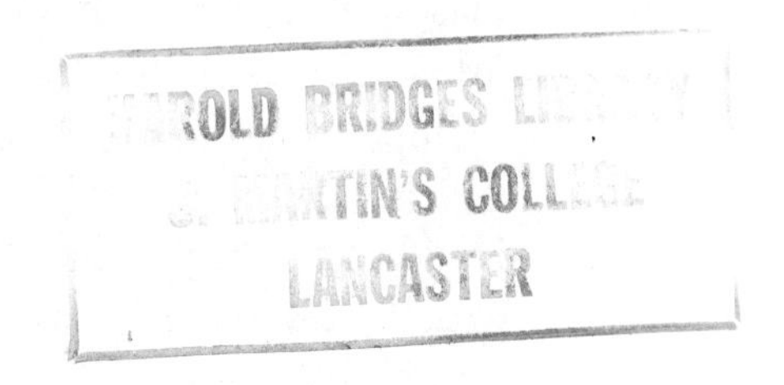

Introduction

Children with a neurological multiple handicap have incurred irreversible damage to the central nervous system (CNS) which may involve a variety of motor and sensory deficits and include disorders of cognition, behaviour and consciousness. In addition there may be secondary biochemical constraints resulting from the primary impairment that further incapacitate the children.

Neurological damage can occur prenatally, perinatally and postnatally. Prenatal causes include genetic abnormalities, congenital malformations and *in utero* infections. Perinatal birth trauma contributes to multiple handicap but improved imaging techniques and recording of apgar scores suggest that this is not common. Infection, vascular insufficiency and postconvulsive problems are potential postnatal factors. In many cases the cause of multiple handicap in children, however, is simply not known (Nelson & Ellenberg, 1986).

Following damage to the CNS, compensatory synaptic formation between neurones can occur within one day. In adults it frequently occurs within five days (Cotman & Nieto-Sampedro, 1985). The catalyst for this process is thought to be the presence of an environmental stimulus. In children, normal maturation is likely to confound these compensatory mechanisms. The timing of neurological damage is crucial as the effect appears to be as dependent on the stage of development at the time of injury as on its specific nature.

The four outstanding biological achievements of humans which separate them from other animals are:

1. Upright posture which facilitates locomotion while leaving the hands free.
2. Finely adjustable vision and flexible digits enabling the construction and use of tools.
3. Spoken language.

4. Structured social behaviour for the benefit of both the individual and the community and for rearing of children who remain dependent for a longer period than in other species (Sheridan, 1973).

It is probably the combination of these four factors plus the intelligence and reasoning powers of humans that mark their superiority. These are the factors often affected in children with multiple handicap.

Impairment in children with multiple handicap refers to the neurological deficit, whereas disability describes the functional effect of the impairment. Handicap is the practical consequences and restriction of social role associated with the disability (WHO, 1980). It has been suggested that the main problem for children with multiple handicap is the restricted nature of maturational change they can expect, which impedes emotional development and remains a lifelong preoccupation of the family (Rang,1982). As children with multiple handicap approach adulthood they may begin to appreciate the future and recognise their own social insecurity and lack of interpersonal skills. There may also be a realisation of the nature of the transition from a protected child to a socially outcast adult.

Physiotherapy for children with multiple handicap in the United Kingdom (UK) is usually provided as a more or less continuous process from the time of identification of risk or diagnosis until school leaving age. It is delivered from the primary care sector by therapists with specialised knowledge in a number of strategies. These approaches target the musculoskeletal system, the CNS, the educational development of the child and the psychological well-being of the child and its family. No conclusive evidence comparing individual approaches or combined strategies exists in the literature. Furthermore, the role of physiotherapy in the care of children with multiple handicap remains unevaluated in the long term.

Development

Development is a process whereby an animal or person grows and becomes more complicated (Sylva & Lunt, 1982). It is in part a genetic process and partly a consequence of interaction with the environment. For centuries there has been controversy concerning the effects of nature and nurture.

The ideas that support nature's influence include inborn biases, maturation and 'canalisation'. An inborn bias can be described as a built-in response pattern. An example of an inborn bias suggested by Buffery (1976) was gender. He suggested that there are consistent differences in verbal and spatial skills between males and females and that this might be ascribed to hormonal differences. In children it is likely that individual development occurs as a result of experiences filtered through the inborn biases.

Maturation (Gesell, 1948) is the genetically programmed sequential pattern of change, as opposed to growth which is a step by step change in quantity. Normal human motor development is variable both in sequence and time of achievement. It may be influenced by early nursing positions, hereditary factors, vision and body dimensions (Illingworth, 1966). Most children progress either through a prone or a supine developmental sequence (Levitt, 1982). Children developing via a prone sequence often crawl before they sit. In contrast, children developing through a supine sequence often sit before they crawl. Some children who bottom shuffle walk late (Robson, 1970), and some do not crawl but progress straight to standing. Most normal children sit by eight months of age, stand between ten and 14 months and walk between 11 and 15 months of age (Illingworth, 1953).

Natural influences may vary in importance at different periods of development. Kagan (1982) has suggested that development is highly 'canalised' in the first two years of life and that built-in biological programmes are very influential. Canalisation seems to be much weaker in later years of childhood. Kagan (1982) cites the anxiety of all infants whatever their cultural background between the ages of eight and 12 months when separated from their mothers as an example of canalisation. There is a time of maximum distress at about 15 months of age but by the third birthday children no longer worry in the same way about maternal separation.

Neuronal development

To what extent nature and nurture are influenced by the pre- and postnatal development of the nervous system is not easy to ascertain. Although the nervous system appears early in gestation, rapid development does not occur until the foetal stage. The neurones and dendrites are then added rapidly (Shepherd, 1983). Neurones are virtually all present at 28 weeks of gestation but glial cells continue to proliferate until two years after birth. At birth the most developed parts of the brain are the medulla and midbrain whereas the cortex is least established (Dobbing & Sands, 1973). Although most of the neurones in the brain are present at birth, those in the cortex are not well connected. Over time the number of dendrites and synapses increases as does the individual neurone size and total brain weight (Nowakowski, 1987). Around two years of age it appears that some pruning of the synapses may take place so as to remove redundant connections and tidy up the 'wiring diagram' (Greenough *et al.*, 1987). It seems that the process of maturation creates some redundant motor and sensory pathways. Experience helps to decide which are most efficient and pruning removes the inefficient ones (Shepherd, 1983). It is an awareness of this process that has led to the justification of various approaches used in the treatment of children with multiple handicap. Myelinisation or the growth of myelin sheaths which encompass axons is most rapid until about three years of age. This process involves insulating individual axons from one another to reduce cross-talk and enables axons to transmit impulses more rapidly and at faster firing frequencies. It is a physiological change facilitating a speedier response and follows the same cephalocaudal and proximodistal pattern followed by muscle development. Purves & Lichtman (1985) suggested firstly that the lower on the evolutionary scale the animal, the more preprogrammed and stereotyped is its nervous system, while more advanced animals have individualised nervous systems. Secondly, the more complex the animal the more drawn out is its neural development and especially the time during which synaptic connections are malleable. Thirdly, the sphere of environmental influences acting on a nervous system enlarges continually.

Environment

The hypotheses that support an environmental role in development include Aslin's models of environmental influence (Aslin, 1981), research undertaken on the timing of experiences, and Bowlby's theory (1951) concerning the internal models of experience.

Aslin suggested that the environment might not have an impact on development, or that environmental input might be necessary to sustain a skill that had already developed. In addition he proposed that a skill might develop earlier than expected as a result of environmental experience and that environmental experience might lead to a higher level of performance, whereas in the absence of environmental experience a particular skill might not develop at all.

Wolf (1943) showed that rats deprived of vision in infancy experienced great difficulty in responding later to visual stimuli. This also applied to those deprived of hearing in early life, suggesting a central environmental influence on development. Illingworth (1966) commented on Wolf's work and suggested that the rats failed when faced with diverse stressful situation when older. In a similar animal experiment, Nissen *et al.* (1951) limited the movement of the limbs of chimpanzees from four weeks to 31 months by encasing their limbs in cardboard cylinders. The abnormality of hand use persisted after release of the limbs, adding support to the environmentalists' hypotheses.

Meanwhile Bowlby (1951) suggested that children deprived of maternal care in the first three years of life displayed physical, intellectual and social retardation. He later, however, suggested that he might have exaggerated the effect (Bowlby *et al.*, 1956). Harow & Harlow (1962) demonstrated that if monkeys were reared in a motherless environment they subsequently displayed problems with socialising, mating and became inadequate parents themselves. If, however, they spent 20 minutes a day with their peers these problems did not seem to occur.

A number of examples of genetic influence on development independent of environmental factors have been highlighted by Illingworth (1966) in the nature versus nurture controversy. For example, Carmichael (1926) kept frog and salamander eggs until the head and tail buds appeared. At this time one group was placed in a dish of plain water and the other group was placed in a weak solution of chloretone. Chloretone, while it does not interfere with growth, results in complete immobilisation and so motion for this group was impossible. These tadpoles remained in this solution until those in the plain water were swimming in a normal manner. At this time the drug was washed from the anaesthetised tadpoles and they were placed in plain water. The first movements appeared within six to 20 minutes and within 30 minutes both the frog and salamander tadpoles were swimming so well that they could not be distinguished from those that had been swimming normally in plain water for five days. Carmichael used this evidence as support for preprogrammed mechanisms in locomotory development.

Dennis (1941) described an experiment in which he and his wife reared two children from the beginning of the second to the end of the 14 month with no stimulation at all. No response was made to them. They were prevented from seeing other children and from playing with toys and they were given no opportunity to practice any skills. Grasping, sitting and weightbearing were consistently retarded, but they rapidly caught up when given the opportunity, although some stimulation was required and it took a little longer (four days) than with the frog and salamander tadpoles (30 minutes). Dennis (1943) found that additional practice had no effect on enabling children to walk early. McGraw (1940) undertook an experiment on two sets of identical twins in which one child in each set was put on a potty hourly for seven hours each day from one month onwards and the other was not allowed to sit on a potty until 17 months and 24 months, respectively. There was no final difference in the age of attainment of continence between the twins in each set. Both these limited studies on children confirm an innate influence on development largely independent of environmental factors.

The extent to which environment can advance or retard development and particularly intellectual development is uncertain. Illingworth (1966) suggests that the general opinion which is based mostly on studies of identical twins reared apart, is that not more than 20–30% of an intelligence test score is likely to be the product of environment, the rest being the product of heredity.

The Wildboy of Averyou, 'L'enfant sauvage' (Itard, 1775–1838) lived in the wilderness until 11 years of age when he was presented as a wild, deaf and dumb idiot. He was trained by Itard and his housekeeper using a reward and punishment system and given plenty of sensory stimulation. He learned to remember, speak albeit abnormally in a high pitched voice, write and count but never became really 'normal'. Studies in this field have shown that poverty, malnutrition, lower social class and a lack of home stimulation and involvement are all adverse influences on development, especially intellectual development (Burt, 1950; Davis & Kent, 1955; Bayley & Schaeffer, 1960; Douglas, 1964).

Time windows in development

Although the environment is of importance throughout childhood, it is considered to be a crucial influence during the first three years (Bowlby, 1951; Knoblach, 1959). One of the interesting ideas that has been expounded in research studies has been the concept of time windows during which an environmental input is necessary for perceptual function to become established. This hypothesis has been borrowed from the study of embryological development.

There is evidence that in animals there are particular periods during their development when learning is easier than at other times. Lorenz (1970) found that there was a time window during a gosling's life when it would 'fix' on a moving figure. This corresponded to the time interval early in life when attachment occurred and was termed a sensitive period. Similarly, there are particular periods of development when the absence of appropriate stimuli will affect the acquisition of skills. Hubel & Weisel (1970) demonstrated that there was a sensitive period during which sensory stimulation was important for the development of normal visual function in kittens by highlighting the effect of deprivation on cortical development.

It seems likely that there are time windows or 'sensitive periods' when skills can be more economically advanced in the development of children too. There are, however, few scientifically proven examples of sensitive periods in human development. One example is the action of teratogens in the prenatal environment, for example the deleterious effects of intrauterine rubella infection in the first trimester of pregnancy but not later in gestation. Illingworth & Lister (1964) have suggested that if babies are not provided with solid foods soon after they are able to chew (usually at six or seven months) it becomes increasingly difficult to introduce solids later. The chronological age may vary between individual children with respect to these sensitive periods. It needs to be stressed that there is no conclusive evidence to assume that if the opportunity is not provided at the sensitive period the skill will never be achieved (McGraw, 1989); however, it is just possible that it becomes more difficult for the child to attain the skill at a later stage.

Sachs (1985) described a patient, Madeleine J, with cerebral palsy who was congenitally blind but whose intelligence was intact. This woman had been totally cared for by her family all the 60 years of her life and had never been encouraged to use her hands. Following entry to a New York Hospital where she was given opportunities and encouragement she initially learnt to feed and care for herself and later became a talented sculptress. He subsequently described a second patient called Simon K with similar impairments but in addition mild intellectual retardation who had not been given the opportunity to use his hands either. This younger man learnt to enjoy simple carpentry. Sachs suggests that these two cases illustrate that the essential component in development is use.

Bowlby (1971) has suggested that experience influences the interpretation by children of subsequent encounters and their responses. For example a 'securely attached' child may have experienced readily available adult affection and attention and thus will expect and create affectionate relationships with new adults.

Bronfenbrenner (1979, 1989) suggests that to describe development properly one needs to look at the total setting or context in which it occurs. Children grow up in a complex social environment which includes people in and out of the home. This ecological approach stresses the importance of understanding interactions between many different environmental influences. Interactionists view the nature/nuture issue by observing the interplay between biology and environment. For example the child's inborn resilience or vulnerability, such as a difficult temperament, may be modified by the facilitativeness of the environment (Horowitz, 1987, 1990). A highly productive environment is one in which the child has loving and responsive parents who provide a rich array of stimulation.

In every aspect of development both hereditary and environmental issues play a role; however, physical development is probably more affected by genetic forces and language seems to emerge with minimal environmental support. Cognitive development seems to fall somewhere in the middle of the continuum, while social and emotional development appears to be determined chiefly by the environment.

Progress during development involves both qualitative advances which refine the execution of a task and quantitative changes that introduce novel activities. The latter employ new neural apparatus. The sequence of quantitative and qualitative changes permeates development in most contexts.

Motor development

Although maturation probably underlies motor development, environmental factors are influential. Sutherland *et al.* (1988) demonstrated, using instrumental gait analysis, that children under two years of age have an immature walking pattern and do not use their tibialis anterior and gastrocnemius muscles. The tibialis anterior is employed during walking after two years of age and the gastrocnemius after five years of age, and the mature walking pattern is achieved by seven years of age. He proposed that this sequence was adopted during childhood to adapt the basic walking pattern to cope with rough ground. Previously Illingworth (1966) suggested that environmental feedback is only able to influence the development within the available potential so that an enriched environment may help children to attain their maximum potential but is not able to expand that potential.

Most of the basic motor skills are accomplished by six or seven years of age. After that age developmental progress is mostly in the quality of performance as children integrate and refine complex movement sequences. The rate of development varies between children but the sequence of progress is virtually always the same. As a general rule children tend to be consistently early, average or late in most aspects of physical development and this is influenced by genetic heritage, for example a child who walks late will often have a parent who walked late.

There have been varying approaches to the description of normal development outlined by Gesell & Armatruda (1947), Griffiths (1954), Illingworth (1953) and Sheridan (1973).

Bobath & Bobath (1975) described the pattern of normal development of children at three, five, seven and nine months of age marking the achievement of certain important abilities that they considered prepared children for new and more complex activities. These patterns were based on many of McGraw's (1943) neuromuscular maturation concepts and the work of Andre Thomas *et al.* (1960). The Bobaths suggested that the observed changes were achieved by a gradual increase in postural control against gravity. As the righting reactions develop and are perfected around the sixth month they are modified and become incorporated into the equilibrium reactions. The developing parachute reactions of the arms are equally important. Together with these developments, changes in motor patterns of the limbs occur from the flexion–adduction pattern of the newborn to flexion–abduction and then towards the extension–abduction pattern of the seven-month-old. From the seventh month onwards the extension–abduction pattern is combined with rotation of the trunk. This was considered to be a necessary prerequisite of normal equilibrium reactions. Bobath & Bobath (1975) complemented this account with a systematic description of the abnormal development in the different types of cerebral palsy.

McGraw (1943) suggested in her description of neuromuscular maturation that training in any particular activity before neuromuscular mechanisms were ready is futile. Her observations on two sets of identical twins and sphincter control (see earlier) illustrated this concept as did the experimental attempts made to train a 12-month-old infant to ride a tricycle. McGraw (1989) states that this infant did not achieve adequate neural maturation for tricycling until he was approximately 19 months old. The daily exposure to the tricycle during seven long months before he was capable of making an appreciable response cultivated an attitude of tolerance which curtailed the natural interest and enthusiasm that would have been obtained had the activity been delayed until the child was more mature.

McGraw also proposed that practising a newly developing function was inherent in the process of growth and if ample opportunity were afforded at the proper time specific achievements could be advanced beyond the stage normally expected. This concept was illustrated by her study with Johnny and the roller skates. Johnny had custom-made ball bearing roller skates put on his shoes every day from the age of 12 months, and by 14 months was totally proficient in their use. She felt that periods of transition from one type of neuromuscular organisation to another are an inherent part of development and are characterised by disorganisation and confusion. This could be illustrated by the fact that when children begin erect locomotion they do not immediately acquire optimum efficiency but go through a period of tumbles and falls while practising. Spurts, regressions, frustrations and inhibitions are an integral part of organic growth and there is evidence that they also function in the development of complex behaviour activities.

This concept was extensively studied in her work on the maturation of bladder control in two sets of twins. There were peak periods of success interspersed with troughs of decline associated with the emergence of other specific skills. This idea of competing patterns of development was also discussed by Milani-Comparetti (1964) in connection with motor development. McGraw also hypothesised that evidence that children are ready for a particular educational subject is supported by certain behavioural signals or syndromes which reflect the maturity of neural mechanisms. This was illustrated by the readiness of the untrained twin for potty training at 24 months which was the age at which the other twin became potty trained despite receiving regular training since the age of one month. McGraw concluded that maturation which is an innate process, and learning which results from environmental stimuli were not different processes but merely different facets of the fundamental process of growth.

A new approach to the development of movement skills has been described by Thelen (1992) and is one of dynamic systems. In this theory movement is considered to be the result of many subsystems working together to accomplish a goal. The components include perceptual, cognitive and motivational attributes together with neural and muscular networks.

Perception

Perception involves the acquisition of knowledge through the senses about the environment. It is mainly concerned with differences and changes that are transmitted through the nervous system by the six sensory systems. The six senses are vision, hearing, taste, smell, touch and proprioception. Proprioception is concerned with the spatial location of the mobile parts of the body especially the limbs and this information is transmitted through receptors situated in muscles, tendons and joints; for example the receptors in the joints record the angles between the activating bones of the joint. Proprioception provides a continuous but unconscious sensory flow from the moveable parts of the body (muscles, tendons and joints) so that their position, tone and motion is continually monitored and adjusted as necessary. Sachs (1985) in a description of a patient, Christina, who suffered from a sudden onset of total loss of proprioception reported that she felt 'disembodied'. Despite there being not a trace of any neurological recovery over a period of eight years this woman achieved functional gains so that she was able to feed herself, talk, walk and take public transport, although in a rather unnatural and too perfect way, and so long as her attention was not unduly diverted from the activity in question. She had largely to use her vision to compensate for the loss of feedback from proprioception but Sachs suggests that in addition she used a feed forward mechanism as characterised by her too perfect learned movements.

Experiments conducted by Fantz (1961) on early visual perception and by Gibson & Walk (1960) on perception of depth at nine months of age indicated that basic perceptual skills were probably innate but became increasingly sophisticated with subsequent experiences.

The senses most closely involved with motor skills are vision, proprioception and probably touch. Impairment of these senses and the consequent loss of feedback will lead to restricted motor functions which may be transient or permanent depending on the severity of the senses involved. For example, children with visual impairments may be delayed in crawling, standing and walking. Children who have severe apraxia or difficulty with motor planning (not using movements appropriate to the task), may be permanently disabled in dressing or writing skills even though they have the motor capacity for each of the individual movements involved in the task. Children with spastic cerebral palsy may have difficulties with spatial relationships including concepts such as up and down, in front and behind, away and near, and left and right. These difficulties may have been accentuated by the paucity of movement experienced by children with spasticity.

Vurpillot (1976) performed experiments in which children had to comment on differences in a series of pictures. He demonstrated that at three and a half years children identify changes in the form or shape and presence or absence of an object and at seven and a half years recognise changes in the size and location or position of an object. Defects in perception produce difficulties in childrens' abilities to appreciate differences in space, depth, form, size, colour and shape, and in discriminating differences in tactile properties. These difficulties can produce problems with feeding, washing, toiletting, playing, social and scholastic activities.

To achieve normal balance reactions during sitting, standing and walking so that these positions can be used dynamically, children require relatively intact tactile, proprioceptive, visual and vestibular functions. The vestibular system largely controls balance and equilibrium, maintaining the extensor tone in the trunk and limbs and ensuring an upright posture against gravity. The ears provide the sensory input for vestibular feedback which monitors their position in space and hence the body's relationship with gravity. The otoliths in the labyrinths of the ears are thus essential for the maintenance of balance and equilibrium which is achieved by modifications of muscle tone.

Shumway-Cook (1992) suggested that to compensate for the loss of one sense requires the intact functioning of other senses in conjunction with central processes that coordinate input from the remaining senses as well as the ability to apply these compensatory mechanisms during active behaviour. Von Hofsten & Rosblad (1988) studied how children develop their ability to utilise vision and proprioception for manual control and Rosblad (1992) questioned whether therapists have taken perception into sufficient account when trying to understand and minimise disturbed or delayed motor abilities and in particular the roles of vision and proprioception.

Recent work by Robertson & North (1994) in adults with neglect has shown that sensory awareness can be improved by generating voluntary movements in the affected area so that the links between motor and sensory function may be mutual ones and not simply from sensory function to motor function.

Cognition

Cognition can be defined as pertaining to the intellect and its development (Sylva & Lunt, 1982). It has been suggested that the development of gross motor function is not affected by mild or even moderate impairment of cognition (Illingworth, 1966; Egan, 1990). Studies have concluded that the mean IQ of children with Down's syndrome is between 25 and 49 (Malzberg, 1950; Oster, 1953). Gesell & Armatruda (1947) observed that children with Down's syndrome sat at a mean age of 12 months and walked at a mean age of 24 months but that their manipulative skills were often permanently immature. Perhaps children with impaired cognition display a delay in motor skills and, in more extreme cases or for advanced skills, a permanent immaturity rather than abnormal or deviant motor skills.

Children with cognitive problems are frequently not interested in eating and have feeding problems. Malnutrition, especially in the first two to three years, can reduce the number of dendrites and synapses between neurones and slows down the rate of myelinisation (Dobbing & Smart, 1973). This would clearly interfere with the normal process of brain maturation and development and would be expected to produce detectable abnormalities of function.

Babies with cognitive impairment often sleep a lot and are described as being 'no trouble' and hence they may receive less attention. A lack of attention and therefore stimulation results in delayed maturation of vision and hearing and in consequence late smiling and problems with parental bonding. These children may also be less interested in their surroundings and have a decreased natural desire to explore so that again their development is adversely affected. Diminished concentration and alertness may produce a similar detrimental effect.

Thinking and feeling

Sylva & Lunt (1982) proposed that Piaget describes the intellectual level at which children think whereas Freud illustrates the subject of the children's thoughts. Piaget's concepts will have a bearing on the children's understanding of the purpose of performing a particular motor skill. Freud's ideas will influence the children's motivation and drive to undertake a task. Some activities are automatic whereas others require opportunity and motivation. The latter involve elements of situational understanding from the children so that if therapists wish to influence the motor development of such skills they also need a comprehensive knowledge of cognitive and emotional development.

Piaget's theories straddle the nature/nurture argument. He suggests that intelligence is a mental activity that enables a child to gradually adapt to the environment in an ever more, complex fashion. Whereas Gesell (1942) established milestones in motor development, Piaget (Ginsburg & Opper, 1979) outlined milestones in intellectual development. These milestone or mental structures Piaget termed schemas which were based on his clinical interviews with and naturalistic observations of many children and are described by Kathy Sylva and Ingrid Lunt in '*Child Development, A First Course*' published by Blackwell, reprinted 1989.

Freud (1962) described the psychosexual development of children from birth to adulthood in five stages (Bee, 1995). Freud was more concerned with the psychological than the reproductive aspects of sexuality. His conclusions were based on the case studies of many patients, for the most part adults. In common with Gesell's motor milestones and Piaget's intellectual schemas, Freud's stages of development were fixed in their sequence. Freud considered that the libido or energy of the sex instinct was the source of all actions or life's motivating energy. He described it to be the dominant force continuous throughout life although the goals of the sex drive change with age.

Freud divided personality into three parts: the id, the ego and the superego. The id is that part of the personality from which impulses of the libido arise. It is the primitive, newborn instinct to satisfy all needs immediately and at all costs and remains with a person throughout life. It is characterised by the pleasure principle, a mental operation, which relieves tension without recourse to reality. The ego deals with the external environment in rational ways. It develops as the child matures and distinguishes fantasy from reality. It is characterised by the reality principle which consists of rational activities directed towards satisfying the needs of the instincts. Learning, thinking, perceiving and evaluating all occur in the ego as does the daily maintenance of the body in terms of hunger, thirst and the escape from pain. The superego is the moral watchdog over the entire personality. It often conflicts with the id but the ego is left to work out an acceptable compromise. The superego is the model of what people ought to be like and is moulded by parental teaching. It can be the origin of both anxiety and irrational behaviour.

Socialisation

Bowlby (1969) suggested that there were three phases in an infant's development of attachment. The first he called non-focused orienting and signalling and suggested that it lasted from birth to three months. During this period babies emit behaviours such as crying, eye contact, clinging, cuddling and responding to caregiving efforts towards any person (Ainsworth & Wittig, 1969). At this stage there is little evidence of a definite attachment although the foundations are being laid. The second phase Bowlby called focus on one or more figures and suggested that this period lasted from about three months to about six months. During this phase children may respond more readily to the person or persons who regularly take care of them. Children show no fear of strangers and no special anxiety of being separated from their parents during this phase. The third phase Bowlby called secure base behaviour and suggested that it began at about six months. At this time children can begin to initiate moving themselves towards the caregivers or parents as well as enticing the caregivers or parents towards them. In addition they use the caregivers or parents as a safe haven from which to explore their surroundings. Object permanence develops around this age and children begin to check their parents expressions before venturing forth. Additional information on the development of the social skills can be found in Helen Bee's book *The Developing Child* published by Harper Collins (7th edition, 1995).

Impact of impairments

Children who are blind from birth usually lack facial expression and early problems often include a lack of communication by facial expression between mother and child. A lack of smiling and visual interaction may in turn produce a paucity of maternal handling of the child with possible consequent socialisation problems. Deaf children often fail to respond at a very early age to mother's voice, footsteps and the noises customarily associated with domesticity. As with visual impairment, hearing loss may produce problems with socialisation.

Children with a hearing deficit may show a delay in speech. Speech problems can also be associated with motor deficits in which case breath control, feeding and expressive speech may also be affected. Communication problems cause a deterioration in behaviour if childrens' intentions are repeatedly not understood. It is difficult to attract people's attention without speech so that the opportunity to express oneself is limited and in consequence so are one's options and experiences. A deficit in communication may result in social deprivation at first between mother and baby and later between the child and its peers.

Babies who move abnormally or insufficiently are often difficult for the mother to nurse or handle so that a barrier to natural interaction and cuddling may be established and the baby may experience deprivation while the mother may feel inadequate. If children cannot move around their environment they may be restricted in their exploration, learning, daily functions and socialisation. If children are unable to sit they may be deprived of the experience of seeing their peers and communicating with them at the same level. Upper limb function may be curtailed leading to a delay or loss of hand and eye coordination and fine motor activities, which in turn may affect self-care activities such as teeth cleaning, feeding and learning activities including holding a pencil or a pair of scissors. Feeding problems may lead to malnutrition which worries both parents and health care professionals. Inappropriate oral feeding may lead to problems with keeping airways and lungs clear. Inappropriate positioning during feeding may result in reflux. Feeding times may become associated with unpleasant experiences in the children and a consequent deterioration in behaviour, all of which may precipitate extra stress in the parents. Sloper & Turner (1995) investigating longitudinal predictors of current functioning in parents of older children with Down's syndrome suggested that high and persistent levels of distress were related to high levels of child behaviour problems, parental personality and coping strategies, and socioeconomic circumstances. Fathers' distress was likely to have increased if the coping strategies used were wishful thinking. Mothers' distress was likely to have increased if they were not employed outside the home and if family relationships were poor.

Growth

Growth is influenced both by nutrition and movement. At birth the lower limbs account for one-third of the child's total body length and the trunk is longer than the legs. At five years the lower limbs account for one-half of the total body length and as an adult they account for more than half of the total body length and the trunk is shorter than the legs. At birth the child's centre of gravity lies above the umbilicus, whereas at five years it lies below and as an adult it lies at the height of the anterior superior iliac spine. Children grow substantially in height and weight in the first five years and then have a growth spurt with an increase in both height and weight around puberty. These changes with age in the relative lengths of different parts of the body and in the position of the centre of gravity probably influence some aspects of the development of mobility in children, for example the progression from sitting and four point kneeling to upright standing.

Bones grow at the epiphyseal plates and muscles enlarge by adding sarcomeres at the musculotendinous junction (Ziv *et al.*, 1984). The stimuli for this growth include the growth factor somatotropin, growth hormone and stretch. Stretch is provided by active movement in normal children so that muscles are stretched over continuously growing bone. (Tardieu *et al.*, 1977). During growth the coordinated activity of agonist and antagonist muscles helps to control alignment across joints. In addition, weight bearing increases bone density (Dalen & Olssen, 1974) and promotes joint modelling (Harris *et al.*, 1975) in weight-bearing bones and joints.

Deterioration in motor function may occur during adolescence as a result of growth, especially at puberty. At this time the strength of persons with movement disorders may not keep pace with their mass.

Abnormal motor development

Children with multiple handicap develop motor skills but their acquisition is likely to be abnormal and may also be retarded. The abnormalities are largely predictable and specific in different types of cerebral palsy (Bobath & Bobath, 1975). There may be a paucity of movement, an excess of purposeless movements or a combination of the two. Bobath & Bobath (1975) have described the abnormal motor development of some children with different types of multiple handicap.

Active movement enables a child to practise and perfect a motor skill through sensory feedback; however, if the active movement is abnormal the feedback will also be and the movement never perfected will be repeated. This will result in deformity and early arthritis with increasing pain and immobility. Deformities may be mobile, fixed or structural. A mobile joint deformity can be defined as a maintained but correctable abnormal posture while a fixed joint deformity is a movement limited in its normal range by soft tissue. In contrast a structural joint deformity is a change in bony shape. Joint deformity in children with cerebral palsy frequently progresses from mobile to fixed to structural over a period of time.

The effect of abnormal posture on the development of joint deformity in cerebral palsy was described by Fulford & Brown (1976). Muscle contractures in CNS dysfunction primarily result from shortened muscle in response to prolonged abnormal functioning (Tarbary *et al.*, 1981) as the structure of muscles is conditioned by their use (Leiber, 1986). Furthermore, Goldspink & Williams (1981) described the part played by protein synthesis in the development of deformity and have suggested that the connective tissues around bones and joints display adaptive changes in response to abnormal positioning.

Spasticity is characterised by excessive and inappropriate involuntary muscular activity in association with an upper motor neurone syndrome. The clinical manifestations include a velocity dependent increase in tonic stretch reflexes with exaggerated tendon jerks (McLellan, 1991). The abnormal tonic stretch reflexes and spasms associated with nervous system dysfunction resist stretch and tend to maintain muscle in contraction. Holly *et al.* (1980) concluded from experiments with chickens that stretch is essential as a stimulus for growth and to maintain optimal muscle size once growth is completed. Further information on abnormal motor development and deformity was described by Ziv *et al.* (1984) following studies on mice with hereditary spasticity resultin from genetic mutation. They found that while bones grow at the epiphysea plates, muscles elongate from the musculotendinous junction (muscle growth plate) by the addition of sarcomeres or muscle cell segments. Two factors control muscle growth; hormonal stimulation mediated by somatotropin, and physical stimuli manifested by muscle stretch over continuously growing bones. The latter assists the coordination of muscle and bone growth allowing function to be preserved during development. Muscle contractures are shortening of muscle fibres which may be caused by abnormal joint positioning, differences in muscle and bone growth rates and dysfunctional contractile properties of muscles (O'Dwyer *et al*, 1994). Contractures in CNS dysfunction may affect the spine leading to scoliosis and impaired respiratory function. They may affect the hips resulting in reduced mobility and weight bearing and later loss of sitting ability, pain and problems with peroneal skin care. Contractures affect the knees, produce pain, loss of mobility and weight bearing. They may affect the feet in which case mobility and the ability to wear shoes can be affected. In the upper limb hand and arm contractures impair functions. Some of the treatment procedures undertaken by physiotherapists are specifically intended to counteract the development of deformities. Bobath & Bobath (1984) hoped to achieve this by manually inhibiting abnormal movement postures and patterns and facilitating more normal movement, postures and patterns. Phelps (1990) aimed to prevent deformities by the more normal positioning of children in both static (furniture) and dynamic (orthoses) equipment and by the use of orthopaedic surgery.

Active and passive movements

Active movements refer to self-induced movements, passive movements are externally produced. Zuck & Johnson (1952) suggested that active movements produce voluntary motor skills whereas passive movements keep joints mobile and help to prevent deformity. Held & Hein (1963) in experiments on kittens and monkeys demonstrated that along with intact sensory feedback, active movement as opposed to passive movement is needed to develop normal coordination and visuomotor adaptation. Young kittens restrained in a 'gondola' apparatus were unable to guide their forelimbs towards an object when freed despite normal unrestricted visual function, although they did later recover. Young monkeys reared in conditions that denied them the sight of their limbs developed deficiencies in grasping visible objects (Held & Bauer, 1967). Furthermore, White *et al.* (1964) emphasised the importance of self-induced movements in accelerating perceptuomotor development in young babies in hospital. The babies were given 'enriched crib environments' and encouraged to look around and to reach out at toys overhanging their cots. It was found that these babies were advanced in their hand regard compared with the norm on the Gesell scale (1947). White & Held (1966) also showed that an extra 20 minutes per day of handling, cuddling and playing with children between the ages of six and 36 days produced an increase in visual attentiveness.

Skill and motor skill acquisition

Many skills are acquired by learning which Sylva & Lunt (1982) defined as a change in behaviour brought about through association, reward and punishment or observation. Learning theorists emphasise the dominant role of experience in the process. Bandura (1989) suggested that human nature was characterised by a vast potential that could be fashioned by direct and vicarious experience into a variety of forms within biological limits. Many of the different schools of physiotherapy based on neurological concepts (Bobath & Bobath, 1984; Ayres, 1972) aim to provide children with experiences which they hope will be carried over into functional usage.

There are three major schools of learning: classical, operant and observational.

Classical conditioning was described by Pavlov in his studies of mature dogs. This type of conditioning is dependent on an association between two events so that the pairing of two stimuli, one a conditioned stimulus and one unconditioned stimulus, produces an involuntary response. In this example, at the first stage if food is the unconditional stimulus and the bell is the conditioned stimulus, food will produce saliva in the dog, but the bell will not produce saliva in the dog. At the second stage, food and the bell will produce salvia in the dog and at the third stage the bell, alone, will produce saliva in the dog. The problem is that extinction can easily occur, the bell alone may not continue to produce saliva in the dog. If young babies are touched on the cheek they will turn towards the touch and begin to suck. This is an early reflex reaction. As the babies begin to associate mother's footsteps or being picked up and held with sucking milk either of these stimuli may trigger the response of head turning and sucking.

Operant conditioning or instrumental learning as described by Thorndike (1919) and Skinner (1968) was carried out by Thorndike with cats and a puzzle box and by Skinner with rats and a tray with a lever. This type of conditioning is dependent on the pairing of a response with a reward. An experimental subject performs a voluntary action and gets a reward for it. For example Thorndike let a cat notice food in a puzzle box. It took the cat ten minutes to open the box and obtain the food on the first day on each successive day it took less time to open the box and obtain the food. Skinner put a rat in a box with a lever that had to be pulled to get at the food tray. The rat learnt to pull the lever and get the food. The food is termed a reinforcer and encourages the animal or child to repeat the process. A smile, a cuddle or a sweet may all be used as reinforcers. The same method can be used to prevent an animal or child performing an unwanted act. The reinforcer in that case being a punishment: a smack, no sweet or put to bed. Reinforcement can be continuous so that it follows each act or intermittent which often produces a higher response rate. Once again extinction can occur when the reinforcer no longer follows the learned response.

Skinner's work (1968) emphasised two main points to educators. Firstly, the importance of positive reinforcement, i.e. reward in the form of success and constant praise for even small achievements, and secondly the frequent necessity of 'breaking down' a learning task into small sequential steps. A further result of Skinner's work has been the development of behaviour modification, whereby children's unacceptable behaviour is altered to make it more compatible with their environment.

Observational learning or modelling was advocated by Freud and Piaget (1950). A child may watch and then copy an activity or notice someone else's behaviour and model their own on it. This is the way in which children frequently acquire skills but such observation is often denied to children with multiple handicap. An example of observational learning in children is the use of eating implements, cutlery or chopsticks, rather than the digits and this is usually accomplished by the children modelling themselves on their mealtime companions. Whereas classical and operant conditioning are fact centred and require a formal programme, observational learning is less formal and is subjective focusing on the individual child. It is relatively easy to measure the effects of programmed learning as described by Pavlov or Thorndike and Skinner but more difficult to gauge the results of observational learning as described by Piaget and Freud.

Developments of these learning strategies include shaping, modelling, guided rehearsal and role playing. The performance of all tasks deteriorates if illness or fatigue are present and if the child is fearful of being separated from the parent.

Both Conductive education (Hari & Tillemans 1984) and Portage (Jesien, 1984) are largely based on learning theories. Schmidt (1982) defined motor learning as a set of processes associated with practice or experience leading to relatively permanent changes in skilled behaviour. Haskell & Barrett (1989) have described three stages in the normal process of motor skill acquisition. The first is the cognitive process in which the child wishing to acquire the particular motor skill is motivated to perform the skill and works out the necessary components required to perform it. This process requires an active role on the part of the acquirer. The second stage is the practice and repetition required to refine and perfect the skill. During this process the acquirer needs feedback in two areas. Firstly, a knowledge of the results (KR), has the task been achieved, and secondly, a knowledge of the performance (KP), i.e. how has the task been performed. Practise requires appropriate rest periods to inhibit boredom and fatigue and thus should be 'distributed practice'. The third stage is the process whereby the ability to perform the skill becomes automatic for everyday use with the development of a motor engram (Granit, 1977). Roland *et al.* (1980) have shown that if a movement sequence is rehearsed by thinking through the complex movements that need to be made but without making any actual movements an increased neural activity occurs in the supplementary motor area. *The Education of Children with Motor and Neurological Disabilities* by Simon Haskell & Elizabeth Barrett (published by Chapman and Hall, 2nd ed., 1989) is recommended for further information on this topic.

A critical analysis of the major schools of therapy for cerebral palsy

Five therapeutic approaches to children with multiple handicap are in common usage:

1. The Bobath school (Bobath & Bobath, 1984; Mayston, 1992) is a neurodevelopmental treatment aimed at normalisation of movement to prevent deformity.
2. Conductive education (Hari & Tillemans, 1984; Cottam & Sutton, 1986) proposes a training programme focusing on learning movement, language and functional skills.

3. The Doman Delacato programme (Doman *et al.*, 1960), based largely on the ideas of Temple Fay (Fay, 1948), is both a neurophysiological treatment and training aimed at minimising the brain impairment and promoting the development of cognition.
4. Portage (Shearer & Shearer, 1972; Jesien, 1984) is a training programme designed to improve general skills and cognition.
5. The Vojta (Jones, 1975; Vojta, 1984) approach combines the ideas of Temple Fay and Kabat (Kabat *et al.*, 1959) and is a neurophysiological treatment aimed at influencing brain impairment so that normal skills are developed.

Rood's concepts (Stockmeyer, 1967) are employed in various sensory stimulation programmes. Children with mild motor symptoms or clumsy children are often treated by sensory integration methods (Ayres, 1972). These methods employed by therapists and teachers are based on the concept that learning is dependent on the ability to gather sensory information from the environment, to process and assimilate the information and to plan and perform tasks. Deficits in this pathway lead to difficulties in executing planned and organised behaviour and consequently a deterioration in motor learning capacity. It is considered that the provision of opportunities for enhanced sensory intake will lead to an improvement in motor learning.

In addition, Kabat's proprioceptive neuromuscular facilitation techniques are incorporated into some eclectic approaches (Levitt, 1966). Many physiotherapists use an approach tailored to the needs of each individual child, and often influenced by the interpretations of Phelps (Phelps, 1990). As a consequence his ideas on diagnosis and assessment using slow motion pictures, team approach, orthopaedic management of the peripheral musculoskeletal problems, aids equipment and exercise are still largely in evidence today.

Voluntary active movement

Voluntary movement enables children to acquire motor skills but this can only occur when the neural mechanisms are mature (McGraw, 1989). The process involves motivation to perform the movement, practice to improve the skill and the neuronal storage of the acquired activity for future use (Haskell & Barrett, 1989). Conductive education and Portage are the two schools which particularly encourage such voluntary active movement.

If the neural mechanisms are not ready for the particular motor skill no amount of practice will speed up their acquisition (Dennis, 1943). Schools such as Conductive education in which groups of children are expected to perform a series of preprogrammed tasks may be wasting the time of some of the children as it is impossible to match all the children perfectly into groups.

Portage may cause frustration to both the child and the parents by expecting a child to master a preprogrammed skill for which the child may not yet be ready without providing adequate guidance to teachers or parents on assessing whether the child has attained the neurological developmental level required to undertake the tasks. Furthermore, there may be insufficient counselling in the event of inability to perform the skills.

If a child has a CNS deficit it is most likely that he or she will use compensatory strategies to perform certain voluntary movements. These are likely to be abnormal movements which encourage the development of deformity as a consequence of the motion and the inappropriate sensory feedback that results. Deformity hinders movement and causes regression in functional skills.

Phelps encouraged the use of active voluntary movement to stretch shortened spastic muscles and to strengthen weak, lengthened muscles in an effort to combat secondary biomechanical constraints. The Danish school of orthopaedics (Plum, personal communication 1967–68) suggested that passive muscle stretching should be emphasised in outer ranges of movement and strengthening in middle and inner ranges of movement. Many therapists use concentric (shortening) and eccentric (lengthening) movements in full range. As the effect of spasticity is individually variable and different according to the manner in which muscles are used (McLellan, 1995), it is difficult to lay down any generalised prescription for treatment. Perhaps it is time to emphasise that spasticity is a symptom and needs to be treated only if function or care are impeded.

Facilitated automatic movement

Different schools of therapy facilitate movement by different methods. Bobath therapists stimulate normal automatic movement having first inhibited any abnormal postures and movements. This process is achieved by the hands of the therapist controlling postures and movements at key proximal points such as the hips and shoulders and facilitating by subtle guidance movement at the more distal points in conjunction with righting, equilibrium and saving reactions. Kabat promotes sensory stimulation of movement in diagonal and rotational patterns from positions of extreme length of the muscles to positions of maximal shortening of the muscles, using particularly, but not exclusively, resisted movement. Rood therapists encourage automatic movement by afferent sensory stimulation of tactile, temperature, pressure and muscle stretch receptors. They consider this in the context of which muscles are performing concentric (light work) contraction and which muscles are performing eccentric (heavy work) contraction. Vojta therapists stimulate automatic movement by afferent sensory stimulation of normal reflex patterns especially crawling and rolling, using manual pressure on identified trigger points or zones. Crawling and rolling are suitable for small, young children.

All these schools hope to facilitate or control automatic movement in such a way as to prevent deformity both from abnormal, voluntary movement and from the abnormal sensory feedback. All the schools hope to achieve carry-over from facilitated automatic movement to functional activity (Bobath & Bobath, 1984). Even though a facilitated movement may look and feel more normal, whether this is actually the case may only be shown by electromyographic testing. It seems unlikely that voluntary actions will be improved by these facilitated automatic movements. The heterogeneous causes of spasticity further complicate treatment (Wright & Rang, 1990). Spasticity can be cerebral and/or spinal in origin and the resistance felt and abnormal movements seen probably have both neural and mechanical components. Cerebral spasticity usually develops slowly following CNS damage and may, for example, be due to a lesion in the internal capsule, in which case the arm flexors may become spastic and the arm extensors weak, whereas the leg flexors may become weak and the leg extensors spastic. In such a case the child might benefit from some degree to elevated tone in the presence of weakness in the leg as the extensor strength of a relatively stiff leg can aid transferring and ambulation and inappropriate lowering of spasticity might result in worsening function. In spinal spasticity which also develops slowly there is considerable individual variation and different forms may be present at different times in the same child. Chapman & Wiesendanger (1982) have suggested that the slow development of spasticity may result from synaptic changes including axonal sprouting following CNS damage. Another suggestion has been an increased chemical sensitivity and a third suggestion that inactive synapses become active (Carr *et al.*, 1995). Bobath & Bobath (1975) proposed that spasticity becomes apparent as the child adopts antigravity postures. If spasticity is relieved by procedures such as selective dorsal rhizotomy abnormal patterns persist. Although there may be an increase in the range of movement, if no structural deformity is present an underlying lack of control may be unmasked which was previously overshadowed by a stability resulting from the spasticity. Spasticity can both benefit and impede functional activity, and even if spasticity is controlled the child is still likely to be left with coordination, sensory and cognitive defects. The three main reasons for controlling spasticity are to control troublesome flexor and extensor spasms, delay muscle contractures and joint deformities and reduce pain.

Passive movement

Passive movement in a phylogenetic sequence with very frequent repetition was advocated for the control of spasticity by Temple Fay and Doman & Delacato with the expectation that there will be carry-over to voluntary, functional activity from the storage of the passive movements administered.

Although full range passive movement without immobilisation may be successful in lengthening connective tissue and muscles and in promoting muscle growth so that the joints are kept more mobile, there appears to be no carry-over from the passive movements administered to voluntary functional action (Zuck & Johnson, 1952; Held & Hein, 1963; Held & Bauer, 1967). How much passive movement may be required to prevent contracture in differing muscles is unknown. Tardieu *et al.* (1988) suggested that a normal child stretches the soleus muscle for six hours out of 24 hours.

Normalisation of the quality of movement

The Bobath school is particularly concerned with the quality of movements and focuses on the normalisation of movement to prevent deformity and to give a child the experience of normal movement. They hope to achieve this manual inhibition of abnormal reactions by the therapist facilitating normal reactions at key points of control on the body of the child. The long-term aim is to develop normal movements useful for daily living functions. As stated above it is unlikely that achieving passive or facilitated automatic movement will lead to mastery of voluntary, active movement. This transformation of abnormal voluntary action to a normal functional movement during daily living tasks and at times when extra concentration is required such as at times of stress would be exceptional (Forssberg, 1992). Furthermore, if a child is deprived of the opportunity to use a skill for which it is developmentally prepared because it is unable to perform it normally it may be more difficult for the child to achieve the action at a later date (Illingworth & Lister, 1964).

Functional activities

Two schools that place a particular emphasis on functional activities are Conductive education and Portage. Conductive education consists of an all embracing, full-time preprogrammed education process including a combination of movement, language and function. Children are selected into groups and these are led by a conductor. Portage consists of a home-education programme comprising 580 developmentally progressive skills for children from birth to six years taught by a visiting teacher to the parents who then practise with their child. Children may acquire skills more easily in familiar situations and these skills are then more readily available for daily use. How much consideration is given to the readiness of individual children to perform the skill taught either in Conductive education preprogrammed groups, or in Portage preprogrammed developmentally sequenced tasks is unclear. A further point of concern regarding Conductive education is whether tasks habitually practised in an artificial environment using specialised pieces of equipment are generalised into daily living, particulary if the tasks demand more effort from either the child or the parents. Walking is the functional task emphasised in Conductive education. The early weight bearing encouraged may help joint modelling and bone density.

Orthopaedic management of secondary biomechanical constraints

The orthopaedic management of multiple handicap was pioneered by Phelps (1990). Today many eclectic physiotherapists still employ serial plaster of paris immobilisation and orthotics for the control of deformity, the improvement of sensory feedback and to give added stability for functional improvement. Orthopaedic management whether surgical, serial plaster of paris immobilisation or orthotic bracing affects primarily the peripheral musculoskeletal system. Consideration by Ziv *et al.* (1984), Williams & Goldspink (1984) and Wright & Rang (1990) has suggested that local musculoskeletal remodelling occurs but that the CNS deficits remain and continue to exert their influences on the musculoskeletal system.

O'Dwyer *et al.* (1989) pointed out that immobilisation may affect the connective tissues, and that any effects of immobilisation on musculature will be reversed once immobilisation is discontinued. Furthermore, they noted that if a muscle is passively immobilised in a shortened position it loses sarcomeres and shortens its fibre length, albeit slowly, while if a muscle is actively shortened by muscle contraction shortening occurs very rapidly. Passive lengthening by immobilisation of growing muscles produces an initial increase in sarcomeres (muscle cell segments) in series followed by a decrease in the number of sarcomeres so that firstly, the length of the overall muscle and tendon may only be maintained by tendon lengthening and secondly the muscle may atrophy and waste. Although an increase in range of joint movement may be initially evident following passive lengthening of muscle by immobilisation this procedure will not alleviate the muscle shortening which is the main cause of contracture and deformity in children with cerebral palsy and hence the problems tend to recur.

Developmental sequence of activities selected for intervention

Most schools of therapy follow a human sequence of development in their selection of activities for intervention. Some schools are more rigorous in this respect than others, for example Rood. As pointed out earlier normal human development is variable both in the method and timing of achievement.

Temple Fay, Doman & Delacato and Vojta follow a 'creature' sequence in which each step (swim, squirm, creep, crawl and walk) has to be perfected before progressing onto the next one; however, normal human physiological development does not follow this evolutionary phylogenetic pattern (Cohen *et al.*, 1970). Conductive education and Portage are the two schools that have most emphasised the formulation of precise goals in very small and simple steps to facilitate successful skill acquisition.

Selection of children for treatment

The only school which specifically selects children for their intervention is Conductive education. The selection criteria employed at the Birmingham Institute have been described by Bairstow *et al.* (1991). Peto (Conductive education) originally suggested the following selection criteria: good situational understanding, adequate vision, no evidence of epilepsy, adequate hearing and no evidence of bodily involvement making walking an eventual total impossibility.

Most children with unilateral involvement walk between the ages of 18 and 21 months (Bleck, 1987), the mean age being 15 months (P. Robson, personal communication, 1992) and most children with unilateral involvement achieve community walking (Hoffer *et al.*, 1973). In general children with mild to moderate bilateral involvement of the legs walk by 48 months (mean age of 24 months) (Bleck, 1987); (P. Robson, personal communication, 1992). The need for walking aids in this group is primarily dependent on whether equilibrium reactions are present (Bleck, 1987), and most children with mild to moderate bilateral involvement of the legs achieve household walking (Hoffer *et al.*, 1973). Walking ability reaches a plateau in children with multiple handicap at seven years of age (Crothers & Paine, 1959).

It is possible that Peto intended to select children who would succeed rather than fail. As selection standards for Conductive education have been lowered internationally to meet public demand, false hopes have probably been raised.

Individual or group treatment

Conductive education is the only school that favours group treatment exclusively. Most professionals consider that children and their families can benefit from both individual and group treatment and preference for one or the other is probably a personal matter. This is appropriate as individual treatment is able to focus on individual problems. The problems that manifest themselves in multiple handicap are individual and may be unique, as is the precise stage of maturation of each child. Group treatment has the advantage of taking the pressure off an individual child. In addition groups may help children to motivate and facilitate each other to progress and may be more fun. Moreover, groups may encourage children and their families to socialise although in the event this will happen primarily among those with similar problems.

Segregation from or integration with normal peers through treatment

Segregation can occur in Conductive education by the nature of the intervention and management at a centre of selected groups of disabled children which can either be residential or for substantial parts of each day. This early segregated intervention is supposed to facilitate later integration. To a lesser extent segregation from normal peers may occur through the intensity of the treatment regimen suggested by Doman & Delacato although those administering the treatment are likely to be teams of volunteering adults.

Phelps suggested management for about five years in a residential institution to facilitate the special care required.

Integration may be combined with most other schools of therapy as management is undertaken individually, can be accommodated in most environments, rarely exceeds an hour and can be arranged by mutual agreement. Segregation from normal peers imposes a different lifestyle which may include increased dependency and decreased initiative and may cause problems with socialisation in the real world which do not become apparent until adulthood.

Involvement of parents in treatment either at a centre and/or at home

Bobath therapists usually treat a child with a parent present and request the parent to supplement their treatment by correct handling and functional management at home. Conductive education expects a parent to work with their child as a pair in the selected group while the child is aged between 18 months and three and a half years after which a parent is no longer expected to be intimately involved, as children over three and a half years are usually able to cooperate with a task or exercise independently. Doman & Delacato centres aim to provide parents with a programme of intensive passive exercises to be undertaken on the child several times daily at home by the parents, often supplemented by teams of voluntary helpers. The progress of the child is monitored regularly at the centre and in the past there have been suggestions that parents have been held responsible for the lack of progress in their child. Portage teachers instruct parents on a weekly basis to become the educators of their preschool child in their home and maximum involvement of the parents is apparently required for success. Vojta therapists expect parents to undertake prescribed exercises regularly with their child but as the children are usually still quite young (it is difficult to perform Vojta exercises on a large child) this may be the time of life when parents expect to spend more of their time with their child. If no significant progress is observed within one year Vojta treatment is terminated.

Individual parents will have different requirements and aspirations concerning involvement in their child's management and they may vary as the child ages.

Intensity and duration of treatment by the professional

Only Conductive education expects professional management sessions to extend habitually beyond one hour. As the children are trained in groups the pressure on each individual child is not likely to be so intensive. Furthermore, both Conductive education and Phelps demand that children attend professional intervention on a daily basis. None of the other schools advocates such intensive professional involvement in the normal course of management. Some parents and therapists have expressed the sentiment that more treatment would achieve more progress but this has not been proven in the long term (Bower *et al.*, 1996) and too much individual intervention may induce behavioural problems in children (Bower & McLellan, 1994*a*).

Use of aids and equipment

Some of the preprogrammed tasks in Conductive education employ specially designed furniture to facilitate compensatory strategies enabling children to carry out functional skills which they could not perform without these aids, for example getting from sitting to standing by pulling up on the bar of a ladder-back chair with both arms and using a positive supporting reaction in both legs for weightbearing. Phelps designed many such aids to daily living such as standing frames, which are still in general use today.

At differing stages most children and their families will require various aids to daily living. These need to be provided either at the time when the child indicates a readiness for the particular task or at the time when management would be eased for the parents by the provision of the aid. One caveat is that therapists have been known to assess a child's needs in relation to daily living aids purely on physical ability without taking into consideration cognitive and social needs.

In view of the suggestion that immobilisation of muscle in a passively lengthened position does not prevent muscle shortening and contracture (O'Dwyer *et al.*, 1989) and the lack of contact between the femoral head and the acetabulum in posterior areas in the sitting position (Rab, 1981) so that hip joint modelling is not enhanced, the desirability of prescribing special seating which exerts rigorous control with the aim of preventing hip deformity may need reconsideration.

The final common purpose of all the schools is to achieve the maximum independence for each child. Whereas some of the schools place more emphasis on training voluntary movement and resultant function, others place more emphasis on the treatment of the quality of movement skills performed in an attempt to prevent the deformity that may result from abnormal movement and defective sensory feedback. Some of the voluntary movements in multiple handicap are likely to be compensatory and abnormal so that over time they will produce deformity that can result in regression of voluntary movement and function and pain. Whether any of these facets can be permanently influenced by therapy still remains largely unproven. As yet no single school of treatment or training has been proven to be more successful than any other (Bower & McLellan, 1994*b*).

The ability to interact socially with success is probably the most important single priority for any person with cerebral palsy; however, this aspect has not achieved a high profile in any of the schools of therapy described.

Physical therapy and its integration with family life and education

Physical therapy in the context of childhood neurological dysfunction has traditionally been concerned with movement problems. Most systems of therapy commence with an assessment by the physiotherapist of the problems followed by a prescription of treatment to be given by the physiotherapist to the patient. In some cases aspects of this treatment are expected to be continued by the patient at home, nursery or school in between visits to the physiotherapist. This pattern of therapy often continues from identification of risk or diagnosis at under one year of age to the transfer to adult services at 16–19 years of age when the patient leaves school.

In the past the reasons for treating children with multiple handicap have usually been related to symptoms and functional disability. There is little point in assessing the symptoms without reference to the associated functional capacity of the child. It may be time to reconsider this hierarchical system of treatment and allow the identification of problems to be transferred to the child, the parents and the relevant nursery or school carers. The likely causes for and possible solutions to these disabilities can then be discussed between the child, the parents, the relevant carers and the physiotherapist. If appropriate treatments are available which are acceptable to the child, family and carers these can be instituted and monitored by all the participants who also participate in judging the success of interventions (Bower & McLellan, 1992). Thus problems which are of immediate concern to the child and its carers are addressed and a gradual comprehension of the core neurological problems may be achieved. This acquisition of knowledge covers the treatment options and prognosis, including realistic goals for each aspect of the individual child's disabilities. This process does however require a physiotherapist who understands the condition and its likely progression, possesses sensitive interpersonal skills and is sufficiently secure to be willing to learn with the child, its family and other carers. Table 15.1 outlines the steps involved in this process. Figure 15.1 illustrates a worked form that can be used for this process. This integrated schedule should illustrate what the child can do, what the child does do, what the child would like to do and what would help the parents and carers in the management of the child.

Bleck (1987) suggested that when a child is diagnosed with multiple handicap the first question asked by the parent is always 'Will he walk?' The second question is 'When?' the third is 'What can we do to make him walk?' He suggests that the real priorities in terms of optimum independent living are different and he ranks them in descending order as:

1. Communication (verbal or non-berbal).
2. Activities of daily living.
3. Mobility (mechanical devices).
4. Walking.

It is suggested that the most important priority is likely to be the ability to interact socially which will be the result of an emotional adaptation to handicap enabling the patient to function in the community giving and taking with grace and dignity.

Table 15.1 *Steps in goal setting and appraisal*

1	A discussion with the child, the family and the relevant school or nursery carer is undertaken concerning their problems, and these problems are documented
2	A joint assessment of the child is carried out with the parents and school or nursery carers over several days if necessary in the relevant environments to establish: (a) The child's likes and dislikes (b) The personality of the child (c) The social skills of the child (d) The daytime activities of the child at home (e) The daytime activities of the child at school (f) The daily living functional abilities of the child (g) The cognitive skills of the child (h) The hearing skills of the child (i) The communication skills of the child (j) The visual skills of the child (k) The fine motor skills of the child (l) The gross motor skills of the child (m) The child's habitual static positions and dynamic movement patterns and the active and passive range of joint movement
3	In the light of the knowledge gained in step 2, the problems documented in step one are jointly categorised into (i) those which physiotherapy may help (ii) those which physiotherapy may not help, and (iii) those which someone else may be able to help. The list is then jointly ranked in order of priority and documented
4	The child, family, school or nursery carer and physiotherapist then agree on useful, realistic, short-term goals understood by the child and a time scale in which they should be achieved. These goals must be specific, measurable and documented
5	The physiotherapist identifies his or her ideas on progression and long-term goals, discusses these with the child, family and school or nursery carers and documents them
6	Realistic methods of treatment are discussed, jointly agreed and documented
7	Realistic frequency and duration of treatment, including who is going to undertake the treatment is discussed jointly, agreed and documented
8	Measuring methods are discussed and documented
9	The child is baselined in the presence of the family and school or nursery carers on the agreed goals by the method agreed in step 8 prior to commencement of treatment. This measurement is documented
10	The treatment is commenced as agreed and progression documented
11	The child is re-measured after the agreed time scale in which the goals were to have been achieved and the results documented
12	Reappraisal by joint discussion is undertaken

Source: Bower for CPO Interlink, 1992.

Name:****

Date: ****

Chronological age:
2½ years

Developmental motor age:
3–6 months

Provisional diagnosis:
Bilateral CP

Problems: *(as identified by child/carers)*
1 Cannot sit on chamber pot for continence training

Reasons: *(as identified by therapist)*
1 Extensor thrust – but can bring hands to midline in flexed position

Short-term goals: *(as negotiated between child/carers)*
1 Sit on chamber pot for three minutes

Long-term goals: *(as identified by therapists)*
1 Child to learn strategies to control extensor thrust enabling functional use of sitting position in various environments
2 Provision of tables at heights to prevent excessive trunk flexion and neck extension for use with chamber pot, feeding chair and nursery chair. If necessary fix grab rails on tables
3 Strengthen trunk extension muscles and lengthen trunk flexion muscles with head controlled in neutral position, movements performed by child at a tempo unlikely to invoke spasticity/spasm to try to delay developmental deformity resulting from compensatory strategies
4 Monitor hips for problems
5 Discuss 1, 2 3 and 4 with child, family and nursery

Treatment means:
1 Encourage child to sit on chamber pot placed between therapist's or carer's legs and to hold onto shoelaces to counteract extensor thrust
2 Encourage child to do this while therapist or nursery carer sings increasingly longer rhymes
3 As child gains confidence replace person with soft mats placed round child
4 As child becomes more proficient encourage holding onto trousers/skirt at knees or thighs instead of shoelaces
5 Prone lying position hands clasped on buttocks, head in line with shoulders lift and lower rhythmically

Frequency:
1 Chamber pot sitting × 2 daily on first day progressing to × 4 daily at end of first week, then as required for continence
Mother and Nursery: Monday to Friday. Father at weekends
Physiotherapist × 1 at Nursery: Monday, Wednesday, Friday
2 Active exercises × 3 weekly each exercise × 3 progressing to × 10 if tolerated
Physiotherapist: Monday, Wednesday, Friday at Nursery.

Duration:
On first and second day replace child on chamber pot × 1 if falls off
On third day replace child × 2 if falls off. Continue for 3 weeks
If child or carers become distressed STOP and investigate cause

Is it being done:
1 *Yes.* Physiotherapist, Mother, Nursery Carers
2 *No*
3 *Some doubt.* Father at weekends

Measures:
1 Stop watch
2 Chart

Has goal been achieved:
1 Yes, sitting on chamber pot for three minutes holding shoelaces surrounded by soft mats: 01 06 1994

Elapsed time:
1 Three weeks

Further action: *(following joint discussion)*
1 Continue for further two weeks ONLY to see if child can improve holding on to trousers/skirt at knees at times when placed on pot for continence
2 Continue with active exercises: physiotherapist once weekly at home until regimen has been established at the nursery. Nursery carer x 2 at school combining the exercise into music and movement sessions – 'catch a fish like a seal'. Add lying with straight legs comfortably abducted and heels raised on a stool 3–6 inches high both hips lift and lower rhythmically: music and movement sessions 'make a tunnel'
3 Check progress re provision of tables required
4 Make date to discuss further problems in eight weeks if requested
5 Leave telephone number for contact

Figure 15.1. Clinical physiotherapy form.
Source: Bower for CPO Interlink, 1992.

Goal setting

Treatment goal-setting is at the centre of attempts to reduce disability and resolve handicaps for children and their families. Therapists can help children and families by steering them towards realistic end-points and by providing a framework for action. A workable goal is an accomplishment that helps the individual manage problematic situations (Herbert, 1987). In this context goals are really achieved when the children and/or their families have acquired the skills, practised them and employed them to solve or manage disabilities. Herbert (1987) suggests that goal setting can help children and parents in four ways:

1. Goals focus attention and action, providing a vision that offers hope and an outlet for concentrated effort.
2. Goals mobilise energy and help pull the children and/or parents out of the inertia of helplessness and depression.

3. Goals enhance the persistence needed for working at problems.
4. Goals motivate all concerned to search for strategies to accomplish them.

Several points need to be considered by the therapist and discussed with the children and caregivers when setting goals:

1. One cannot change a child from 'can't do' to 'can do' if the neural mechanisms are not ready, in other words you cannot change or normalise the neurological impairment.
2. One may be able to help a child to change from 'can do' to 'does do' if and when the child displays a wish to do so.
3. If one misses the time window during which a child wants to achieve a skill, and have not provided the necessary environment or compensatory mechanical devices at that time, it may be more difficult for the child to achieve that skill at a later date.
4. Children achieve skills in stages, and so goals should be formulated in simple small steps which are achievable, allowing the child to experience success instead of failure.
5. The secondary biomechanical impairments which result from compensatory strategies used by the child and the strategies that may combat these further impairments are valuable goals to assist in development.

Careful though needs to be given to the reason for physical intervention. The priority should not be the satisfaction of the physician, the therapist or even the family but should be the possibility of helping the child to become more acceptable to the rest of society. Factors which should be discussed with children, parents and nursery or school carers include:

1. The realistic aims and rationale of treatment.
2. The appraisal of therapy at regular intervals so that it can be stopped if not successful.
3. Access to appropriate information including predictions of outcomes.
4. Provision of adequate and sympathetic support.
5. An identification of the child's abilities and likely objectives.
6. Methods of integrating treatment with the academic and social goals of education.

If this process is completed the effects of physical therapy on family relationships, childrens' abilities to integrate socially and their scholastic attainments will have been more carefully considered than has often been the case in the past.

References

Ainsworth, M. D. S. & Wittig, B. A. (1969). Attachment and exploratory behaviour of one year olds in a strange situation. In *Determinants of Infant Behaviour* ed. B. M. Foss vol. 4, pp. 113–16, London: Methuen.

Aslin, R. N. (1981). Experiential influences and sensitive periods in perceptual development: a unified model. In *Development of Perception: Psychobiological Perspective*, ed. R. N. Aslin, J. R. Alberts & M. R. Peterson, vol. 2, *The Visual System*, pp. 45–93. New York: Academic Press.

Ayres, A. J. (1972). *Sensory Integration and Learning Disorders.* Los Angeles: Western Psychological Services.

Bairstow, P., Cochrane, R. & Rush, T. (1991). Selection of children with cerebral palsy for conductive education and the characteristics of children judged suitable and unsuitable. *Developmental Medicine & Child Neurology*, **33**, 984–93.

Bandura, A. (1989). Social cognitive theory. *Annals of Child Development*, **6**, 1–60.

Bayley, N. & Schaeffer, E. S. (1960). Relationships between socio-economic variables and the behaviour of mothers towards young children. *Journal of Genetic Psychology*, **96**, 61.

Bee, H. (1995). *The Developing Child*, 7th ed. New York: Harper Collins.

Bleck, E. (1987). Orthopaedic management in cerebral palsy. *Clinics in Developmental Medicine*, 99–100.

Bobath, B. & Bobath, K. (1975). *Motor Development in the Different Types of Cerebral Palsy*. London: Heinemann.

Bobath, K. & Bobath, B. (1984). The neurodevelopmental treatment. *Clinics in Developmental Medicine*, **90**, 6–19.

Bower, E. & McLellan, D. L. (1992). Effect of increased exposure to physiotherapy on skill acquisition in children with cerebral palsy. *Developmental Medicine and Child Neurology*, **34**, 25–39.

Bower, E. & McLellan, D. L. (1994*b*). Assessing motor skill acquisition in 4 Centres for the Treatment of Children with Cerebral Palsy. *Developmental Medicine and Child Neurology*, **36**, 902–9.

Bower, E. & McLellan, D. L. (1994*a*). Measuring motor goals in children with cerebral palsy. *Clinical Rehabilitation*, **8**, 198–206.

Bower, E., McLellan, D. L., Arney, J. & Campbell, M. J. (1996). A randomised controlled trial of different intensities of physiotherapy and different goal setting procedures in 44 children with cerebral palsy. *Developmental Medicine and Child Neurology*, **38**, 226–38.

Bowlby, J. (1951). Maternal Care and Mental Health Bulletin, *WHO* **3**, 357.

Bowlby, J. (1969). *Attachment and Loss*, vol. 1, *Attachment*. New York: Basic Books.

Bowlby, J. (1971). *Attachment and Loss*, vol. 1, *Attachment*. Hammondsworth: Penguin.

Bowlby, J., Ainsworth, M., Boston, M. & Rosenbluth, D. (1956). Effects of mother–child separation: follow-up study. *British Journal of Medical Psychology*, **29**, 211.

Bronfenbrenner, U. (1979). *The Ecology of Human Development*. Cambridge, MA: Harvard University Press.

Bronfenbrenner, U. (1989). Ecological systems theory. *Annals of Child Development*, **6**, 187–249.

Buffery, A. W. H. (1976). Sex differences in the neuropsychological development of verbal and spatial skills. In *The Neuropsychology of Learning Disorders: Theoretical Approaches* ed. R. M. Knights & D. J. Bakker, pp. 187–205. Baltimore: Baltimore University Park Press.
Burt, C. (1950). *The Backward Child.* London: University of London Press.
Carmichael, L. (1926). The development of behaviour in vertebrates experimentally removed from the influence of external stimulation. *Psychological Review*, **33**, 57.
Carr, J. H., Shepherd, R. B. & Ada, L. (1995). Spasticity: research findings and implications for intervention. *Physiotherapy*, **81**, 421–9.
Chapman, C. E. & Wiesendanger, M. (1982). The physiological and anatomical basis of spasticity: a review. *Physiotherapy, Canada*, **34**, 125–36.
Cohen, H. J., Brick, H. & Taft, L. T. (1970). Some considerations for evaluating the Doman Delacato pattering method. *Pediatrics*, **45**, 302–14.
Cotman, C. W. & Nieto-Sampedro, M. (1985). Cell biology of synaptic plasticity. In *Neuroscience* ed. P. H. Abelson, E. Butz & S. H. Snyder, pp. 74–8. Washington: American Association for the Advancement of Science.
Cottam, P. J. & Sutton, A. (1986). *Conductive education: a System for Overcoming Motor Disorder*. London: Croom Helm.
Crothers, B. & Paine, R. (1959). *Natural History of Cerebral Palsy*. Cambridge, MA: Harvard University Press.
Dalen, N. & Olssen, E. K. (1974). Bone mineral content and physical activity. *Acta Orthopaedic Scandinavica*, **45**, 170–4.
Davis, D. R. & Kent, N. (1955). Psychological factors in educational disability. *Proceedings of the Royal Society of Medicine*, **48**, 993.
Dennis, W. (1941). Infant development under conditions of restricted practice and minimum social stimulation. *Genetic Psychological Monographs*, **23**, 143.
Dennis, W. (1943). On the possibility of advancing and retarding the motor development of infants. *Psychological Review*, **50**, 203.
Dobbing, J. & Sands, J. (1973). Quantitative growth and development of the human brain. *Archives of Disease in Childhood*, **48**, 757–67.
Dobbing, J. & Smart, L. (1973). Early under-nutrition, brain development and behaviour. In *Ethology and Development*, ed. S. A. Barnet. Clinics in Developmental Medicine, **47**, London: Heinemann.
Doman, R. J., Spitz, E. B., Zuckman, E., Delacato, C. H. & Doman, C. (1960). Children with severe brain injuries: neurological organisation in terms of mobility. *Journal of the American Medical Association*, **174**, 257–62.
Douglas, J. W. B. (1964). *The Home and the School.* London: MacGibbon & Kee.
Egan, D. F. (1990). Developmental examination of gross motor skills. In *Developmental Examination of Infants and Preschool Children.* Clinics in Developmental Medicine, no. 112, pp. 71–4. London: Blackwell.
Fantz, R. (1961). The origin of form perception. *Scientific American*, **204**, 66–72.
Fay, T. (1948). The neurophysical aspects of therapy in cerebral palsy. *Archives of Physical Medicine*, **29**, 327–34.
Forssberg, H. (1992). A neural control model for human locomotion development. In *Movement Disorders in Children*. ed. H. Forssberg & H. Hirschfeld. Medicine and Sports Science, Basel, Karger 36. pp. 174–81.
Freud, S. (1962). Three essays on the theory of sexuality. Standard Edition of the *Complete Psychological Works of Sigmund Freud*, vol. 7. London: Hogarth Press.

Fulford, G. & Brown, K. (1976). Position as a cause of deformity in children with cerebral palsy. *Developmental Medicine and Child Neurology*, **18**, 305–14.
Gesell, A. (1942). *The First Five Years of Life*. London: Methuen.
Gessell, A. (1948). *Studies in Child Development*. New York: Harper.
Gesell, A. & Armatruda, C. S. (1947). *Developmental Diagnosis*. New York & London: Hoeber.
Gibson, E. & Walk, R. D. (1960). The visual cliff. *Scientific American*, **202**, 64–71.
Ginsburg, H. & Opper, S. (1979). *Piaget's Theory of Intellectual Development*. New Jersey: Prentice Hall.
Goldspink, G. & Williams, P. E. (1981). Development and growth of muscle. In *Mechanism of Muscle*. Adaptation to Functional Requirements ed. F. Gube, G. Marechal & O. Takacs, *Advances in Physiological Sciences*, vol. 24, pp. 87–98, New York: Pergamon Press
Granit, R. (1977). *The Purposive Brain*. Cambridge , MA: The MIT Press.
Greenhough, W. T., Black, J. E. & Wallace, C. S. (1987). Experience and brain development. *Child Development*, **58**, 539–59.
Griffiths, R. (1954). *The Abilities of Babies*. London: University of London.
Hari, M. & Tillemans, T. (1984). Conductive education. *Clinics in Developmental Medicine* **90**, 19–36.
Harlow, H. F. & Harlow, M. K. (1962). Social deprivation in monkeys. *Scientific American*, **203**.
Harris, N. H., Lloyd Robert, G. C. & Gallien, R. (1975). Acetabular development in congenital dislocation of the hip. *Journal of Bone and Joint Surgery*, **57B**, 46–52.
Haskell, S. H. & Barrett, E. K. (1989). *The Education of Children with Motor and Neurological Disabilities*, 2nd edn. New York: Nichols Publishing.
Held, R. & Bauer, J. A. (1967). Visually guided reaching in infant monkeys after restricted rearing. *Science* **155**, 718–20.
Held, R. & Hein, A. (1963). Movement produced stimulation in the development of visually guided behaviour. Journal of Comparative Physiological Psychology **56**, 872–6.
Herbert, M. (1987). *Behavioural Treatment of Children with Problems. A Practice Manual*, 2nd edn. London: Academic Press, Harcourt Brace.
Hoffer, M. M., Fiewell, E., Perry, R., Perry, J. Bonnett, C. (1973). Functional ambulation in patients with myelomeningocele. *Journal of Bonea nd Joint Surgery*, **57A**, 137–48
Holly, R. G., Barnett, J. G., Ashmore, C. R., Taylor, R. G. & Mole, P. A. (1980). Stretch-induced growth in chicken wing muscles: a new mode of stretch hypertrophy. *American Journal of Physiology* **238** (Suppl) C62–C71.
Horowitz, F. D. (1987). *Exploring Developmental Theories: Toward a Structural/Behavioural Model of Development*. Hillsdale, NJ: Erlbaum.
Horowitz, F. D. (1990). Developmental models of individual differences In *Individual Differences in Infancy: Reliability, Stability, Prediction* ed. J. Colombo & J. Fagen, pp. 3–18. Hillsdale, NJ: Erlbaum
Hubel, D. H. & Weisel, T. N. (1970). The period of susceptibility to the physiological effects of unilateral eye closure in kittens. *London Journal of Physiology*, **206**, 418–36.
Illingworth, R. S. (1953). *The Normal Child*. London: Churchill.
Illingworth, R. S. (1966). *The Development of the Infant and Young Child, Normal and Abnormal*, 3rd edn. Edinburgh and London: Churchill Livingstone.

Illingworth, R. S. & Lister, J. (1964). The critical or sensible period, with special reference to certain feeding problems in infants and children. *Journal of Pediatrics*, **65**, 839.
Itard, J. (1962). 'The Wild Boy of Aveyrou', translated by G. Humphrey & M. Humphrey. New York: Appleton-Century-Croft.
Jesien, G. (1984). Home based early intervention: a description of the Portage Project Model. *Clinics in Developmental Medicine*, **90**, 36–49.
Jones, R. B. (1975). The Vojta method of treatment of cerebral palsy. *Physiotherapy*, **61**, 112–13.
Kabat, H., McLeod, M. & Holt, C. (1959). The practical application of proprioceptive neuromuscular facilitation. *Physiotherapy*, **45**, 87–92.
Kagan, J. (1982). Canalization of early psychological development. *Pediatrics*, **70**, 474–83.
Knoblach, H. (1959). Pneumoencephalograms and clinical behaviour. *Pediatrics*, **23**, 175.
Levittt, S. (1966). Proprioceptive neuromuscular facilitation techniques in cerebral palsy. *Physiotherapy*, **52**, 46.
Levitt, S. (1982). *Treatment of Cerebral Palsy and Motor Delay*, 2nd edn. Oxford: Blackwell.
Lieber, R. L. (1986). Skeletal muscle adaptability: 1: review of basic properties. *Developmental Medicine and Child Neurology*, **28**, 390–7.
Lorenz, K. (1970). *Studies in Animal and Human Behaviour*. vol. I, Cambridge, MA: Harvard University Press.
Malzberg, B. (1950). Some statistical aspects of mongolism. *American Journal of Mental Deficiency*, **54**, 266.
Mayston, M. (1992). The Bobath Concept Evolution and Application. In *Movement Disorders in Children*. 36. ed. H. Forssberg & H. Hirschfield. pp. 1–6. *Medicine and Sports Science*, **36**. Basel: Karger.
McGraw, M. (1940). Neural maturation as exemplified by the achievement of bladder control. *Journal of Pediatrics*, **16**, 580–90.
McGraw, M. (1943). *The Neuromuscular Maturation of the Human Infant*. New York: Columbia University Press.
McGraw, M. (1989). The neuromuscular maturation of the human infant. *Clinics in Developmental Medicine*, **4**. Oxford: Blackwell.
McLellan, D. L. (1991). Functional recovery and the principles of disability medicine. In *Clinical Neurology*, ed. M. Swash & J. Oxbury, pp. 781. London: Churchill Livingstone.
McLellan, D. L. (1995). Lecture at *Symposium on Spasticity* at Society for Rehabilitation Research meeting at Southampton, July.
Milani-Comparetti, A. (1964). Spasticity versus patterned postural and motor behaviour in spastics. Exertia Medica International Congress Series 107. *Proceedings of the IVth International Congress of Physical Medicine*, Paris, 6–11 September.
Nelson, K. B. & Ellenberg, J. H. (1986). Antecedents of cerebral palsy: 1. Univariate analysis of risks. *New England Journal of Medicine*, **315**, 81–6.
Nissen, H. W., Chow, K. L. & Semmes, J. (1951). Effects of restricted opportunity for tactile kinaesthetic and manipulative experience on the behaviour of a chimpanzee. *American Journal of Psychology*, **64**, 485.
Nowakowski, R. S. (1987). Basic concepts of CNS development. *Child Development*, **58**, 568–95.

O'Dwyer, N., Neilson, P. & Nash, J. (1989). Mechanisms of muscle growth related to muscle contracture in cerebral palsy. *Developmental Medicine and Child Neurology*, **3**, 1543–52.
O'Dwyer, N., Neilson, P. & Nash, J. (1994). Reduction of spasticity in cerebral palsy using feedback of the tonic stretch reflex: a controlled study. *Developmental Medicine and Child Neurology*, **36**, 770–86.
Oster, J. (1953). *Mongolism*. Copenhagen: Munksgaard.
Phelps, W., A. (1990). Cerebral birth injuries: their orthopaedic classification and subsequent treatment. *Clinical Orthopaedics and Related Research*, **253**, 4–12.
Piaget, J. (1950). *The Psychology of Intelligence*. London: Routledge & Kegan Paul.
Purves, D. & Lichtman, J. W. (1985). *Principles of Neural Development*. Sunderland, MA: Sinauer Associates pp. 13; 301–27.
Rab, G. (1981). Preoperative roentgenographic evaluation for osteotomies about the hip in children. *Journal of Bone and Joint Surgery*, **63A**, 305–9.
Rang, M. (1982). *The Easter Seal Guide to Children's Orthopaedics*. Ontario, Canada: Easter Seal Society.
Robertson, I. H. & North, N. T. (1994). One hand is better than two: motor extinction of left hand advantage in unilateral neglect. *Neuropsychologia*, **32**, 1–11.
Robson, P. (1970). Shuffling, hitching, scooting or sliding: some observations in 30 otherwise normal children. *Developmental Medicine and Child Neurology*, **12**, 608.
Roland, P. E., Larsen, B., Lassen, N. A. & Skinhoj, E. (1980). Supplementary motor area and other cortical areas in organisation of voluntary movements in man. *Journal of Neurophysiology*, **43**, 118–36.
Rosblad, B. (1992). Perceptual determinants of precise manual pointing in children with motor impairments. In *Movement Disorders in Children* ed. H. Forssberg & H. Hirschfield, Medicine in Sport Science, vol. 36, pp. 137–43. Basel: Karger.
Sachs, B. (1985). *The Man Who Mistook His Wife for a Hat*. UK: Picador.
Schmidt, R. A. (1982). *Motor Control and Learning: a Behavioural Emphasis*. Illinois: Human Kinetics Publishers, p. 438.
Shearer, M. S. & Shearer, D. (1972). The Portage Project: a model for early education. *Exceptional Children*, **39**, 210–17.
Shepherd, G. M. (1983). *Neurobiology*. Oxford: Oxford University Press.
Sheridan, M. D. (1973). *From Birth to Five Years. Children's Developmental Progress*. Windsor, Berks: Nfer-Nelson, pp. 12–13.
Shumway Cooke, A. (1992). Role of the vestibular system in motor development: theoretical and clinical issues. In *Movement Disorders in Children*, ed. H. Forssberg & H. Hirschfeld. Medicine in Sports Science, vol, 36, pp. 209–17. Basel: Karger.
Skinner, B. F. (1968). *The Technology of Teaching*. New York: Appleton-Century-Crofts.
Sloper, T. & Turner, S. (1995). Longitudinal Predictors of Current Functioning in Parents of Older Children with Down's Syndrome. Abstract, *European Academy of Childhood Disability* Meeting, Stockholm. Sweden, June.
Stockmeyer, S. A. (1967). An interpretation of the approach of Rood to the treatment of neuromuscular dysfunction. *American Journal of Physical Medicine*, **46**, 900–56.

Sutherland, D. H., Biden, E. N. & Wyatt, H. P. (1988). *The Development of Mature Walking. Classics in Developmental Medicine*. London: Blackwell, pp. 104–5.
Sylva, K. & Lunt, I. (1982). *Child Development: a First Course*. Oxford: Blackwell.
Tarbary, J. C., Tardieu, C., Tardieu, G. & Tabary, C. (1981). Experimental rapid sarcomere loss with concomitant hypo-extensibility. *Muscle and Nerve*, **4**, 198–203.
Tardieu, C., Lespargot, A., Tabary, C. & Bret, M. D. (1988). For how long must the soleus muscle be stretched each day to prevent contracture? *Developmental Medicine and Child Neurology*, **30**, 3–10.
Tardieu, C., Tarbary, J., Heut de la Tour, E., Tabary, C. & Tardieu, G. (1977). The relationship between sarcomere length in the soleus and tibialis anterior and the articular angle of the tibia calcaneum in cats during growth. *Journal of Anatomy*, **124**, 581–8.
Thelen, E. (1992). Development as a dynamic system. *Current Directions in Psychological Science*, **1**, 189–93.
Thomas, A, Chesi, A. T. & Dargassies St Anne, Y. (1960). The neurological examination of the infant. *Little Club Clinics in Developmental Medicine*. I.
Thorndike, E. L. (1919). *Educational Psychology*, vol. I. *The Original Nature of Man*. New York: Columbia University Press.
Vojta, V. (1984). The basic elements according to Vojta. *Clinics in Developmental Medicine*, **90**, 75–86.
Von Hofsten, C. & Rosblad, B. (1988). The integration of sensory information in the development of precise manual pointing. *Neuropsychologia*, **20**, 461–71.
Vurpillot, E. (1976). *The Visual World of the Child*. London: Allen & Unwin.
White, B. L. & Held, R. (1966). Plasticity of sensorimotor development in the human infant. The causes of behaviour. In *Readings in Child Development and Education Psychology*, ed. W. Allinsmith & J. F. Rosenblith. Boston: Allyn & Bacon.
White, B. L., Castle, R. & Held, R. (1964). Observations on the development of visually directed reaching. *Child Development*, **35**, 349–64.
Williams, P. E. & Goldspink, G. (1984). Connective tissue changes in immobilised muscle. *Journal of Anatomy*, **138**, 343–50.
Wolf, A. (1943). The dynamics of the selective inhibition of specific functions in neurosis. *Psychosomatic Medicine*, **5**, 27.
World Heath Organization. (1980). *International Classification of Impairments, Disabilities and Handicaps*. Geneva: WHO.
Wright, J. & Rang, M. (1990). The spastic mouse, and the search for an animal model of spasticity in human beings. *Clinical Orthopaedics*, **253**, 12–19.
Ziv, L., Blackburn, N., Rang, M. & Koreska, J. (1984). Muscle growth in normal and spastic mice. *Developmental Medicine and Child Neurology*, **26**, 94–9.
Zuck, F. & Johnson, M. K. (1952). Progress of cerebral palsy patients, under in-patient circumstances. *American Academy of Orthopaedic Surgeons Instructional Course Lectures*, **9**, 112–18.

16

The transition to adult life

P. JANE LONES

Introduction

The teenage years are a time of adjustment for all young people but for those with disabilities it is also a time of heightened awareness of individual problems and a growing realisation of possible implications for the future. While their non-disabled peers are taking major steps in independence they often experience a sense of being left behind.

Besides having to make considerable emotional adjustments, young people with disabilities have more to learn than their peers to cope with life in general. Much education may have been lost for medical reasons and their disabilities may slow them down, yet the expectation is that maturation and education attainment will be achieved in the same time as their non-disabled contemporaries.

Education in the UK, as in the majority of countries, is organised by age and McGinty & Fish (1992: 38) point out that for pupils with special needs the end of the school stage should not be strictly timed to this but more to the individual's readiness to move on to the next stage. It follows, too, that more time is needed to complete further and higher education. The Further and Higher Education Act (1992) recognises this by permitting education up to 25 years; however, it remains to be seen how freely this will be funded and implemented.

The transition to adulthood can be defined as a period of time between the teens and early twenties when a young person acquires the skills necessary to function as an adult. It can also be regarded as the process whereby the individual grows through adolescence to reach a balanced state of independence and dependence which a particular community expects of its adult members McGinty & Fish (1992: 6).

Recently a greater awareness of disability in society has resulted in much goodwill but provision remains patchy and, for those most severely affected, choice and opportunities are limited.

Education

Education in the United Kingdom

Education has undergone much change in the early 1990s. With the introduction of the National Curriculum for children up to 16 years of age there is greater uniformity of approach. Broadly speaking most attend local coeducational comprehensive schools where education is free but there is a parallel and small system of independent provision where parents pay fees. There are many variations in both areas, some schools are single sex, some have selective intake on academic grounds and others have a particular religious ethos. Children with special needs are catered for in normal classes with support, in units attached to comprehensive schools or in special schools.

Education is compulsory to the age of 16 years but increasingly young people are choosing to remain in education through the transition years. This may take place in a 'Sixth Form' attached to a school or in a separate Further Education College. In the past the former concentrated on advanced academic courses in preparation for university entrance whereas the Colleges were vocationally orientated. With the introduction of new vocational qualifications there is greater parity of levels of attainment and both types of courses are being offered in the same setting. Education at sector Further Education Colleges is free to young people and most attend a local College. Few have residential provision and students do not have the freedom of selecting their education from what is available nationally until they attain university level. Some independent schools have boarding provision; the so-called public schools, many of whom have existed for centuries, traditionally have prepared the sons (and in a few cases, the daughters) of the aristocracy and the professional classes for lifestyles consistent with family expectations. Intake has changed in recent years but there remains a sector of the British public who regard boarding education as providing the best opportunity for the all round development of their sons and daughters.

The education of young people with special needs has undergone many changes during the past 20 years. The 1981 Education Act which followed the Warnock Report (1978) includes a requirement for assessment of special needs to be recorded in a document called the Statement, which has to be agreed by parents and reviewed annually; appropriate provision must be made in accordance with identified needs. The 1993 Education Act and the Code of Practice detail the procedures for assessments, statementing and appeals to the

Special Educational Needs Tribunal. Statements cease to apply if a young person proceeds to a Further Education College at 16 years of age.

Mainstream or special provision

The issues

The Swedish Institute (1990) stated that an effort must be made above all to integrate disabled pupils into the regular compulsory and upper secondary schools. Other countries profess similar intentions but few, if any, have found that they can dispense with special provision altogether.

A survey by Lones (unpublished survey, 1992) determined that many countries placed young people with severe physical sensory disabilities into special provision for at least part of their education. All claimed to be working towards total integration but the type of educational provision and cultural and environmental differences varied so much from country to country that direct comparisons were inappropriate. Mitchell (1985) determined that a ten-year-old boy suffering from muscular dystrophy and confined to a wheelchair was more likely to be educated in a special school in at least six out of 13 European countries.

Ward *et al.* (1994) surveyed the attitudes of teachers, resource teachers, school psychologists, principals and preschool directors to mainstreaming young people with 30 disability conditions in New South Wales. Preschool directors were positive in their attitudes to 27 conditions while teachers showed greater uncertainty, recording positive attitudes to only seven conditions.

Lectures and papers advocating total integration are often the work of educationalists and policy makers far removed from the classroom. Those working directly with young people have few opportunities to express their views and influence policy. Ward *et al.* also recorded the attitudes of preschool directors in Canada and the UK with those in New South Wales. The latter were the least positive with Canada scoring between the two. There is so much variation in resource provision both within and between countries, however, that direct comparisons could be misleading.

In many developing countries children who are disabled do not have the luxury of any form of education. The South African Department of National Health and Population Development (1987) identified that at least 10% of their children were disabled. Their right to the same education as their non-disabled peers was affirmed but as yet few received any education at all and certainly not the specialised services needed.

In the UK many arguments are used against special provision, some ideological, others based on the belief that the quality of special education is inferior because of a limited curriculum and low academic expectations. Previously small special schools catered for a wide range of needs, ages and abilities with few specialist subject staff but since the Education Reform Act (1988) detailing the requirement that the National Curriculum should be delivered to all pupils, changes have occurred to comply with this. The National Curriculum, however, is not the panacea for all students as it was not developed with special needs foremost. Warnock (1978) recognised that school failure may be caused by faults in the curriculum or the ways in which it is delivered as much as by the limitations of the disability.

Most special schools today have high expectations but the teachers recognise the needs of the student for therapy, treatment, independence training and counselling in addition to the academic programme. Their students may take much longer to complete their academic work, and it can be impossible to fit everything in. Setting priorities is never easy, educationalists look for academic success, doctors and therapists feel that health issues must take precedence. Parents naturally desire everything but teenagers want their priorities recognised and resent leisure time being taken up by the surgery and treatment. Often the optimum time for surgery is during the transition years when examinations feature. There is a need for a better understanding of the different priorities by all concerned.

Integrationalists feel that normal friendships will exist if education takes place in local mainstream provision. Integration, however, does not happen just because a disabled pupil is placed in such a school and the transition years are a time when young people become increasingly active and mobile and a disabled colleague can be left out and left behind.

It is often debated whether integration is a process or a goal (Daunt, 1991). The issue must be the whole needs of the individual and family at a particular time. This will change over the years hence, financial implications apart, there is value in having a range of quality provision both mainstream and special and to offer real choices to the family. The debate as to whether either is best is then irrelevant. Schools and Colleges would stand on their merits providing families receive information and support to choose what they feel is appropriate. Professional advice is important but it is sad when it becomes dictatorial against the wishes of the family.

During the past decade the language used in relation to special educational needs has undergone many changes. Undoubtedly words are important, affecting the self-esteem of those with disabilities. Corlett (1994) points out that they are only one factor in influencing changes in attitude to disability. Unfortunately, excessive preoccupation with political correctness inhibits the people who could do much through speaking and writing to bring about a better understanding of disability. There is confusion and terms that are acceptable in one country are deemed inappropriate in another. No offence is intended in any terminology used in this chapter.

Disability grouping

Warnock (1978) counselled against grouping young people by disability; instead their special educational needs should be identified. Special schools usually cater for one of the broad categories of visual impairment, deafness, physical disability or learning difficulty. There is a certain commonality of need and it is easier, and more economical, to develop equipment and expertise in one setting rather than try to respond to all special requirements in all special schools. This assumes that individuals fit neatly into these groups but many young people are multi-disabled, hence there must be a flexibility of response.

Hidden disabilities

In educational settings, it is easy for expertise and other resources to be concentrated on the outward signs of disability. There may be additional problems, however, that are not immediately obvious yet have wide-reaching effects. A young person with cerebral palsy may have such severe perceptual problems that these affect the ability to learn and to lead an independent lifestyle far more than their physical problems. Indeed they can be so severe that body language is not understood and social interaction is affected.

Sequencing skills are often impaired in young people with spina bifida and hydrocephalus and give rise to difficulties with problem solving and the organisation of daily tasks. Such specific learning difficulties are not easily understood by parents and mainstream teachers but they require early identification so that the classroom programme takes account of these issues.

With some disabilities pain can be present intermittently, or in varying intensity most of the time. These young people need sympathetic encouragement and understanding if their educational programme is to have any degree of continuity.

Slowly declining intellectual functioning can be difficult to recognise in progressive conditions particularly by those working with the student every day. Teachers need to be alerted to the possibility because the situation needs to be handled sensitively and tasks given must be achievable so that morale is sustained. Repeated epileptic seizures can have a similar affect. Petit mal 'absences' are easily missed by the teacher and may occur hundreds of times a day (Besag, 1993). The discontinuity experienced leads to confusion and can be misconstrued as poor concentration unless teachers are fully informed. It is usual for medical information to be directed to 'the class teacher' yet, commonly, a teenager may be taught by 12 or more tutors who change from year to year. Regular case conferences ensure sharing of knowledge and a unified approach.

Residential special education

Special schools with boarding facilities offer comprehensive medical, therapy and counselling services so that a much wider programme is offered through the 'twenty-four hour curriculum'. While residential education is seen as normal by some sectors of the British public it is anathema to others who feel it is isolating and over-protective even though many establishments promote links with sector provision and interaction with the local community. Positive role models and peer group pressure help motivate individuals to achieve more and parental absence encourages greater self-reliance and maturation in the years of transition.

By focusing entirely on the young person it is easy to forget the needs of the family where severe disability causes great strains. Parents become excessively tired, particularly when night care is required, and siblings face a restricted lifestyle. Residential placement may give some respite; it may support a marriage and make for better relationships overall.

The dying adolescent

Death is rare in mainstream education but with deteriorating conditions such as Duchenne muscular dystrophy there is a possibility that death will occur during the transitional years. Usually the wish is for life to be normal for as long as possible with continuity of education. Some parents want their child to live life as fully as possible, ignorant of the prognosis, but inevitably, the truth is discovered and then the young person feels there is a barrier to the subject being discussed at home. Parents, siblings and friends need help to work towards accepting the situation so that they can offer the support required. Teachers and other professionals need support too, as except in special schools, death is rarely discussed in in-service training.

The tendency to ignore spiritual matters in education is a reflection of society's fear and denial of the unknown. At the very least the young person should have easy opportunities to explore his spirituality or to receive secular counselling if it is desired. If parents focus all their time and resources on their dying child, providing expensive gifts and holidays, siblings experience jealousy and the young person can become spoilt and demanding. Sometimes signs of deterioration are not acknowledged and parents can make unrealistic demands for continued progress.

Education following medical rehabilitation

Returning to education following trauma

The usual expectation after the completion of medical rehabilitation is that the young persons will return to their previous school. Sometimes this is successful, particularly if the time away from education has been short but if the disability is severe or hospitalisation has lasted many months, many factors should be considered to find the most appropriate place:

1. Physical accessibility of the buildings.
2. Access to the full curriculum.
3. Availability of individual teaching to catch up with work.
4. Availability of support for specific learning difficulties.
5. Other factors which may affect social integration such as changes in behaviour or appearance.

Harrison (1987) found that the worst effect of becoming tetraplegic was its destruction of spontaneity of action. Returning to the previous setting emphasises this loss as activities once enjoyed may not be possible.

Inappropriate placement can be disastrous for the young person and the family. Medical rehabilitation is built on a series of successes but re-entering education confronts the student with reality and, if failure is experienced, self-confidence is lost with serious consequences. Those with head injuries have difficulty in rejoining their former school, even when overall physical disability is minimal.

Catching up months of missed education is impossible without individual teaching and a reduction in the curriculum. Joining a lower class may have damaging social implications.

Specific problems concerning head-injured young people

The consequences of head injury affect the return to education as any or all of the following may be present:

1. Memory deficit.
2. Other cognitive impairment.
3. Facial disfigurement.
4. Speech difficulties.
5. Visual problems.
6. Disinhibition, aggression or other behavioural problems.

1. *Memory deficit*: A pupil who may return to school with his previous knowledge intact, may discover that new information is quickly forgotten. An uninformed teacher may chastise the student for poor attention. The student may resort to distracting behaviour and try to cover up the difficulty and alienation from his or her peers may result in non-attendance. Reintegration will fail if a young person returns to education without appropriate preparation and support and when this occurs the consequences are not easily overcome (Lones, 1985).
2. *Other cognitive impairment*: Stevens (1992) found that poor insight, a lack of motivation and slowness in sorting information are common sequelae to head injury. Poor concentration and distractibility are common. Wilson & Moffat (1984) emphasise the need of head-injured individuals and their families to receive help to gain strategies to assist in alleviating their memory problems, yet acknowledge that it is not easily obtained.
3. *Disfigurement*: Facial damage or deformity can cause others to stand back or show shock. Teenagers are highly sensitive to their appearance and on receiving a negative reaction the perception of disfigurement is heightened. Former friends need to be prepared particularly for changed facial appearance.
4. *Speech problems*: Normal peer group interaction can be alienated if there is difficulty in communicating. Re-establishing a good means of communication must be the priority and it takes time to assess, acquire equipment and teach the new method. Until this is complete educational progress will be limited.
5. *Visual problems*: Tunnel vision, double vision or poor perception may be overlooked causing distress and confusion both in and out of class.
6. *Behavioural changes*: These cause the greatest problems in the reintroduction of the young person to education. Some reaction is to be expected; anger, frustration, sadness and despair may be displayed in school particularly if the young person senses that the family discourages such reactions. Someone willing to listen may be all that is required but professional counselling should be sought if there is much distress. Grieving responses usually fade with time but other behavioural changes may persist.

   Violent outbursts of temper cause teachers to consider the safety of others. Firm and consistent standards and an opportunity for 'time out' assist in regaining control but the incidents can be frightening to peers and worry parents. Friends often say that the young person is 'not the same as before' and inappropriate remarks, loud laughter at the wrong time and excessive swearing may lead to social isolation. Where there is disinhibited sexual behaviour families can be too embarrassed to seek help.

Further and higher education

For some time teachers involved with students with disabilities have been emphasising the need for extended time so that attainment goals can be reached. In the USA the issue has been controversial and Lucht & Kaska (1991) summarised attempts by the Courts to address the matter. In 1982 a Court concluded that the state is not required to provide disabled children with educational programmes designed to allow them to reach their *maximum* potential in every respect. Subsequently there have been moves to amend this and to extend the year beyond the statutory 180-day school year. In this country the solution is seen as allowing the young person to have extra years in education and the Further and Higher Education Act (1992) opens up this possibility.

The former Further Education Unit (FEU, 1990) stated there was a necessity for partnership in planning special educational needs beyond the confines of the Local Education Authority (LEA) and its institutions with the aim of effectively bridging the transition from school. Recently more students overall have enrolled in Further Education Colleges where prevocational and vocational courses, as well as academic courses, have been developed to suit a broader range of cognitive ability and presenting also increased opportunities for those with disabilities. When such students are educated in sector provision support is needed not only for the student but also for the tutors and when planning the curriculum.

In the UK the tuition element of further and higher education is funded from government or local resources. In 1993 the funding for students in further education was transferred to the Further Education Funding Council (FEFC) which specifies that courses must lead to academic or vocational qualifications or prepare students to access these courses in the future Sector colleges receive extra funding for students with disabilities.

Complementing mainstream sector provision is a relatively small area of residential special college provision, mainly in the independent sector which is able to deliver individual programmes to those with more severe disabilities. Many of these students have lived sheltered lives within their families and a period of residential education can assist in developing a degree of physical and emotional independence, thereby aiding the transition to adult life. These colleges offer a range of courses similar to those in sector colleges but the pace of work is suited to the student's capabilities and alternative means are devised for individual students to achieve assessment objectives. These too may be funded by the FEFC.

Universities and Colleges of Higher Education try to accommodate students with special needs; however, not all older buildings are fully accessible and stringent fire precautions may prohibit their use by those in wheelchairs. Departments experiencing an application from a disabled student for the first time sometimes require a little encouragement but often rise to the challenge. SKILL offers advice to students (1991) and to staff working in higher education establishments (1992*a*). The Royal National Institutes for the Blind and Deaf give disability related information too.

Selecting the right course is the first priority but a student should consider the size, topography and overall access of the campus and its proximity to local facilities. There are differing approaches to residential accommodation. Some universities have specially built provision, some will make minor adaptations to ground floor rooms in existing hostels, while a few rely on local purpose-built accommodation run by charities for those with disabilities.

Many students requiring help in lectures or with their personal care use Community Service Volunteers whereas others prefer qualified assistants. Silver & Silver (1991) stated that the crucial difference between those institutions that are able to provide a coherent, welcoming approach to students with disabilities, and those who are not, appears to be the existence of a coordinator or adviser or other coordinating machinery for offering support.

Students with disabilities may qualify for funding to meet the cost of equipment which is needed to access the course and for non-medical assistance (SKILL, 1992*b*). The considerable financial support required by students needing 24-hour care and assistance is paid usually by Social Services but funds are limited and can be difficult to obtain.

Applicants are expected to achieve the usual qualifying grades but reports mentioning any special problems the disability has caused the student during his education and at the time of the examinations will be taken into account. Obtaining a place is not easy in all cases, particularly for those whose disability is severe. Hurst (1993: 162–215) recounts the experience of these students receiving rejection letters and the anxiety caused by institutions leaving decisions until very late. He also cites figures (Hurst, 1993: 399) showing the lower percentage of students in wheelchairs studying science and of deaf students studying arts subjects. This suggests certain preconceptions by the students, teachers or university personnel and perhaps an inflexibility of approach. Once a degree is achieved there are many openings in most disciplines where disability would not be limiting. Corlett (1993) suggests that there may be a residual 'culture' in Fine Arts departments that works against talented disabled people. Clearly there are issues in higher education requiring investigation and disability equality and awareness training needs furthering.

Failure to complete a course is infrequent but generally results from insufficient preplanning for support. All students find life tiring at first, particularly if they are catering and caring for themselves for the first time. A disabled student taking much longer to complete work and daily living tasks soon becomes exhausted and health can be affected. Organising care, medical matters and repairs to equipment adds to the burden, hence a support system is vital and ideally someone should share the organisational tasks.

If illness causes a serious interruption to the course it may be impossible for the student to attend lectures at the same time as catching up with work, particularly during convalescence. There should be a simple mechanism for requesting and gaining extra time and funding.

Examinations

At the age of 16 years the majority of students sit the General Certificate of Secondary Education (GCSE). In recent years much progress has been made in standardising special arrangements to allow disabled candidates to fulfil the objectives of the assessments. The integrity of external examinations must not be jeopardised but as far as possible the usual method of working by each individual is permitted. From school-based National Curriculum assessments to vocational, professional and degree examinations there is recognition that such arrangements should be allowed.

Most countries have a similar approach to assessment and aim to prevent disabled candidates being handicapped by the testing procedures providing that the candidate receives no unfair advantage and that the resulting certification does not mislead others. Not all countries permit special arrangements for candidates with dyslexia.

Technological and other support

Modern technology provides access to new opportunities in education and employment (Vincent, 1989). Computers with word processing packages can be accessed using expanded keyboards, miniaturised keyboards, joy sticks, head switches or mouthsticks and others can be voice activated. Speech synthesisers and other communication equipment allow participation in class and social interaction. None of these will ever *replace* the hand or voice, however. When a student's handwriting is impossible, illegible or excessively slow a word processor may help but keyboard skills will be slow too. It takes time to communicate using a speech synthesiser, wordboards are limited to words and phrases chosen by someone making assumptions as to what is appropriate. Teenagers need to interact using peer group terminology and to have the vocabulary to complain and communicate problems. As some of the most vulnerable members of society they *must* be able to call for help and report abuse or assault.

Students need advice before purchasing expensive equipment. Too often it is bought before the requirements of the course are known, and sometimes a well-meaning donor funds something that is inappropriate. Regional-based Access Centres can assess students and provide opportunities to try the most modern equipment. Once a student becomes dependent on a piece of equipment, a rapid response repair and modification service is a priority because all work becomes impossible if it is out of use.

There is no common source of funding for technological equipment, although most local educational authorities provide it on loan for school-based students. While means tested funding is available through the disabled student allowances for higher education, other school leavers may have to find their own means to purchase such equipment. Vincent (1989) reported that for Further Education College students there is a perceived lack of collaboration between, and within, government departments in relation to schemes and initiatives in the area of new technology for disability and special educational needs.

Non-teaching assistants often help in class to set up equipment and attend to personal needs, take notes and act as 'hands' to be directed in practical work. This is a difficult role as too much help hinders the acquisition of independence skills and discourages normal interaction with peers. If there are severe communication problems the assistant may prompt the student for expediency and compromise the independence of the student's work.

A requirement for physiotherapy or speech therapy is indicated on the Statement although the quantity required is seldom specified. In mainstream schools therapy support is variable and seldom is it possible to fit in sessions that avoid crucial lessons, leading to a clash of priorities. Sometimes parents are asked to carry out prescribed daily exercises necessitating a very early start to the day, and in the evening the time for homework and social activities may be affected. Except in *special* further education establishments there is rarely any on-site therapy provided.

Teachers value the services of occupational therapists, educational psychologists and other advisers to ensure an optimum programme is arranged and to ensure that the aids and adaptations are supplied to access it.

Preparation for the transition to adult life

The needs

Bennet (1990) recognised that there are two elements in education, one which teaches us to earn a living, the other teaches us how to live.

The Department for Economic Cooperation and Development/Centre for Educational Research and Innovation (OECD/CERI) study (1986) identified four main areas in which adulthood is achieved:

1. Employment, useful work and valued activity.
2. Personal autonomy, independent living and adult status.
3. Social interaction, community participation, leisure and recreation.
4. Adult roles within the family including marriage.

While academic and vocational subjects are taught through courses to all young people, knowledge in the other areas is gained by interaction within the family and with peers. With greater freedom increased responsibility is expected and as family dynamics change so the maturing adolescent is gradually accorded adult status. The passage is rarely smooth but there is an underlying expectation that a degree of separation will be achieved leading to an autonomous lifestyle.

Those with disabilities may find it much harder to reach this status within the family. Opportunities to gain and practise independence may have been limited in childhood. They may have been protected from failure and risk-taking or they may have been accorded a central place in the family with their needs taking precedence so that they have not learnt the give and take necessary to make and sustain relationships. If adulthood is to be attained in the four areas identified, a broader training will be needed in addition to the academic or vocational programme.

Where there is a significant learning difficulty, in addition to physical and/or sensory disability, the risk of the individual being kept in an *eternal childhood* is greater, and planned and positive efforts will be needed to achieve a reasonable quality of adult life (Open University, 1986).

Vocational Training

In the Warnock Report (1978) 'Significant living without work' was propounded for those with severe disabilities but this has become an unacceptable concept to most young people who see work as vital, giving them status, independence and choice (McGinty & Fish, 1992: 69). Vocational training must offer equal opportunities to those with disabilities so that work can be the expectation.

Recently a more coherent programme of vocational training in this country has been introduced leading to National Vocational Qualifications (NVQ) or General National Vocational Qualifications (GNVQ).

The attainment of vocational skills is insufficient on its own. To sustain employment other qualities must be acquired such as motivation, responsibility, reliability and conscientiousness. There must be an ability to travel to work, to understand and carry out instructions, to relate to colleagues appropriately and to have acceptable standards of personal hygiene and self-presentation (Griffiths, 1989).

Work experience is a valuable part of vocational training for disabled students providing both the tasks given and the evaluation of the performance are realistic. The employer's report must be equally honest or false hopes of employment prospects will be raised.

Independence training

The degree of overall independence attained will depend on the effects of the disability and on the motivation, determination and courage of the individual. The aim should be to achieve all that is possible before a choice is made to accept some help in order to have time and energy to devote to areas that give a quality to life.

Even when there is total dependency for personal care it is possible for the individual to exert independence through decision-making, self-advocacy and the direction of carers. Such skills have to be learnt and the consequences must be understood before decisions and choices are made. Hence many students benefit from a programme of independence training tailored to their individual needs.

Special schools and colleges regularly include such programmes and residential colleges emphasise that independence training is best learnt in real situations within the 24-hour curriculum. In sector colleges students with learning difficulties receive lifeskills training but students following academic or vocational courses rarely get this special help.

At a personal level the aim is to acquire independence in dressing, washing and the management of bodily functions. Acceptable standards of eating in public, use of the telephone and social skills of all kinds may have to be taught. Devereux (1982) points out that social learning is not easy to teach as it depends on the reaction of others in the social group. Young people with disabilities sometimes behave inappropriately because of their limited participation in social situations. If much of their time has been spent with parents and other adults they may not know *how* to interact with their peers or how to make and sustain friendships.

Young people have a right to receive sex education but sometimes those with disabilities miss out or their particular needs are not addressed. Ideally the programme should have commenced by early adolescence but their knowledge and understanding needs checking in the transitional years as these young people can be very vulnerable and trusting in their relationships.

There is a need to learn how to perform practical daily domestic tasks and the management of money and time. Those with specific learning difficulties may find problems in the sequencing of tasks and may require strategies to help with memory and perceptual deficits or their progress will be limited. A high level of independence in a given setting may be achieved but the individual may lack the ability to transfer these skills to a new environment and help will be needed to build up new routines.

Mobility, road safety and the use of transport are equally important issues. In this country young people with disabilities can start driving lessons at 16 years of age and some special colleges arrange for assessments and tuition as part of the student's programme. Being able to drive greatly increases the freedom and employability of the individual. Darnborough & Kinrade (1995: 168–200) give practical advice on all matters concerning driving assessment, tuition, car purchase and the Motability Schemes.

Self-advocacy

In preparing young people for adulthood they must be empowered, so that they can advocate confidentially on their own behalf. Wertheimer (1989) stated that self-advocacy is said to include one or more of the following objectives:

putting forward and defending your own views
communicating your needs and wishes to other people
making choices for yourself
making decisions about things which affect your life
being assertive
having autonomy

Williams & Shoultz (1982) and Crawley (1988) emphasised that it also involves the individual taking *action* to achieve what is desired and Crawley pointed out that even those with the most severe level of cognitive disability can take part in self-advocacy at some level. If a young person is to self-advocate successfully, however, it requires an acceptance by others that all human beings are of equal value and deserving of respect. Without this attitude professionals give negative messages about the value and competence of individuals (Clare, 1990).

The greater the degree of disability of a young person the harder it is for parents and carers to grant the right of self-advocacy. Grant (1988) recognised that self-advocacy caused instability in the lives of carers of young people with learning difficulties.

It is unrealistic to expect many of these young people to be capable of autonomous living at the same age as their non-disabled peers. Many have become conditioned in childhood to parents, doctors, teachers and others making all the decisions. Compliance is rewarded by praise, assertiveness can lead to labelling as being *difficult*, and not surprisingly some young people need encouragement and even permission to take on the adult role. Without such help it can be more comfortable to remain passive and uninvolved.

Where oral communication is absent or limited it is much harder for the individual to develop self-advocacy, as much depends on the versatility of the communication equipment. Time and patience are required if the young person's views and wishes are to be heard.

The responsibilities of services, organisations and individuals at the time of transition

Parents

Most young people start leaving the parental home towards the end of the transition years; however, if the young person is disabled this is not the usual expectation. Society assumes that parents will continue to be the carers even though the economic, emotional and physical demands on them may be too much. In subtle ways neighbours, relatives and professionals sometimes cause guilty feelings if they suggest otherwise. Yet it may be in the best interests of all concerned, and with positive planning and support, separation can take place without guilt or bad feelings and relationships are preserved.

Many young people with disabilities qualify for certain benefit payments. Sometimes the family may become so dependent on this extra income that it mediates against the young person being able to establish an independent lifestyle.

Local Education Authorities and the Further Education Funding Council

In the UK until the age of 16 years the LEA are totally responsible for the education of the child. They assess and record the special educational needs in the Statement and it is then their responsibility to provide and finance the services required. The progress of the pupil is monitored through compulsory annual reviews.

At the age of 16 years the situation becomes more complex as *most* of the finance for further education courses is provided by the Further Education Funding Council (FEFC) and LEA involvement with the student lessens and the Statement may no longer apply. It remains the duty of the LEA, however, to recommend student placements to the FEFC and students and parents are concerned that others, largely unknown to them, are responsible for directing the future and fear that financial considerations may be the deciding factor.

The role of the LEA educational psychologist in the school years is invaluable in identifying specific learning difficulties, advising teaching programmes and supporting teachers with the handling of emotional and behavioural problems. They also provide evidence of the need for special arrangements in examinations. Such support is not readily available in further education.

Careers service

For many years young people with disabilities have been well served by Careers Officers who specialise in guiding those with disabilities. Their wide knowledge of provision in all sectors of training and of employment possibilities locally proved invaluable and they built up goodwill with employers and colleges by offering advice and support, thus easing the transition from school to further education or employment. Many have been involved in the development of alternative programmes for young people with severe disabilities or when paid employment is unavailable and they have encouraged the introduction of courses to meet the needs of those with learning difficulties.

Warnock (1978) recommended that a named person should act as a guide and mentor to parents and to the young person. Although never named as such the Careers Officer has often acted in this role during the transition years. As there is some overlap of responsibilities between professionals, the Career's Officer may be the best person to coordinate planning and advocate on behalf of the parents and the young person, if this is so desired. Hegarty *et al.* (1981) recount an incident when a specialist careers officer showed a lack of awareness about deafness but while perhaps this individual criticism was valid, it highlights the vast amount of knowledge that is needed about the whole field of disability if an adviser is to be effective. It is hard to see how the interests of special needs students can be served if the trend continues towards all Careers Officers becoming *generic*.

Social Services

There will have been Social Services involvement with many of the families throughout childhood. As the end of education approaches, however, the DP

Act Social Worker, appointed as the result of the Disabled Persons (Services, Consultation and Representation) Act (1986) has the duty of assessing the needs of the young person at least three months before the proposed leaving date. This date is not always easy to predict, as frequently requests for extensions of funding in education are not decided until very late in the academic year.

The National Health Service and Community Care Act (1990) together with the previous legislation is designed to see that the services so identified, are met but demand for services exceeds the financial resource available.

Voluntary bodies

With so much recent legislation affecting the disabled it might be assumed that all the needs of the young person are being addressed. This is not so and in some areas there remain matters of apparent injustice. For example, when someone loses a leg an artificial one is supplied but for someone who has no effective speech there is no automatic funding for a speech synthesiser. Young people have to approach charities and other bodies to seek help to purchase and maintain such equipment.

Voluntary bodies do more than just provide funds. Their work includes broad issues affecting disabled people and undoubtedly many lives would be very bleak without their interest and assistance. Specific disability support groups offer advice and promote research while others are involved with education, housing, disability awareness, mobility, aids research and development. Darnborough & Kinrade (1995: 366–444) list more than 300 UK-based associations, largely voluntary, who may provide the help or support needed by an individual and his or her family.

Parental concerns during transition

Any parent with a child, disabled from birth or subsequently, wishes above all for their son or daughter to be restored to full health, and normal mobility, cognitive functioning and behaviour. At the very least they want progress made in all these areas and hence they press for more and more therapy and education. Once these cease it is seen as professionals giving up and there can be a relentless pursuit for further treatment, however unorthodox, particularly where the disability is the result of traumatic injury. In extreme cases the professionals may be delivering treatment, therapy and teaching in ignorance of the many others involved. Parental pressure for the young to improve and achieve can become excessive and quite damaging.

The transition years can be painful to parents as they have to face the reality that their son or daughter will have to live with the consequences of disability for the foreseeable future. Unfortunately all parents are affected by the bureauc-racy that accompanies applications for the services they require. Acrimonious encounters with officialdom leave their mark and parents sometimes show aggression to those trying to help with transitional planning as they anticipate resistance. They carry so many concerns and worries and it is regrettable when such encounters become confrontational. At times a conspiracy of silence is suspected as information, particularly about the choices available, is not volunteered except in response to direct questions. This is apparent particularly when there are financial implications. In Australia, the New South Wales Department of School Education issues a clear, comprehensive guide for parents explaining rights, options and services available and the procedures for obtaining them. Contact names and addresses are listed for further information and help. There is now a *user friendly guide* to education and other services in the UK entitled Special Educational Needs – A Guide for Parents (DFE 1994).

Parents *feel* that no one really listens or addresses *their* feelings and *their* needs. Professionals concentrate on their own area of expertise and tend to avoid painful emotional issues. It must be remembered that when all the professionals have exhausted their input it is the parents who are left to carry the burden of emotional and often physical care, and their determination and tenacity must be valued and supported by society. Cubitt (1993) recounts the great number of distressed and angry parents that he witnessed in outpatient clinics, who showed through their body language so much stress, frustration and grief, yet these signs were ignored by the clinicians.

The pat on the shoulder when a mother is trying to explain that she can no longer cope is not helpful and clearly there is an unmet need for support. Parents can be overwhelmed and intimidated by professionals and the quiet, acquiescent parent is regarded as cooperative but the angry, questioning one as *difficult*.

This is not to deny that parents can make unrealistic demands on professionals and fail to understand that employers cannot afford to give jobs to young people unable to profit the company or to those whose presence adversely affects fellow employees.

As the years of transition proceed parents' worries focus more and more on the future. They press for employment and fear any alternative. The financial, physical and social problems of looking after a disabled son or daughter is daunting but equally difficult is obtaining a place in a residential establishment. Parents worry what will happen when they die, particularly if their son or daughter's self-advocacy skills are limited. If there are associated learning difficulties they fear that their child will be vulnerable to exploitation unless life-long support can be guaranteed.

Parents resent the frequent criticism that they are too protective and feel that others do not understand their worries for their child's safety and that no one takes into account the family situation. It is unrealistic to suggest that their son should be left to dress himself if this takes an hour as other family deadlines have to be met.

Services tend to focus *only* on the specific needs of the young person. Hutchinson & Tennyson (1986) emphasised the need for a multi-disciplinary service and stated that no matter how hard it was to achieve or how many different service providers there were it was *essential* that they worked together. This would allow a more beneficial and holistic approach to be taken, particularly if the decision also included the needs of the parents and siblings.

Teenage concerns and worries

It is easy to ascribe all behavioural problems to the disability, ignoring the fact that the majority of teenagers pass through very turbulent stages of development. Rejection of parental values, rebellion, an outrageous appearance, reluctance to wash, untidiness and disorganisation are common features of this stage of maturation, and the young person requires understanding and some tolerance rather than professional intervention. The disability *is* an extra dimension adding to teenage worries, particularly about employment prospects, the acquisition of boy or girl friends and the future. Those whose physical dependency is high, worry about who will care for them when parents cannot cope. They fear being trapped in a setting they dislike or being moved as a pawn for the convenience of others. It is difficult to reassure young people when resources and choices are so limited.

More immediate issues concern relationships within the family. They resent not being allowed the same freedom at the same age as their siblings and that frequently decisions are made for them. They wish to take some risks and not always be protected from failure. Many are only too aware of the strain their disability has caused and the limitations it has placed on family outings and holidays. This can result in siblings leaving home early, parental careers curtailed and sometimes it leads to marital breakdown. The knowledge of this is a hard burden to be carried by the young person who can be reluctant to seek an independent lifestyle because it will be seen as ungratefulness and a rejection of the family's help and support.

Sexual issues are hard to discuss and there may be difficulty in obtaining the precise information and advice required when normal physical relations are impossible. In the transition years the right to privacy becomes very important and those requiring intimate care find it embarrassing if this is carried out by the parent of the opposite sex. Society in the UK remains uneasy in its attitude to sexual relationships involving those with disabilities.

The years of transition are a time when society's values and procedures are challenged and it is not surprising that disability rights become an important issue when prejudice is experienced in the adult world. Worthy of consideration is the resentment of attempts to 'normalise' people. Reiser & Mason (1990) expressed this as society regarding the human being as flexible and society as unalterable. Thus the disabled must adapt to the hostile world. They feel disempowered by the medical model where they are expected to 'try' to get better. They would rather function within a social model of disability where disabled people are valued fully as are the able bodied and as part of society and where society is prepared to adapt to ensure that this is possible.

Discussion topics

1. The skills needed to achieve adult status and how these can best be taught effectively.
2. Integration: a process or a goal?
3. Ways in which professionals can learn to understand and value the priorities and expertise of other disciplines and work together for the benefit of the young person.
4. Listening skills and dealing with emotional issues. Are the supporting and facilitating systems addressing the real issues?
5. The medical and social models: are changes needed in the attitudes of professionals and society in general to those with disabilities?
6. Self-advocacy, is it an ideal or a right? How to empower young people with disabilities and their parents and the consequences this will have on relationships with professionals.

References

Acts

The Disabled Persons (Services, Consultation and Representation Act) (1986)
The Education Act (1981)
The Education Reform Act (1988)
The Further and Higher Education Act (1992)
The Education Act (1993)
The National Health Service and Community Care Act (1990)
Code of Practice on the Assessment of Special Educational Needs (DFE, 1994)
All the above published by HMSO, London.

Articles and books

Bennett, K. (1990). *Supported Work Experience enhancing the Employability of Special Needs Students*, pp. 14–24. Ontario, Canada: Industry-Education Council (Hamilton Wentworth).

Besag, F. M. C. (1993). The brain and behaviour: organic influences on the behaviour of children. *Education and Child Psychology*, **10**, p. 41.

Crawley, B. (1988). *The Growing Voice*: A Survey of Self-Advocacy Groups in Adult Training Centres and Hospitals in Great Britain. Lincoln: Community Mental Handicap Team.

Clare, M. (1990). *Developing Self-Advocacy Skills with People with Disabilities and Learning Difficulties*,15–16. London: FEU.

Corlett, S. (1994). Special language and political correctness. *British Journal of Special Education*, **21**, 17–19.

Corlett, S. (1993). Students with disabilities on Fine Arts Degrees. *Educare*, **46**, 24–8.

Cubitt, T. (1993). Crying out for succour. *British Medical Journal*, **306**, 800.

Darnborough, A. & Kinrade, D. (1995). *Directory for Disabled People* 7th edn. Hemel Hempstead, UK: Prentice Hall Harvester Wheatsheaf.

Daunt, P. (1991). *Meeting Disability : A European Response*, pp. 39–40. London: Cassell Educational.

Department for Education. (1994) Special Educational Needs: A Guide for Parents, pp. 1–49. London: HMSO.

Devereux, K. (1982). *Understanding Learning Difficulties*, pp. 105–114. Milton Keynes: Open University Press.

FEU. (1990). *Planning F.E. Equal Opportunities for People with Disabilities or Special Education Needs*. London: FEU.

Grant, G. (1988). *Stability and change in the Care Networks of Mentally Handicapped Young Adults Living at Home*. University College of North Wales: Centre for Social Policy Research and Development.

Griffiths, M. (1989). *Working Together? Enabled to work*, pp. 24–38. London: FEU.

Harrison, J. (1987). *Severe Physical Disability: Responses to the Challenge of Care*, pp. 41–4. London: Cassell Educational.

Hegarty, S., Pocklington, K. & Lucas, D. (1981). *Educating Pupils with Special Needs in the Ordinary School*, pp. 347–8. Windsor, UK: NFER-Nelson.

Hurst, A. (1993). *Steps Towards Graduation*. Aldershot: Avebury, Ashgate Publishing.

Hutchinson, D. & Tennyson, C. (1986). *Transition to Adulthood: A Curriculum Framework for Those with Severe Disability*, pp. 72–3. London: FEU.

Lones, P. J. (1985). Some educational consequences of spinal and head injuries in the teenage years. *Educare*, **23**, 19–23.

Lucht, C. L. & Kaska, S. B. (1991). *Extended Year Special Education Planning Critical Issues in the Lives of People with Severe Disabilities*, pp. 459–65. Baltimore, MD: Paul H. Brooks.

McGinty, J. & Fish, J. (1992). *Learning Support for Young People in Transition*. Milton Keynes: Open University Press.

Mitchell, P. (1985). *Report of a Comparative Study of People with Similar Disabilities in Thirteen European Countries* 7. London: RADAR.

OECD/CERI Study, (1986). *Young People with Handicaps. The Road to Adulthood.* Paris: OECD.

Open University. (1986). Mental Handicap. *Patterns for Living*. Multi-media Study Pack, Milton Keynes: Open University Press.

Reiser R. & Mason, M. (1990). *Disability Equality in the Classroom: A Human Rights Issue*, pp. 14–15. Inner London Education Authority.

Silver, H. & Silver, P. (1991). *Students with Disabilities in Higher Education Unpublished Report 11*. Oxford: Nuffield.

South African Department of National Health and Population Development. (1987). *Disability in the Republic of South Africa.*

SKILL. (1991). *A Guide to Higher Education for People with Disabilities.*
Part I Making your Application.
Part II A Guide to Universities.
Part III A Guide to Polytechnics, Institutes and Colleges of Higher Education.
National Bureau for Students with Disabilities, London: SKILL.

SKILL (1992*a*) *Students with Disabilities in Higher Education. A Guide for all Staff* ed. D. Cooper & S. Corlett. National Bureau for Students with Disabilities, London: SKILL.

SKILL (1992*b*) *Financial Assistance for Students with Disabilities in Higher Education* ed. E. Delap. National Bureau for Students with Disabilities, London: SKILL.

Stevens, C. (1992). *The Journey Back (after Head Injury)*, pp. 23–37. Mansfield: Portland College.

Swedish Institute. (1990). *Support for the Disabled in Sweden. Fact Sheet on Sweden.* Stockholm: The Swedish Institute.

Vincent, T. (1989). *Working Together? New Technology, Disability and Special Educational Needs*, pp. 1–26. London: FEU.

Ward, J., Center, Y. & Bochner, S. (1994). A question of attitudes: integrating children with special needs into regular classrooms? *British Journal of Special Education*, **21**, 34–9.

Warnock Report, (1978). *Special Educational Needs.* London: HMSO.

Wertheimer, A. (1989). *Working Together? Self-Advocacy and Parents.* London: FEU.

Williams, P. & Shoultz, B. (1982). *We Can Speak for Ourselves*. Souvenir Press: Human Horizons Series.

Wilson, B. A. & Moffatt, N. (1984). *Clinical Management of Memory Problems*, pp. 1–4. London: Croom Helm.

Recommended Reading

Bell, L. & Klenz, A. (1981). *Physical Handicap : A Guide for the Staff of Social Service Departments and Voluntary Agencies*. Cambridge: Woodhead Faulkener.

Clare, M. (1990). *Developing Self-Advocacy Skills with People with Disabilities.* London: Woodhead Faulkener.

Cole, T. (1986). *Residential Special Education : Living and Learning in a Special School.* Milton Keynes: Open University Press.

Corlett, S. & Cooper, D. (1992). *Students with Disabilities in Higher Education.* National Bureau for Students with Disabilities, London: SKILL.

Darnborough, A. & Kinrade, D. (1995). *Directory for Disabled People*, 7th edn. London: Woodhead Faulkener.

Daunt, P. (1991). *Meeting disability : A European Response*. London: Cassell Educational.

Dwyfor Davies, J. & Davies, P. ed. (1989). *A Teacher's Guide to the Support Services*. Windsor: NFER-Nelson.

Haskell, S. H. & Barrett, E. K. C. (1989). *The Education of Children with Motor and Neurological Disabilities* 2nd edn. London: Chapman and Hall.

Hurst, A. (1993). *Steps Towards Graduation*. Aldershot: Avebury-Ashgate Publishing.

McConkey, R. (1985). *Working with Parents : A Practical Guide for Teachers and Therapists*. London: Croom Helm.

McGinty, J. & Fish, J. (1992). *Learning Support for Young People in Transition*. Milton Keynes: Open University Press.

OECD/CERI. *Working Together*? A Series of Studies carried out for the UK contribution to the OECD/CERI Disabled Action Programme.

(a) Vincent, T. (1989). New Technology, disability and Special Education Needs.

(b) Griffiths, M. (1989). Enabled to Work: Support into Employment for Young People with Disabilities.

(c) Wertheimer, A. (1989). Self-Advocacy and Parents: Self-Advocacy and its Impact on the Parents of Young People with Disabilities. London: FEU.

Stevens, C. (1992). *The Journey Back (after a Head Injury)*. Mansfield: Portland College.

Sutcliffe, J. (1992). *Integration for Adults with Learning Difficulties*. Leicester: National Institute of Adult Continuing Education (England & Wales).

Reiser, R. & Mason, M. (1990). *Disability Equality in the Classroom: A Human Rights Issue*. Inner London Education Authority.

Philp, M. & Duckworth, D. (1982). *Children with Disabilities and their Families*. A Review of Research. Windsor: NFER-Nelson.

SKILL (1991) *A Guide to Higher Education for People with Disabilities*.
Part 1 Making your Application.
Part 2 A Guide to Universities.
Part 3 A Guide to Polytechnics, Institute and Colleges of Higher Education.
National Bureau for Students with Disabilities, London: SKILL.

17

Factors specific to disabled elderly people

ROGER BRIGGS

Introduction

Throughout the world, populations are ageing rapidly. Elderly people experience not only a decline in physiological function, but they are also more prone to a range of diseases. In developed countries older people already comprise the majority of those who suffer from disability, and developing countries are set to face a similar challenge in years to come. This chapter explores the effects of ageing on populations and individuals, some of the key age-related diseases such as stroke, dementia and hip fracture, and how services may be organised to cope with ensuing disabilities.

Ageing populations

Until recent times, great old age in human populations was a relative rarity. Families were large, and deaths in infancy, childhood and early adulthood were commonplace. Most people spent the whole of their lives rooted to the environment into which they were born, so that those few who survived into old age could rely on a strong network of support. The role of the extended family was paramount, the passing of knowledge from one generation to another relied largely on the spoken word, and so elders could claim pride of place within their communities. In terms of the history of the human race, the situation has changed with extraordinary speed.

Following the industrial revolution in Western countries, improvements in housing sanitation, nutrition, education and the like led to a gradual reduction in premature deaths. Figure 17.1 shows 'survival curves' for the population in England in the years 1901, 1946 and 1975. It can be seen that in 1901, 25% of people died before reaching their mid-twenties (largely from infectious diseases), and only half the population reached their late fifties. Since then, the

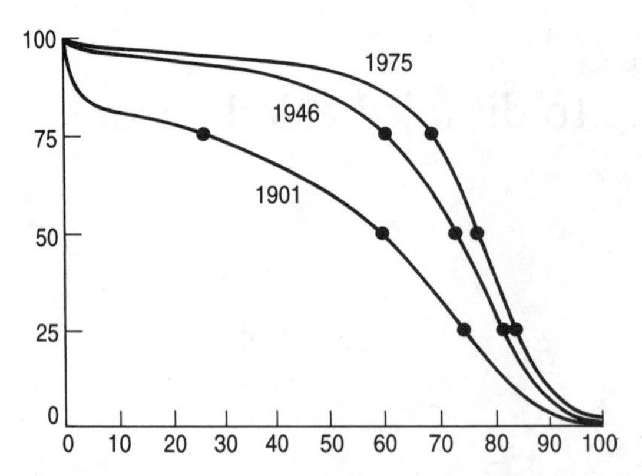

Figure 17.1. Survival curves for the population in England in 1901, 1946 and 1975. The solid circles show the ages at which 75, 50 and 25% of the population were still alive.

proportion of early deaths has progressively reduced so that the majority of people can now expect to reach 75 years of age. This 'rectangularisation of the survival curve' means that deaths, instead of being distributed through all stages of life, are now compressed into old age and are often associated with chronic disabling conditions.

Much of the current health policy in developed countries is based on the assumption that medical and social interventions to promote health and fitness in middle age will decrease the impact of chronic diseases in later life (Fries, 1980). The promotion of healthy lifestyles at any age has obvious appeal, as for an individual it is preferable to be alive and well than ill or dead. It may prove, however, that increased survival into great old age will bring with it an increasing burden of chronic disease and disability, so that societies will have to care for large numbers of dependent, elderly people (Brody, 1985).

In countries such as the United Kingdom (UK), the change in the pattern of survival has evolved over a century or two. The rapid industrialisation of developing countries, however, has brought about changes in their population structure over a much shorter period. Figure 17.2 shows population 'pyramids' during the 1980s from Pakistan, Brazil and the UK. Pakistan still has a classical pyramid: the combination of high birth rates and poor survival rates determines that most of the population are young, with only 2–3% over 65 years of age. Brazil is a country in transition, with a combination of poor rural areas and large industrialised urban centres. The UK demonstrates the effects of increased survival and reduced birth rate, with the proportion of people over 65 years (some 16%) roughly matched by children under 15 years. Rapidly developing countries, for example Singapore and Thailand, are

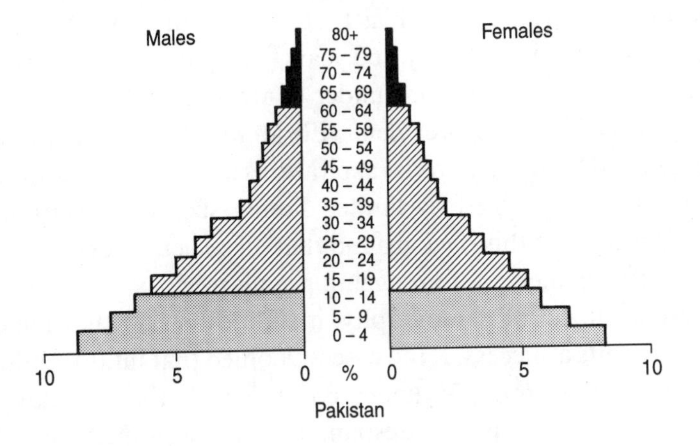

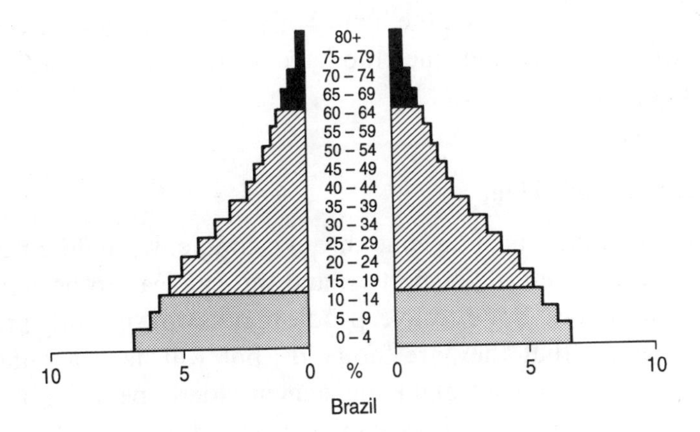

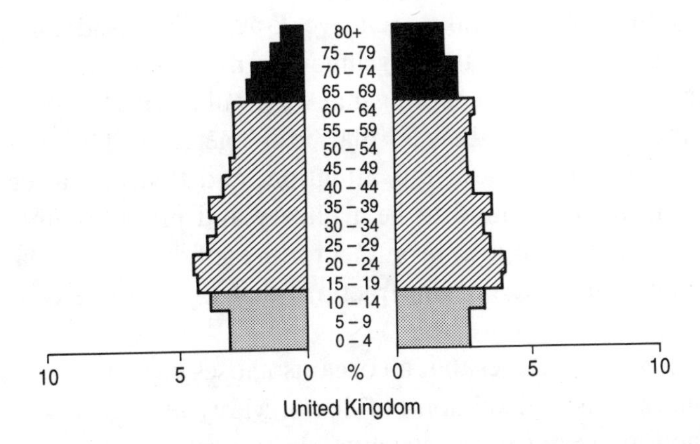

Figure 17.2. Population 'pyramids' for Pakistan, Brazil and the United Kingdom during the 1980s. The percentage of the population in each five-year band is shown.

moving from population structures such as that of Pakistan to those resembling the UK over periods as short as 50 or 60 years. The pattern of morbidity is shifting as infectious disease is brought under control and 'Western' degenerative conditions become more prevalent (Ebrahim, 1992). Fertility rates decline in response to education, material aspirations and access to contraception. Social networks are strained by limited family size, urbanisation and changing values. It is against this background that all societies sooner or later have to face up to the challenge of an ageing population.

Before leaving the subject of demography, it should be said that the challenge of ageing represents a success. It must be welcomed that infant, child and maternal mortality can be brought under control such that we have the opportunity to live out our natural lifespan. It is to be hoped that those African countries currently facing such terrible hardships of drought and famine will also one day be allowed the luxury of developing services for the elderly, because this will mean that they too have dealt with the basic health need of preventing premature death.

Ageing and the individual

Most of us derive our concepts of 'ageing' through contact with older people rather than from any theoretical perspective, and this can lead to both negative and positive stereotypes. For example, people may say of sprightly grandparents in their eighties that they are 'not old', but will have a different viewpoint if they work daily with highly dependent elderly people suffering from end-stage dementia. Biological, psychological and sociological theories of ageing shed different lights on the ageing process which should be seen as complementary rather than mutually exclusive. One of the disadvantages of the traditional 'medical model' is that 'ageing' is seen as an inevitable decline in function, whereas 'disease' is something that we should strive to prevent and treat. In this chapter I shall take the view that both 'ageing' and 'disease' may give rise to disabilities which merit our attention, and that any attempt to distinguish between them is bound to be arbitrary and probably unhelpful. Some 'age-related diseases' are such prominent causes of disability in later life (for example stroke, dementia and hip fracture) that they will be dealt with specifically.

Ageing (or 'senescence') implies that an organism loses its capacity to adapt over time, with an increasing likelihood of death. Many biological studies of physiological function or anatomical structure have compared young and old animals or insects by following the progress of change over the organism's lifespan. Given a short-lived fruit fly or mouse, such *longitudinal studies* are relatively simple to carry out, at least in theory. In studies of human ageing there are a number of difficulties. To study people over their lifespan would by definition take a lifetime, so that longitudinal studies in humans are of relatively short duration. Even then, methods deemed appropriate at the beginning of a study (for example, the measurement of muscle strength or blood cholesterol) might be obsolete by the end of it (advances in electronics or laboratory methods). Longitudinal studies of psychological or sociological variables may also be perturbed by major upheavals such as war or economic depression.

Most studies of human 'ageing' are *cross-sectional*, and look at the differences between groups of people in different age groups (for example 20-year-olds, 50-year-olds and 80-year-olds as representing 'young', 'middle-aged' and 'old'). Such studies, however, make a number of assumptions that must be borne in mind. Thus muscle strength would be greater in the young than the old; some of the decline in muscle strength would be a result of ageing, but some could be attributed to the fact that 20-year-olds are now better nourished, larger and more powerful than they were 60 years ago. Similarly, young people today are better educated than in the past, so that any difference seen in 'intelligence' in a cross-sectional study may reflect the different experiences of the age groups rather than a real decline from ageing. Such 'cohort effects' can be extremely powerful.

Elderly groups in cross-sectional studies may also be atypical, performing better than expected (because only the fittest are left in the cohort, so called 'selective survival') or worse (because a number are ill as well as old), and selection criteria are crucial. Are the study samples drawn at random (both healthy and ill) or excluding the ill? Longitudinal studies in humans are so time-consuming and expensive, and cross-sectional studies are so problematic, that the best compromise is often a 'cross-sequential design' in which cohorts of different ages are followed up over time.

Biological ageing

Ageing processes have been defined as 'those which render individuals more susceptible as they grow older to the various factors, intrinsic or extrinsic, which may cause death' (Maynard-Smith, 1962). This definition recognises that death may arise from the individual organism's inability to maintain its intrinsic function in the face of an extrinsic stressor such as 'accident' or disease. Strehler's (1962) widely quoted criteria for 'true' ageing (as opposed to disease) stated that the process must be universal (occurring in all individuals), progressive, intrinsic and deleterious (rather than developmental or 'maturational'). It should be noted that 'primary ageing' is maladaptive, i.e. it has an adverse effect on an individual's ability to survive the rigours of life. Some differences seen in old age may be the result of 'secondary ageing' and represent an adaptive response, for example behaviours such as obsessional making of lists or sticking to routines may be ways of coping with impaired memory. This is an important distinction during rehabilitation, as one is often trying to ameliorate the effects of primary ageing and this may involve reinforcing (rather than 'correcting') secondary adaptations.

Extrinsic factors include many environmental agents or 'lifestyle' components (including diet, smoking and exercise) that are open to manipulation. The benefits of education and health promotion may extend into late life, and much of current preventative strategy is based on lifestyle interventions. For example, exercise may have beneficial effects on cardiorespiratory fitness, muscle strength and bone mass not just in middle age but well beyond. The cumulative effects that we recognise as 'ageing', 'disease' or their associated disabilities represent the interaction between extrinsic processes and intrinsic processes, which are genetically determined. Knowledge of cellular biochemistry has grown at an explosive rate in recent years, and there are a large number of theories that attempt to explain intrinsic ageing at the molecular level. An understanding of these individual theories would not enlighten the practice of rehabilitation, but it is perhaps worth asking why do we age at all? Evolutionary theories of ageing attempt to answer this question in a way that unifies the various underlying genetic, molecular and cellular processes. The most comprehensive so far is the 'disposable soma theory' (Kirkwood, 1977; Kirkwood & Rose, 1991). All organisms, be they microbes or men, can be thought of as 'bodies' (the 'soma') whose function is to house the genetic material (the 'genome') which they contain; evolution is concerned with the increasingly effective transfer of the genome through reproduction. The organism has to allocate resources such as food and energy between different activities (such as growth, defence, maintenance and repair) as well as reproduction. It can be shown mathematically that the optimum investment in maintenance and repair processes is always less than would be required for indefinite somatic survival; an organism which adopted the latter strategy would be overrun by others which sacrificed a faultless repair system for more efficient reproduction. In fact, even given a perfect repair and maintenance system an organism could not survive for ever in the real world, because sooner or later it would fall victim to accident or predation.

We should not be surprised, therefore, if the human frame is not particularly well adapted to great old age, as evolutionary pressures will have been directed at the earlier stages of life when most reproduction occurs. Even though the processes of intrinsic ageing may be controlled by a relatively small number of

Table 17.1. *Difficulty with hearing among elderly people*

Age (years)	65–69 (%)	70–74 (%)	75–79 (%)	80–84 (%)	85+ (%)	All 65+ (%)
Wears an aid	4	8	10	14	22	8
Does not wear an aid but has difficulty	20	22	28	31	34	24
Does not wear and aid, has no difficulty	76	70	63	56	44	68

Source: Office of Population, Censuses and Surveys (1982).

genes, it is unlikely that we will be able genetically to manipulate human ageing at least in the foreseeable future.

Ageing organ systems

All organ systems show structural change and declining physiological function across the lifespan, often starting in early adulthood. While these changes are universal, some systems deteriorate faster than others and ageing affects different individuals at different rates. Many ageing changes, however, are such frequent causes of disability and handicap in the elderly that they warrant specific mention, as they often complicate the process of rehabilitation.

Hearing

Deafness is very common in old age, although not inevitable. The gradual deterioration in hearing ability associated with ageing is known as *presbyacusis*, and results from degeneration of the neuronal cells in the inner ear. The process is progressive, bilateral and starts at about the age of 40 years. The causes are uncertain, and genetic factors are probably involved, but excessive exposure to noise earlier in life may predispose to later hearing loss. Up to one-third of the population aged over 65 years suffers from hearing impairment of sufficient degree to have unfavourable social consequences (Table 17.1).

The hearing loss of presbyacusis is greater for high frequency than low frequency sounds. Normal conversation consists of sounds over a wide spectrum of frequencies, with consonants generally having higher frequency than vowels. Presbyacusis results in poor *speech discrimination* as there is a disproportionate loss of the ability to hear consonants which convey much of the meaning. An additional problem is *loudness recruitment*: sounds become disproportionately louder to the sufferer as they increase in intensity, so that there is only a small difference between a sound loud enough to hear and one that causes acute discomfort. Many old people find a normal, quiet speaking voice inaudible but experience pain when shouted at, and for the same reason cannot tolerate a hearing aid. Presbyacusis also causes impaired *sound localisation*, so that a deaf person may not be able to tell from where the noise is coming.

Although deafness is common, it is often neglected; it is a major cause of social deprivation and may be associated with significant depressive illness (Gilhome-Herbst & Humphrey, 1980). Communication with hearing-impaired people is improved by sitting facing them in a good light, raising one's voice slightly (not shouting), and speaking slowly and clearly. Consonants are relatively easy to lipread, but in institutions the deaf person can often not see the speaker and high levels of background noise make speech discrimination worse. Hearing aids, which amplify sound, may be helpful to some provided that they have realistic expectations. Many old people find a hearing aid difficult to use, and up to half those prescribed are not worn. Adequate training, encouragement and after-care, preferably run by specialist hearing therapists, are cost-effective means of ensuring that those who are given hearing aids derive some benefit from them.

Vision

Light enters the eye through the pupil, the diameter of which is determined by the iris. With age, the iris becomes more fibrous, the pupillary diameter constricts, and so less light is able to enter the eye. Elderly people thus require higher levels of lighting for optimal vision, often double that needed by younger people.

Young people are able to focus on objects at varying distances from the eye because the lens is elastic and its shape can be altered by the action of the ciliary muscles from which it is suspended. The lens grows throughout life by the addition of new layers, so that by the age of about 50 years it is invariably less elastic and focusing becomes more difficult. Clarity of distant objects usually remains, but close vision (such as reading) becomes blurred. This is a usual feature of ageing known as *presbyopia*, and most people will eventually require glasses (Table 17.2).

In some elderly people the centre of the lens is compressed and forms a hard, opaque *cataract*. Initially this may disperse light, so that vision is particularly

Table 17.2 *Difficulty with eyesight among elderly people*

Age (years)	65–69 (%)	70–74 (%)	75–79 (%)	80–84 (%)	85+ (%)	All 65+ (%)
Wears glasses, still has difficulty	18	20	30	32	45	24
Wears glasses, then has no difficulty	78	77	68	65	51	73
Does not wear glasses	4	3	3	4	4	3

Source: Office of Population, Censuses and Surveys (1982).

affected in bright light; this is the reason that some older people wear eye-shades or peaked caps. Once the cataract is obscuring vision such that it interferes with normal activities, only surgical removal can restore vision. After such an operation, an artificial lens must be implanted in the eye or the patients must wear corrective spectacles or a contact lens. People with diabetes are especially prone to cataract formation.

The most common cause of intractable blindness in the elderly is *senile macular degeneration*, in which the specialised retinal cells (on which central vision depends) degenerate gradually, for reasons unknown. No satisfactory treatment is generally helpful, although magnifying aids may be of some use to the patient.

Heart and lungs

Heart disease, as in other age groups, remains a major killer in later life, particularly ischaemic heart disease. Atherosclerotic damage to the coronary arteries and to peripheral vessels predisposes to angina and myocardial infarction, stroke and ischaemic problems in the legs. Such diseases are the major causes of death and disability in the Western world, and have rapidly increased in developing countries with industrialisation and urbanisation. The main hope for the future is that changes in lifestyle may prevent much of the morbidity and mortality consequent upon arterial disease; however, such benefits may take a long time to become evident. Recent findings suggest that good maternal, foetal and infant nutrition is associated with lower rates of cardiovascular disease in the next generation. The associations between early growth and adult disorders are strong, and are independent of the influence during adulthood of factors such as cigarette smoking or obesity. They are thought to reflect the long-term 'programming' of abnormal physiology and metabolism through impaired development of tissues and organs (including blood vessels) at critical stages during early life (Barker, 1992). The implications of these findings are worrying, particularly in parts of the world where malnutrition is commonplace. Not only will malnourished women bear children who carry greater risk of cardiovascular disease into later life, but their daughters in turn (already affected by impaired development) will be less equipped to provide a satisfactory intrauterine environment for the succeeding generation.

By comparison, the effects of 'intrinsic ageing' on the cardiovascular system appear relatively minor. Cardiac output falls slightly with age, and the ability to increase heart rate in response to stress is diminished. Blood pressure tends to rise with age, at least in societies adopting 'Western' urban habits. Disturbance of cardiac rhythm, particularly atrial fibrillation, becomes more common. In the absence of overt cardiac disease, however, the ageing heart is unlikely to present a barrier to rehabilitation.

With advancing years the elasticity of the lung declines, similar to the changes seen in emphysema. The chest wall becomes more rigid, kyphosis more common, and respiratory muscles weaker. These structural changes produce the functional results which one would expect: forced expiratory volume, peak flow rate and vital capacity all decline, more markedly in smokers. Pulmonary reserve capacity in the very elderly may be diminished to the extent that breathlessness limits exertion, but training may be able to mitigate these effects, probably by conditioning respiratory muscles.

Bone, joint and muscle

Peak bone mass is achieved in the late twenties and early thirties. Gender, race and body build are important determinants, influenced by nutrition and exercise during maturation. After middle age, bone density declines in both sexes but the loss is more marked in women after the menopause. Although the bone retains its normal composition, there is too little of it (osteoporosis) so that fractures become more common. Fractured neck of femur is now reaching epidemic proportions in elderly Western women, and will be addressed later in this chapter. Exercise has a protective effort on bone, particulary load-bearing and non-repetitive exercise, such as climbing stairs, shopping and gardening, are better at preventing osteoporosis than marathon running or swimming. It is important that exercise programmes be tailored for their desired outcomes, as programmes which achieve cardiovascular fitness will not necessarily add to bone strength. Hormone replacement therapy in women after the menopause is known to reduce bone loss, but there is considerable debate amongst health professionals as to which women to target, and among women themselves in weighing up the possible risks and benefits. Cyclical vaginal bleeding (analogous to menstruation) and side-effects such as weight gain and breast tenderness may be troublesome, particularly for the older woman. There has been some concern over the possibility of an increased risk of breast cancer in women treated for many years, although this has to be set against a reduced risk of cardiovascular disease. The widespread acceptance of hormone replacement therapy in North America, however, suggests, that it can be both safe and effective.

For people in private households, arthritis is the commonest cause of disability (Young, 1991). Lack of mobility and the loss of personal independence are volunteered by sufferers as of greater consequence than pain. Although rheumatoid arthritis may present late in life, osteoarthrosis is far more common and affects the majority of people over 75 years of age. Repetitive overuse and age itself are established risk factors for osteoarthrosis, but the underlying causes are uncertain. The joints worst affected tend to be in the spine, hips and knees, and it may be that osteoarthrosis is the evolutionary price of adopting an upright, bipedal gait.

Muscle strength declines after early middle age. The diminution of muscle bulk results from reduction in both the number and size of fibres, probably consequent on the loss of spinal anterior horn cells. Particularly in women, muscle weakness in the very elderly may have significant functional consequences. For example, some may find it impossible to rise from a chair without using their arms, or even to support their body weight if they have been ill in bed for any length of time. Even in great old age, training can lead to significant improvement (Fowlie, 1991); only a small (10–15%) increase in muscle strength can be of great functional advantage if it takes the patient across the threshold between being chairfast and being able to stand up.

There are many other examples of biological ageing, for example in the endocrine and immune systems, the kidney and the alimentary tract. The above selection has been made as representing those changes that are most likely to impinge on the rehabilitation process, and also because several key principles are illustrated. Firstly, some ageing changes are inevitable, but others may be modified in their onset by 'lifestyle' interventions during growth, development and middle age. Secondly, some ageing changes are inevitable, but their consequences for the individual can be mitigated by 'prosthetic' interventions such as hearing aids for deafness or glasses for visual impairment. Thirdly, some age-related deterioration (for example in muscle strength) can be ameliorated by 'therapeutic' intervention. For each intervention, even if the absolute improvement is small, the benefits to individuals can be significant if they cross a functional threshold and are enabled to carry out a necessary task that was previously beyond them.

Psychological ageing

In many instances, biological ageing changes in humans have parallels in laboratory animals, so that there is supporting evidence even though much of the human data is derived from cross-sectional studies. Psychological changes in ageing humans are more difficult to interpret, as cross-sectional studies are easily confounded by cohort effects, and animal studies are of limited relevance. This section begins with a description of the effect of ageing on cognitive functions (intelligence, learning and memory) before moving on to consider ageing and personality. It is important for us to understand how people adjust to the changing circumstances and many losses of late life if we are to help older people to maintain their morale and self-esteem, and to achieve goals that are consonant with their aspirations rather than our own. Although these areas of inquiry are now actively pursued by researchers in psychological and social gerontology, most of our knowledge and theory derives from studies in North America and Western Europe. It should be remembered that many developing countries (where some 60% of the world population over 60 years of age now live) do not yet share Western concepts of retirement, still less pensions, and have very different religious and cultural values.

Cognitive ability

Although the interaction between age and 'intelligence' has been extensively studied, it is a complex field and the research needs careful interpretation. Intelligence may be defined as a general ability to think, to solve problems and to learn new tasks. Broadly based 'intelligence tests' measuring 'IQ' span a number of cognitive functions, which may be differentially affected by ageing. There are also very large secular trends from cohort effects, as demonstrated by a steady rise of mean IQ scores during this century in the general population of Western nations (Flynn, 1984). By definition, biological ('primary') ageing in individuals would be reflected by deterioration in measured IQ, but performance on such tests may not reflect the ability to cope in the real world: the integration of experience and knowledge over a long period may lead to greater 'wisdom' in later life ('secondary ageing'). Some individuals experience less cognitive decline than others ('differential ageing'), and substantial change in the mental ability of an older person may indicate that they are seriously ill or approaching death ('terminal decline'). It is thus an oversimplification to accept the intuitive belief that intelligence declines with age.

Even mild degrees of chronic illness (including raised blood pressure or hearing loss) can adversely affect performance on cognitive testing over time. In studies confined to healthy elderly people many aspects of cognitive function remain remarkably stable until at least the age of 70 years, and possibly beyond. Tests relying on vocabulary or verbal skills decline much less than those concerned with non-verbal or performance skills. In particular, older people perform less well on tasks measuring speed of response or when put under time pressure. These changes cannot be accounted for solely by the ageing of sensory organs or peripheral neuromuscular function, and suggest that the primary decline is in central information processing ability (Holland & Rabbit, 1991). Even in this domain secondary effects cannot be ruled out, as older people may be more concerned with accuracy than the speed of response. Elderly people also find it difficult to divide their attention between competing tasks and to ignore irrelevant information, with practical consequences for everyday living and for rehabilitation.

Many older people complain that their memory is not as good as it used to be, although simple measures of learning show little or no decline. The nature and extent of the effects of 'normal ageing' on learning and memory are debated; part of the difficulty lies in the various test batteries employed and their underlying cognitive theories. Again, a general age-related decline in information processing has been postulated to lead to reductions in recognition and recall abilities (Craik & McDowd, 1987). In general, it would appear that 'immediate memory' (by which incoming information is held for a few seconds before it is discarded or stored) is little affected by age; however, the consolidation of memory into some form of permanent 'store' and its retrieval show clearer differences between younger and older people. Whether this puts the healthy elderly at any real social disadvantage is arguable. For example, they may approach tasks differently or be more willing to discard information that is meaningless. Performance on formal psychological tests does not necessarily reflect competence in the natural environment. In those who are physically frail or suffering from dementia, the situation is obviously quite different and cognitive impairment is a major cause of disability and handicap.

Although improvement of memory is unlikely in most older people with cognitive impairment, various strategies may be helpful during rehabilitation. Information should be limited and simplified; it is better to prevent the subject from making mistakes rather than allow 'trial and error' learning (Wilson, 1995).

Personality

Intellectual function is one aspect of human behaviour; 'personality' refers to the many other characteristics by which we distinguish one person from another in the types of social and emotional behaviour that they display. There are many theories of personality and associated measurement instruments, and this brief overview will only attempt to highlight some major themes. Some researchers, using detailed personality inventories, have claimed that personality is very stable with age; at the other extreme, adopting a more phenomenological approach (exploring the world in terms of events and assumptions commonplace in everyday life), are authors who suggest that there is considerable psychological development in later years.

Evidence from personality inventories is consistent with increasing introversion with ageing: older people become more preoccupied with their own inner thoughts and feelings and less with the external world. Initial studies in the United States showed that withdrawal from social activities and diminished personal involvement by older people was associated with high levels of life satisfaction (Cumming & Henry, 1961). This led to the formulation of 'disengagement theory', in which withdrawal from major roles and responsibilities in life was seen as a normal and necessary component of ageing. Disengagement theory was the focus of great sociological debate, because (or so it was inferred) the theory implied that social withdrawal was desirable, and this conclusion might condone indifference towards the problems of the elderly. In fact, disengagement is not universal; it is seen in some older people in response (adaptive or inflicted) to various losses such as retirement, bereavement or ill-health. Longer term follow-up (including longitudinal studies of the original sample giving rise to the theory) suggested that people maintain previous activities into old age unless they are forced by circumstances to redirect their energies. Thus an opposing 'activity' theory was adopted by some sociologists, arguing that 'successful ageing' was achieved by carrying through into old age the activity patterns and values typical of middle age. A criticism of such general sociological theories is that they fail to take into account the wide differences between individuals.

At present, a fruitful approach to ageing appears to be in the context of lifespan developmental psychology. To understand people in late life, one must see them in terms of the successes and failures of their whole life. Ageing persons are moving towards a stage of 'integrity', in which they achieve an acceptance of their life and the way it has been lived, and come to terms with the prospect of death (Erikson *et al.*, 1986). Some psychologists regard such an approach as too ambitious, as it is not firmly grounded in empirical observations; however, lifespan psychology may be a useful framework in which to consider our interactions with older people. Firstly, we should recognise that people have widely different experiences, that this diversity will if anything be more pronounced over a long life, and thus to expect great variety among elderly people: any generalised theory concerning the 'ageing personality' is bound to be imprecise. Secondly, we should expect elderly people to adapt to their situation in their own way, and to select goals that are appropriate to their aspirations and not ours. Why should all old people wish to participate in group activities? Why is it unreasonable for a sick old man to prefer a long-term catheter rather than endure repeated painful struggles to reach a lavatory? When survival is compromised, choices have to be made, and the best persons to establish priorities in late life are older people themselves.

Adjustment

Throughout life we have to adjust to many changes in circumstance: starting work, getting married, having children and so forth. We tend to regard these examples in a positive light whereas old age is a time of repeated and unwanted losses such as a fall in income, the death of loved ones or the onset of physical frailty. Depressive symptoms, sometimes serious enough to warrant treatment, become more prevalent in the elderly, and adverse life events may well play a part in the genesis of depressive illness in older people (Murphy, 1982). Younger people also suffer from depression; they too may endure unwanted (and often unexpected) tragedies such as bereavement, divorce or redundancy but they often find ways of coping and coming to terms with such events. Thus although up to one in seven people over 65 years of age have significant depressive symptoms, rather than concentrate on the negative aspects it is informative to ask how the majority of older people successfully adjust to loss. Many measures of 'well-being' have been developed relating to life satisfaction, morale and self-esteem. These may sometimes be as relevant to the assessment of services provided for elderly people as measures of outcome based on disability, but they may also enlighten the study of adjustment in normal ageing. There is some overlap between the study of adjustment and the theories of personality change discussed in the previous section. For example, disengagement theory was explicitly formulated as a functional theory of ageing, in which older people could prepare society for their impending death by withdrawing into themselves. Adjustment to death and dying in any age group has been the subject of much inquiry, various stages of preparation being described in terminally ill patients. A degree of 'denial' is common in older people, and (unless taken to extremes) may help them to battle on to maintain independence in the face of mounting difficulties. The majority of people appear to be able to reach a stage of 'acceptance' regarding both old age itself and dying. In the context of lifespan psychology, this can be seen as the stage of 'integrity', coming to terms with one's life as a whole.

Part of the process of adjustment centres on reviewing one's life, and for those older people who value their memories reminiscence is helpful. Some elderly remain well-adjusted without a need to reminisce, but those who are troubled by the past or try to avoid painful memories are least likely to adjust (Coleman, 1986). The maintenance of self-esteem would appear to be central: those who value themselves and see their lives as having meaning are more likely to cope with the stresses of old age, yet avoid developing depressive symptoms. An important element of self-perception is the notion of being in control of events. It is crucial that elderly people retain a sense that they are responsible for their own lives, particularly in institutional settings.

Although standardised tests and questionnaires have their place in understanding the psychology of ageing, they have their limitations in considering the process of adjustment: what makes an individual life worth living and gives it meaning? Systematic case-study methods in individuals may reveal more subtle information about human problems than generalised inquiry in large samples; both are amenable to scientific and rational interpretation (Bromley, 1986).

Ageing and disease

It is likely that therapists, in common with other health professionals, will become increasingly involved in the prevention of disease and disability; however, most health workers are predominantly involved with patients who already have overt needs for care or treatment. The major neurological and musculoskeletal causes of disability increase almost exponentially with age, and occur on a background of the ageing changes already described. The process of rehabilitation in the elderly is not markedly different from that in the young, but some general considerations are worthy of emphasis.

The incidence of so many diseases rises with age, and so most elderly patients have several pathologies. Each may contribute to a complex pattern of disability, and one problem may interfere with the solution of another. Many of the diseases of late life are chronic, degenerative conditions that will progress. In younger persons with a head or spinal injury, the therapist is dealing with a relatively fixed disability, and it is better to spend time finding optimal and durable solutions rather than making do with stop-gap, temporary measures. On the other hand, old people with serious illness may be reaching the end of their life; if there are only a few months left, is it worth spending most of them in hospital undergoing 'rehabilitation' or is it better to lead a restricted life at home? In the face of a progressive disease such as dementia, if one takes too long solving a problem one is overtaken by events: the patient who could just about live alone six months ago is now needing constant supervision. Rehabilitation of older people is sometimes 'quick and dirty' and this is not necessarily a cause of concern but more an acceptance of reality. For example, one would not try to mobilise a bilateral above-knee amputee in their eighties onto artificial limbs: a patient at this age is biologically unable to manage the muscular effort required. It is important to negotiate achievable goals (such as, in this case, wheelchair independence).

Elderly people frequently manifest illness by non-specific presenting symptoms such as the development of falls and immobility, incontinence or an acute confusional state. Virtually any disease can present in this way, including chest and urinary tract infections, gastrointestinal haemorrhage or myocardial infarction. Such presentation is analogous to 'failure to thrive' in childhood: it is vital that in any elderly person with the sudden onset of disability an underlying medical condition be sought and treated. In most instances the associated disability will resolve with appropriate diagnosis and therapy. An old lady who was fit and active a week ago but is now confused, falling about and incontinent of urine needs antibiotics for her urinary tract infection, not a walking frame and a catheter. Most so-called 'social admissions' to hospital, precipitated by an inability to cope at home, are rooted in organic disease. Elderly people often suffer from multiple diseases, and they may be taking several medications. Inappropriate prescribing for older patients is common, and frequently the most effective intervention in a disabled elderly person is the careful and considered alteration or withdrawal of drugs (Gosney & Tallis, 1984).

Age-related disease

The prevalence of stroke, dementia, fractured neck of femur, osteoarthritis and Parkinson's disease all rise dramatically with age, so that the disability rates roughly double every five years after age 65 years. It is assumed that the reader is familiar with the principles and modalities of rehabilitation appropriate to such conditions, and so no comprehensive account of management will be attempted. Some specific aspects of the first three conditions, however, are reviewed as they illustrate factors germane to elderly patients.

Stroke

Three out of four strokes occur in people over 65 years of age. Although age-specific stroke incidence has been declining in Western countries of late (partly through better control of hypertension, but also for reasons that are not understood), this is more than offset by the increase of the age group at risk, so that the absolute numbers of stroke victims are rising in developed and developing countries alike. In the UK, for example, approximately 100 000 first-ever strokes occur per year (two per 1000 population); about 20% die in the first month and a further 10% in the first year, so that stroke is the third commonest cause of death (accounting for 12% of all mortality). Of those that survive, half suffer from significant disability and a quarter remain dependent on others. Most recovery takes place in the first three months, regardless of whether the patient receives formal rehabilitation. There are very few well designed and reliable randomised controlled trials assessing the effectiveness of rehabilitation after stroke, and it is doubtful if 'no rehabilitation' control groups would now be deemed ethical. Rehabilitation has become a recognised part of treatment following stroke, with the general acceptance of what constitutes 'good practice' (Fullerton, 1991). A number of questions remain unanswered.

Rehabilitation services following stroke vary considerably in their organisation, content and availability, and it is difficult to compare these different 'packages'. It is also difficult to compare studies using a variety of outcome measures (some inadequately validated or insensitive) in samples of patients who are not matched for age, sex or characteristics known to influence survival or spontaneous recovery. Despite these limitations, there is some evidence that formal rehabilitation after stroke is effective and that it is best provided by well organised multidisciplinary teams, both in hospitals and after discharge. It is less certain when such rehabilitation should be provided, by whom and how often. Improvements that occur have to be offset against the 'opportunity cost' (therapists could have been employed doing something else of greater benefit) and personal costs to individual patients (in terms of their time and discomfort). Short-term benefits to both providers of health care (such as shorter hospital stay) and recipients (increased rate of improvement) may not be sustained in the long term. There is a lack of recent studies assessing the cost-effectiveness of stroke rehabilitation, despite the considerable resources allocated to it. Evidence is needed from research on adequate numbers of representative patients and controls, using clearly defined rehabilitation protocols and appropriate measures of cost and outcome, with long-term follow-up. Such statements are easy to make; carrying out the necessary studies is time-consuming, difficult and expensive.

Dementia

As has already been stated, healthy elderly people do not suffer from marked cognitive decline and acute confusional states are a marker for systemic illness. A proportion of elderly people suffer from 'senile dementia', perhaps only 2–3% of those aged over 65 years, but rising to 20% of those in their eighties. Some cases result from multi-infarct dementia, essentially a form of stroke disease, but the majority are caused by a degenerative condition known as Alzheimer's disease. The underlying cause of Alzheimer's disease is uncertain but is genetically based in some cases. The course of the disease is relentlessly downhill over five to ten years, starting with gradual impairment of memory, progressing through increasing behavioural disturbance until finally the patient is mute, incontinent and bedridden. Current research tends to concentrate on the basic mechanisms underlying the development of the characteristic pathology of Alzheimer's disease, at molecular and cellular level and in terms of neuronal organisation within the brain, in the hope that drug therapies or preventative strategies may be developed. For the time being, however, we are faced with the prospect of looking after the many sufferers from Alzheimer's disease and their carers. How can therapists help in this enterprise?

It is important to realise that people in the early stage of dementia may reveal considerable self-awareness and insight. Although much research and practical effort is devoted to carers in need of support, the subjective experience of dementing people themselves has received relatively little attention. A lifespan perspective may help us to understand an individual's behaviours and the cues to which he or she responds in terms of habits developed through earlier experience. Dementia is an existential plight of persons, not simply a problem to be investigated and managed through technical skill (Kitwood, 1988). The mainstay of the management of dementia in the community is the support of caring relatives, aiming to sustain their morale and the capacity to cope by responding flexibly to their needs before crises develop. Community care, however, may not be enough, particularly when the carer had a poor relationship with the sufferer even before the onset of dementia. Old people with dementia who live alone are difficult to support and dementia is now the principal reason for admission to long-term institutional care in Western countries.

The most prominent problems encountered by carers are behavioural (Argyle *et al.*, 1985). Accurate and timely information concerning the nature of dementia and the support services available enables carers to deal with their situation much better; knowing that a service such as respite care exists may help them to carry on, even if the service is not used. Practical solutions (such as providing a laundry service for incontinence) may seem obvious for some problems, but efficient provision to help depends on proper assessment of need. For example, difficulty with dressing is common in Alzheimer's disease but can reflect a number of underlying impairments: not being able to remember what to wear, not being able to work out the right movements to put the clothing on, or straightforward physical limitations. Those who suffer from dementia have a reduced ability to learn, so therapists often need to teach the carer strategies to overcome such difficulties. It may be that even in advanced dementia it is possible to improve the patients' function by suitable rehabilitation techniques, for example directed at mobility skills. Such approaches require careful evaluation and the development of specific assessment instruments designed for use with cognitively impaired elderly people (Pomeroy, 1990).

Fractured neck of femur

The association between ageing and osteoporosis was addressed earlier in this chapter, together with the possible means of prevention (directed particularly at middle-aged women). The relationship between osteoporosis and hip fracture is complex, and other factors play a part (Cooper *et al.*, 1987). Falls on the unprotected hip are an important determinant of fracture in the elderly: ageing and disease lead to an increase in the prevalence of falls, loss of soft tissue covering the hip, and impaired neuromuscular protective responses. Thus older people may not be able to put out their arm in time to break a fall. Most femoral neck fractures occur indoors, and measures to prevent falls or even to provide external hip protection may prove as important as measures targeting osteoporosis (Lauritzen *et al.*, 1993).

The incidence of fractured neck of femur has doubled in the UK since the 1950s in both sexes, and may still be rising in women. The reasons for this increase are unclear, but the rate cannot be explained by the ageing of the population alone. Although age-specific incidence is only about twice as high in women as in men, the larger number of elderly females surviving in the population mean that four-fifths of cases occur in women. It may be that poor levels of physical fitness and mobility are the basis of this 'epidemic', which has enormous consequences in terms of mortality, disability and economic costs. Up to one in five patients die in the first year after hip fracture, particularly those with other concomitant illnesses and with mental impairment, and only the minority of those who survive regain their former mobility.

No detailed considerations of rehabilitation after hip fracture will be attempted, but some general principles and unanswered questions will be highlighted (Sainsbury, 1991). The treatment of fractured neck of femur should be tackled with a sense of urgency; preoperative delay contributes to poor outcome, and the aim of surgery should be to enable the patient to weight-bear so that rehabilitation can begin soon after operation. Many of the patients already suffer from other physical illness or disability, and this has led to the development of combined 'orthogeriatric' units in some places. There is dispute about the effectiveness of such units; a team approach in an atmosphere where the elderly patient is the priority is probably the most important factor in reducing length of hospital stay (Hempsall *et al.*, 1990); however, many patients with hip fracture never recover full function. Pain and limited mobility remain significant problems even many months after discharge, with reduced numbers being able to live independently. Most studies have concentrated on hospital stay and early discharge, but there is increasing interest in community rehabilitation after patients return home as a significant proportion continue to gain further mobility for up to a year.

Organisation of services

Throughout the world health services operate under a variety of cultural, economic and political constraints and influences. No one pattern of services for the elderly can be suitable for all circumstances, but in this chapter I have tried to illustrate those needs that any health care system must address. We have looked at the impact of ageing on populations, and on the physical and psychological abilities of individuals. The three age-related diseases discussed above were selected not just because they are common causes of disability in the elderly, but because they represent different kinds of problem. Stroke is an acute illness, but may lead to permanent and complex disability. Dementia is progressive, the pattern of disability changing over time and requiring constant reappraisal. Fractured hip is an acute event which, in an uncomplicated patient, ought to be readily amenable to rehabilitation; the difficulties arise because many of the patients are very old and frail, suffering from a number of concomitant physical and mental impairments. It is important to note that the subjective experience of 'good health' is not synonymous with the absence of disease. Only 10% of English people over 75 years of age admit to no physical symptoms; on average such people have five complaints each. The most common examples are shown in Table 17.3.

Many of these symptoms are well tolerated by the majority of older people, and do not interfere greatly with their lives. A large survey of people over 65 years of age found that 93% believed their health to be 'fair or good', and the

Table 17.3 *Proportion of people aged 75 years or more suffering from various complaints*

Complaint	Percentage
Arthritis, rheumatism	58%
Unsteady on feet	49%
Forgetfulness	44%
Poor eyesight	42%
Hard of hearing	36%
Backache	36%
Breathless after any effort	35%
Swelling of feet, legs	33%
Giddiness	31%
Indigestion, flatulence	29%

Source: Abrams (1978).

number unable to perform a range of activities of daily living was relatively small (Luker & Perkins, 1987). It is thus unjustified to see 'the elderly' as a homogeneous group of frail, dependent people. On the other hand, although the 'young elderly' are predominantly fit and active, the 'old old' are increasingly affected by disease and disability. Defining disability as the inability to exist at home without help, and dependence as a further degree of incapacity for self-care, the prevalence of disability rises from 12% at age 65–69 years to over 80% above the age of 85 years; dependence occurs in only 2% below 85 years of age but in 25% of those who are older (Akhtar *et al.*, 1973). It is among the increasing numbers of very elderly people that the greatest needs will be found.

Health workers (including therapists) are likely to be increasingly involved in strategies aimed at the prevention of premature disease and disability. Some of these efforts will be directed at modifying the lifestyle of whole populations, for example reduction in smoking or promotion of exercise. Other approaches include the identification of individuals at risk, through screening programmes. Some countries are adopting protocols to identify unmet need in the elderly, although there is some doubt as to whether this will be effective in preventing future disability towards the end of life.

For the foreseeable future, most rehabilitation resources will be applied to the treatment of perceived disability. Great effort is put into therapeutic rehabilitation in which the aim is to improve function, but in most instances we do not have sufficient information to enable us to deploy resources in the most efficient and effective way. Much research and evaluation is required to establish which aspects of rehabilitation should be provided (and which should fall into disuse). There is a danger that elderly people will increasingly be supplied with prosthetic services that simply compensate for disability (such as home help or provision of meals). Such services may be needed if therapeutic measures have failed, but also tend to confirm disability, lead to further decline in function, and reinforce dependence.

Most old people wish to remain living at home, and rehabilitation services should reflect this emphasis on the community. Most carers of dependent elderly people are spouses or close family, and support of these carers is an essential element of service provision. Factors such as migration, reduced family size and marital breakdown are reducing the pool of available carers, so that increasing numbers of elderly people have no relatives living near them. Some form of institutional care will be needed by a proportion of old people. As in any other age group, the needs and aspirations of older people themselves should be central to the planning of services, but ageing populations will put governments under economic pressures that necessitate difficult choices. The falling proportion of younger people means that skills may be in short supply, including among health professionals. Nations need to plan well in advance, including the provision of education and training programmes to ensure a supply of competent therapists.

In developed countries services for the elderly have usually grown haphazardly, on the basis of existing systems responding to problems as they arise. A number of organisational models are available, all of which have advantages and disadvantages. For example, do the problems of the elderly merit specific 'geriatric' services designed for their special needs? This has some attractions, but may result in the elderly receiving a second-class service when resources are rationed. An alternative is to provide a 'seamless' service irrespective of age, but this runs the risk that the elderly are not seen as requiring any particular skills, knowledge or expertise in those who provide their care. Should services be 'disease-based', for example stroke units, orthogeriatric services and the like? If so, what happens to people who have several diseases and disabilities, and who will coordinate their treatment? At least developing countries have a chance to address these questions when planning the services that they will soon need. Managerial and logistic considerations also have to be taken into account: it is no use having services which have an admirable philosophy but are too unwieldy to deliver effective care.

The future

'The present package consists of half-hearted attempts at physical reintegration of the patient in the environment (aids, appliances, etc.); half-hearted attempts at psychosocial rehabilitation (a bit of support, a bit of counselling, sporadic provision of carers' groups etc.); and quarter-hearted attempts at reversing impairments' (Tallis, 1992). There are obviously no grounds for complacency. Rehabilitation must become more effective and to do this a more rigorous scientific approach will have to be adopted. Although it is common to emphasise a 'holistic' approach to the elderly (and this chapter is no exception), research looking into the effects of whole packages of care on global outcomes such as quality of life is difficult to carry out and the results are often even more difficult to interpret. It may be that we would do better to focus on discrete impairments and their treatment before moving on to consider disability and handicap. Certainly there will be increasing pressure to justify the use of scarce resources to meet the growing number of elderly people. I do not envisage a shortage of work for any members of the rehabilitation team.

Key points

1. Increased survival into old age and reduced birth rates fundamentally change the structure of populations. This has already occurred in developed countries, and is fast happening in developing nations.
2. Elderly people suffer from intrinsic, genetically determined effects of ageing that are deleterious to function and which cannot be prevented in the present state of knowledge. They also suffer from extrinsic causes of ageing and disease which are amenable to a range of therapeutic and preventative strategies including lifestyle interventions.
3. Cognitive decline is not marked in ageing in the absence of significant disease, although there is considerable variation between elderly people. Personality is also relatively stable, although inner thoughts and feelings assume greater importance. Adjustment to loss and coming to terms with past life are important features of successful psychological ageing.
4. The major neurological and locomotor causes of disability increase almost exponentially with age, particularly stroke, dementia and fractured neck of femur. Rehabilitation in the elderly is often complicated by multiple pathology, the non-specific presentation of illness, and the progression of disability.
5. Freedom from symptoms is not synonymous with health: many old people have a number of symptoms yet perceive their health as good and remain independent, particularly up to the age of 75 years. In those over 85 years, rates of disability and dependence are high.
6. All the above factors need to be considered in planning rehabilitation services for the elderly. Services may be organised along many lines, but the needs and aspirations of elderly people themselves should be central. In many instances,

too little evidence for the effectiveness of rehabilitation is available to allow informed choices to be made.

References

Abrams, M. (1978). *Beyond Three-Score and Ten: a First Report on a Survey of the Elderly*. Mitcham: Age Concern.

Akhtar, A. J., Broe, G. A., Crombie, C., McLean, W. M. R., Andrews, G. R. & Caird, F. I. (1973). Disability and dependence in the elderly at home. *Age and Ageing*, **2**, 102–11.

Argyle, N., Jestice, S. & Broom, C. P. B. (1985). Psychogeriatric patients: their supporters' problems. *Age and Ageing*, **14**, 355–60.

Barker, D. J. P. (ed). (1992). *Fetal and Infant Origins of Adult Disease*. London: British Medical Journal.

Brody, J. A. (1985). Prospects for an ageing population. *Nature*, **315**, 463–6.

Bromley, D. B. (1986). *The Case-Study Method in Psychology and Related Disciplines*. Chichester: Wiley.

Coleman, P. G. (1986). *Ageing and Reminiscence Processes: Social and Clinical Implications*. Chichester: Wiley.

Cooper, C., Barker, D. J. P., Morris, J. & Briggs, R. S. J. (1987). Osteoporosis, falls and age in fracture of the proximal femur. *British Medical Journal*, **295**, 13–15.

Craik, F. I. M. & McDowd, J. (1987). Age differences in recall and recognition. *Journal of Experimental Psychology: Learning, Memory and Cognition*, **13**, 473–9.

Cumming, E. & Henry, W. (1961). *Growing Old: the Process of Disengagement*. New York: Basic Books.

Ebrahim, S. (1992). Ageing in developing countries: challenges and solutions. *Geriatric Medicine*, **22**, 55–61.

Erikson, E. H., Erikson, J. M. & Kirnick, H. Q. (1986). *Vital Involvement in Old Age: the Experience of Old Age in Our Times*. New York: Norton.

Flynn, J. R. (1984). The mean I.Q. of Americans: massive gains 1932–78. *Psychological Bulletin*, **95**, 29–51.

Fowlie, S. (1991). Aging, fitness and muscular performance. *Reviews in Clinical Gerontology*, **1**, 323–36.

Fries, J. F. (1980). Aging, natural death and the compression of morbidity. *New England Journal of Medicine*, **303**, 130–5.

Fullerton, K. J. (1991). Rehabilitation in stroke. *Reviews in Clinical Gerontology*, **1**, 385–401.

Gilhome-Herbst, K. R. & Humphrey, C. (1980). Hearing impairment and mental state in the elderly living at home. *British Medical Journal*, **281**, 903–5.

Gosney, M. & Tallis, R. C. (1984). Prescription of contraindicated and interacting drugs in elderly patients admitted to hospital. *Lancet*, **1**, 564–7.

Hempsall, V. J., Robertson, D. R. C., Campbell, M. J. & Briggs, R. S. J. (1990). Orthopaedic geriatric care: is it effective? *Journal of the Royal College of Physicians of London*, **24**, 47–50.

Holland, C. A. & Rabbit, P. (1991). The course and causes of cognitive change with advancing age. *Reviews in Clinical Gerontology*, **1**, 81–96.

Kirkwood, T. B. L. (1977). Evolution of ageing. *Nature*, **270**, 301–4.

Kirkwood, T. B. L. & Rose, M. R. (1991). Evolution of senescence: late survival sacrificed for reproduction. *Philosophical Transactions of the Royal Society of London, Series, B.* , **332**, 15–24.
Kitwood, T. (1988). The contribution of psychology to the understanding of senile dementia. In *Mental Health Problems in Old Age* ed. B. Gearing., M. Johnson & T. Heller, pp. 123–30. Chichester: Wiley.
Lauritzen, J. B., Peterson, M. M. & Lund, B. (1993). Effect of external hip protectors on hip fractures. *Lancet*, **341**, 11–13.
Luker, K. A. & Perkins, E. S. (1987). The elderly at home: service needs and provision. *Journal of the Royal College of General Practitioners*, **37**, 248–50.
Maynard-Smith, J. (1962). Review lectures on senescence, 1. The causes of ageing. *Proceedings of the Royal Society of London, Series B*, **157**, 115–27.
Murphy, E. (1982). Social origins of depression in old age. *British Journal of Psychiatry*, **141**, 135–42.
Office of Population, Censuses and Surveys (1982). General Household Survey, 1980. London: HMSO.
Pomeroy, V. (1990). Development of an ADL oriented assessment-of-mobility scale suitable for use with elderly people with dementia. *Physiotherapy*, **76**, 446–8.
Sainsbury, R. (1991). Hip fracture. *Reviews in Clinical Gerontology*, **1**, 67–80.
Strehler, B. L. (1962). *Time, Cells and Aging*. New York: Academic Press.
Tallis, R. C. (1992). Rehabilitation of the elderly in the 21st century. *Journal of the Royal College of Physicians of London*, **26**, 413–22.
Wilson, B. A. (1995). Dealing with memory problems in rehabilitation. *Reviews in Clinical Gerontology*, **5**, 457–63.
Young, J. B. (1991). Rheumatological rehabilitation. *Reviews in Clinical Gerontology*, **1**, 283–96.

Further reading

Andrews, K. (1987). *Rehabilitation of the Older Adult*. London: Edward Arnold.
Bennett, G. J. & Ebrahim, S. (1995). *The Essentials of Health Care in Old Age*, 2nd edn. London: Edward Arnold.
Birren, J. E. & Schaie, K. W. (1996). *Handbook of the Psychology of Aging*, 4th edn. San Diego: Academic Press.
Bond, J., Coleman, P. & Peace, S. (1993). *Ageing in Society: an Introduction to Social Gerontology*, 2nd edn. London: Sage.
Kane, R. L., Grimley Evans, J. & MacFadyen, D. (1990). *Improving the Health of Older People: a World View*. Oxford: Oxford University Press.
Lincoln, N. (1991). Specialized techniques in rehabilitation. *Reviews in Clinical Gerontology*, **1**, 171–84.
Tout, K. (1989). *Ageing in Developing Countries*. Oxford: Oxford University Press.

Index